T0338393

SYSTEMS BIOLOGY IN DRUG DISCOVERY AND DEVELOPMENT

Wiley Series on Technologies for the Pharmaceutical Industry
Sean Ekins, Series Editor

Editorial Advisory Board

SYSTEMS BIOLOGY IN DRUG DISCOVERY AND DEVELOPMENT

Edited by

Daniel L. Young
Seth Michelson

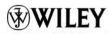

A JOHN WILEY & SONS, INC., PUBLICATION

Published by John Wiley & Sons, Inc., Hoboken, New Jersey
Published simultaneously in Canada

For general information on our other products and services or for technical support, please
contact our Customer Care Department within the United States at (800) 762-2974, outside the
United States at (317) 572-3993 or fax (317) 572-4002.

Wiley also publishes its books in a variety of electronic formats. Some content that appears in
print may not be available in electronic formats. For more information about Wiley products,
visit our web site at www.wiley.com.

Library of Congress Cataloging-in-Publication Data:
Systems biology in drug discovery and development / edited by Daniel L. Young,
Seth, Michelson.
   p. ; cm.
  Includes bibliographical references.
  ISBN 978-0-470-26123-1 (cloth)
 1. Drug development.   2. Systems biology.   I. Young, Daniel L., editor.
II. Michelson, Seth., editor.
  [DNLM: 1. Drug Discovery–methods.   2. Models, Biological.   3.
Pharmacokinetics.   4. Pharmacological Processes.   5. Systems Biology–methods.
QV 744]
  RM301.25.S97 2011
  615'19–dc22
                                   2010043475

Printed in the United States of America

oBook ISBN: 978-1-118-01643-5
ePDF ISBN: 978-1-118-01641-1
ePub ISBN: 978-1-118-01642-8

10   9   8   7   6   5   4   3   2   1

■ CONTENTS

Despite the wealth of data describing mechanisms underlying health and disease in living systems, health care costs continue to rise, and there is a growing need for improved and more affordable treatments. Efficient drug discovery and development requires methods for integrating preclinical data with patient data into a unified framework to project both efficacy and safety outcomes for new compounds and treatment approaches.

In this book we present the foundations of systems biology, a growing multidisciplinary field, applied specifically to drug discovery and development. Systems biology formally integrates knowledge and information from multiple biological sources into a coherent whole by employing proven engineering and mathematical modeling approaches. The integrated system allows rapid analysis and simulation that can inform and optimize the drug research and development processes, by formalizing, and testing, the set of acceptable hypotheses *in silico*, thereby reducing development time and costs and ultimately improving the efficacy of novel treatments.

This book is the first systems biology text to focus on how systems biology can be specifically applied to enhance drug discovery and development, with particular emphasis on real-world examples. Other texts on systems biology to date have focused on particular subdisciplines of systems biology (such as cellular networks) and have not specifically addressed drug discovery and development. This book introduces key methodologies and technical approaches for helping to solve many of the current challenges facing the pharmaceutical and biotechnology industries.

The target audience for the book includes those training or currently involved in all phases of drug discovery and development. Specific examples include life scientists, pharmacologists, computational and systems biology modelers, bioinformaticians, clinicians, and pharmaceutical/biotech management. The methods and case studies presented here will help researchers understand the diverse applications of the systems approach and integrate these technologies into their drug discovery and development programs. Those who incorporate these approaches successfully should increase their organization's competitiveness to address unmet market needs as well as more complex diseases and therapies.

The book is divided into four complementary parts. Providing a foundation for the techniques of systems biology, Part I provides an introduction to engineering and mathematical methods employed to characterize biological systems. In particular, Chapter 2 overviews model construction and analysis, focusing on model building, parameter estimation, model validation, and sensitivity analysis. Chapter 3 presents general statistical modeling approaches as well as methods for representing and analyzing nonlinear dynamical biochemical networks, of which feedback and feedforward loops are central players. In addition to modeling fundamental biological interactions and dynamics, an essential element of the systems biology approach is the study and simulation of population-level variability. To this end, Chapter 4 presents how drug pharmacokinetics is affected by variations in drug absorption, distribution, metabolism, and excretion, illustrating methods for predicting interindividual variability essential for rationale compound evaluation.

Part II highlights systems biology techniques aimed at enhancing the drug discovery process. An essential component of drug discovery is target identification and validation. To tackle many of the challenges inherent in these processes, Chapter 5 introduces a variety of complementary systems approaches, including text-mining, disease and therapeutics modeling, large multicontext data sets, regression modeling, and network and dynamic pathway modeling. In Chapter 6, systems biology approaches are applied to lead identification and optimization disciplines. In particular, systems approaches are shown to enable building bridges between compounds' chemical and biological activities. In this way, lead identification and optimization are enhanced by the systematic quantification of the optimal pharmacokinetic and pharmacodynamic compound profiles, defined potentially for specific patient populations. Chapter 7 addresses drug safety by exploring the role of biological motifs, in particular switchlike circuits, critical for dose–response models. Such models help uncover complex emergent behaviors and reveal factors driving variable patient responses to drugs that could limit efficacy or even lead to low-incidence adverse responses. Finally, Chapter 8 presents the use of mechanistic systems models for the study of pharmacokinetics and pharmacodynamics during discovery and early development. These models integrate a mechanistic understanding of biology and disease processes into a framework to aid in the selection of lead compounds, evaluation of dosing regimens, and support of optimal study design for specific patient populations.

Part III addresses particular applications of systems biology to drug development. Illustrating practical drug development challenges, Chapter 9 details the development and validation of a multiscale mathematical model for angiogenesis, integrating molecular and tissue-level processes. Here the exemplary model is applied for treatment personalization, and results suggest that an arrested drug candidate can be efficacious if applied in combination with current standards of care. Chapter 10 presents methods for applying systems biology to candidate biomarker identification. In particular, the chapter highlights the biomarker discovery process, its application to drug development, and the utility of mechanistic systems modeling to biomarker development in cardiovascular disease and rheumatoid arthritis. Finally, to aid in the design and execution of costly clinical programs, essential aspects of clinical trial simulations are presented in Chapter 11, where both clinical efficacy and safety are essential considerations.

In the final section of the book, Part IV, we address how systems biology technologies can synergize with other approaches. To this end, Chapter 12 presents how biological pathway analysis can be integrated into drug discovery systems approaches. Chapter 13 addresses aspects of personalized medicine and how functional mapping aimed at understanding genes and genetic networks can be used to help predict drug responses in patients. The book concludes in Chapter 14 with a broad overview of opportunities and challenges in systems biology that should ultimately help to extend both its reach and its acceptance, thereby further enhancing pharmaceutical productivity and the success of drug discovery and development for the benefit of patients.

In addition to the contributing authors of this book, we would like to thank our collaborators and colleagues throughout the years who have helped develop and apply systems biology approaches to drug discovery and development. We look forward to future advances and successes in the coming years as these approaches are applied and extended by dedicated researchers for enhanced drug discovery and development and ultimately, better care for patients.

Palo Alto, California   Daniel L. Young

Redwood City, California   Seth Michelson

CONTRIBUTORS

Zvia Agur, Institute for Medical Biomathematics, Bene-Ataroth, Israel

Kwangmi Ahn, Department of Public Health Sciences, Pennsylvania State College of Medicine, Hershey, Pennsylvania

Melvin E. Andersen, Division of Computational Biology, The Hamner Institutes for Health Sciences, Research Triangle Park, North Carolina

Sudin Bhattacharya, Division of Computational Biology, The Hamner Institutes for Health Sciences, Research Triangle Park, North Carolina

Naamah Bloch, Optimata Ltd., Ramat-Gan, Israel

Peter Chang, Chemical Engineering Department, University of California, Santa Barbara, California

Pascale David-Pierson, Modeling and Simulation Group, Drug Metabolism and Pharmacokinetics Department, F. Hoffmann–La Roche Ltd., Basel, Switzerland

Francis J. Doyle III, Chemical Engineering Department, University of California, Santa Barbara, California

Kapil Gadkar, Theranos, Inc., Palo Alto, California

Kalyan Gayen, Chemical Engineering Department, University of California, Santa Barbara, California

Boris Gorelik, Optimata Ltd., Ramat-Gan, Israel

Hans Peter Grimm, Modeling and Simulation Group, Drug Metabolism and Pharmacokinetics Department, F. Hoffmann–La Roche Ltd., Basel, Switzerland

Bart S. Hendriks, Merrimack Pharmaceuticals, Cambridge, Massachusetts

Wei Hou, Department of Epidemiology and Health Policy Research, University of Florida, Gainesville, Florida

Ananth Kadambi, Entelos Inc., Foster City, California

Marina Kleiman, Optimata Ltd., Ramat-Gan, Israel

Yuri Kogan, Institute for Medical Biomathematics, Bene-Ataroth, Israel

Eric Kwei, Chemical Engineering Department, University of California, Santa Barbara, California

Thierry Lavé, Modeling and Simulation Group, Drug Metabolism and Pharmacokinetics Department, F. Hoffmann–La Roche Ltd., Basel, Switzerland

Yao Li, Quantitative Genetic Epidemiology, Fred Hutchinson Cancer Research Center, Seattle, Washington

Seth Michelson, Genomic Health Inc., Redwood City, California

Henry Mirsky, Chemical Engineering Department, University of California, Santa Barbara, California

Ying Ou, Modeling and Simulation Group, Drug Metabolism and Pharmacokinetics Department, Roche Palo Alto LLC, Palo Alto, California

Tom Parke, Tessella plc, Oxfordshire, UK

Micaela Reddy, Modeling and Simulation Group, Drug Metabolism and Pharmacokinetics Department, Roche Palo Alto LLC, Palo Alto, California

Yael Ronen, Optimata Ltd., Ramat-Gan, Israel

Yael Sagi, Optimata Ltd., Ramat-Gan, Israel

D. Sidransky, The Johns Hopkins University School of Medicine, Baltimore, Maryland

Peter Wellstead, The Hamilton Institute, NUIM, Maynooth, Republic of Ireland

Olaf Wolkenhauer, Systems Biology and Bioinformatics, University of Rostock, Rostock, Germany

Rongling Wu, Center for Statistical Genetics, Pennsylvania State University, Hershey, Pennsylvania

Jiansong Yang, Simcyp Ltd., Sheffield, UK

Daniel L. Young, Theranos Inc., Palo Alto, California

Theresa Yuraszeck, Chemical Engineering Department, University of California, Santa Barbara, California

Anton Yuryev, Ariadne Genomics Inc, Rockville, Maryland

Qiang Zhang, Division of Computational Biology, The Hamner Institutes for Health Sciences, Research Triangle Park, North Carolina

Wei Zhao, Department of Biostatistics, St. Jude Children's Research Hospital, Memphis, Tennessee

PART I

INTRODUCTION TO SYSTEMS BIOLOGY IN APPROACH

CHAPTER 1

Introduction to Systems Biology in Drug Discovery and Development

SETH MICHELSON

Genomic Health Inc., Redwood City, California

DANIEL L. YOUNG

Theranos Inc., Palo Alto, California

Summary

Over the last several decades, medical and biological research has opened vast windows into the mechanisms underlying health and disease in living systems. Integrating this knowledge into a unified framework to enhance understanding and decision making is a significant challenge for the research community. Efficient drug discovery and development requires methods for bridging preclinical data with patient data to project both efficacy and safety outcomes for new compounds and treatment approaches. In this book we present the foundations of systems biology, a growing multidisciplinary field applied specifically to drug discovery and development. These methods promise to accelerate time lines, to reduce costs, to decrease portfolio failure rates, and most significantly, to improve treatment by enhancing the workflow, and thus the competitiveness, of pharmaceutical and biotechnology organizations. Ultimately, these improvements will improve overall health care and its delivery.

SYSTEMS BIOLOGY IN PHARMACOLOGY

Discovering a new medicine is a multistep process that requires one to:

- Identify a biochemically based cause–effect pathway (or pathways) inherent in a disease and its pathophysiology

Systems Biology in Drug Discovery and Development, First Edition.
Edited by Daniel L. Young, Seth Michelson.
© 2012 John Wiley & Sons, Inc. Published 2012 by John Wiley & Sons, Inc.

- Identify those cells and molecular entities (e.g., receptors, cytokines, genes) involved in the control of those pathways (typically termed *targets*)
- Identify an exogenous entity that can manipulate a molecular target to therapeutic advantage (typically termed a *drug*)
- Identify, with some level of specificity, how manipulation modulates the disease effects (termed the *mechanism of action* of the drug)
- Identify that segment of the patient population most likely to respond to manipulation (typically through the use of appropriate surrogates termed *biomarkers*)

Given these challenges, pharmaceutical drug discovery and development is an extremely complex and risky endeavor. Despite growing industry investment in research and development, only one in every 5000 new drug candidates is likely to be approved for therapeutic use in the United States (PhRMA, 2006). In fact, approximately 53% of compounds that progress to phase II trials are likely to fail, resulting in amortized costs of between $800 million and $1.7 billion per approved drug (DiMasi et al., 2003; Gilbert et al., 2003; Pharmaceutical Research and Manufacturers of America, 2006). Clearly, the crux of the problem is the failure rate of compounds, especially those in late-stage clinical development. To solve this problem, one must clearly identify the most appropriate compound for the most appropriate target in the most appropriate subpopulation of patients, and then dose those patients as optimally as possible. This philosophy forms the cornerstone of the "learn and confirm" model of drug development suggested by Sheiner in 1997.

For example, to address these three issues specifically, the Center for Drug Development Science at the University of California–San Francisco has developed a set of guidelines for applying one particular *in silico* technology, biosimulation, to the drug development process (Holford et al., 1999).

These guidelines define a three-step process. During step 1, the most relevant underlying biology describing the pathophysiology of the disease is characterized, as are the pharmacokinetics of any candidate compound aimed at its treatment. In step 2, the various clinical subpopulations expected to receive the compound are identified and characterized, including measures of inter-patient variability in drug absorption, distribution, metabolism, and excretion, and compound-specific pharmacodynamics are established. Once steps 1 and 2 are complete, this information is used in step 3 to simulate and thus design the most efficient clinical trial possible.

We believe that the general principles outlined above should not be restricted to only one methodology (i.e., biosimulation) but should be extended to the entire spectrum of *in silico* technologies that make up the generic discipline called *systems biology*. Systems biology is a rapidly developing suite of technologies that captures the complexity and dynamics of disease progression and response to therapy within the context of *in silico* models. Whether these models and their incumbent analytical methodologies represent explicit physiological models and dynamics, statistical associations, or a mix thereof, *en suite* they provide the pharmaceutical researcher with access to the most pertinent information available. By definition, that information must be composed of those data that best characterize the disease and its pathophysiology, the compound and its mechanism of action, and the patient populations in which the compound is most likely to work. With the advance of newer and faster assay technologies, the gathering of those data is no longer the rate-limiting process it once was. Rather, technologies capable of sampling the highly complex spaces underlying biological phenomena have made the interpretation of those data in the most medically and biologically reasonable context the next great hurdle in pharmaceutical drug discovery and development.

To address these challenges adequately, the pharmaceutical or clinical researcher must be able to understand and characterize the effects of diverse chemical entities on the pathways of interest *in the context of the biology they are meant to affect*. To accomplish that, research scientists and clinicians must have at their disposal the means to acquire the most pertinent and predictive information possible. We believe that systems biology is a particularly attractive solution to this problem. It formally integrates knowledge and information from multiple biological sources into a coherent whole by subjecting them to proven engineering, mathematical, and statistical methodologies. The integrated nature of the systems biology approach allows for rapid analysis, simulation, and interpretation of the data at hand. Thus, it informs and optimizes the pharmaceutical discovery and development processes, by formalizing, and testing, the most biologically relevant family of acceptable hypotheses *in silico*, thereby enabling one to reduce development time and costs and improve the efficacy of novel treatments.

REFERENCES

DiMasi, J.A., Hansen, R.W., and Grabowski, H.G. (2003). The price of innovation: new estimates of drug development costs. *J Health Econ 22*, 151–185.

Gilbert, J., Henske, P., and Singh, A. (2003). Rebuilding big pharma's business model. *In Vivo 21*, 1–10.

Holford, N.H.G., Hale, M., Ko, H.C., Steimer, J.-L., Sheiner, L.B., and Peck, C.C. (1999). Simulation in drug development: good practices. http://bts.ucsf.edu/cdds/research/sddgpreport.php.

PhRMA (2006). *Pharmaceutical Industry Profile 2006*. Pharmaceutical Research and Manufacturers of America, Washington, DC.

Sheiner, L.B. (1997). Learning versus confirming in clinical drug development. *Clin Pharmacol Ther 61*, 275–291.

CHAPTER 2

Methods for *In Silico* Biology: Model Construction and Analysis

THERESA YURASZECK, PETER CHANG, KALYAN GAYEN, ERIC KWEI,
HENRY MIRSKY, and FRANCIS J. DOYLE III

University of California, Santa Barbara, California

2.1. INTRODUCTION

Despite increasing investment in research and development, the productivity of the pharmaceutical industry has been declining, and this unfortunate phenomenon necessitates novel approaches to drug discovery and development. Systems biology is an approach that shows great promise for identifying and validating new drug targets and may ultimately facilitate the introduction of personalized and preventive medicine. This interdisciplinary field integrates traditional experimental techniques from molecular biology and biochemistry with computational biology, modeling and simulation, and systems analysis to construct quantitative mathematical models of biological networks in order to investigate their behavior. The utility of such models depends on their predictive abilities. Although constructing models that can predict all phenotypes and perturbation responses is not feasible at present, it is tractable to develop models of sufficient detail and scope to predict behavioral responses to particular perturbations and to perform sensitivity analyses. Model building, validation, and analysis are usually iterative processes in which the model becomes successively closer to the reality of the biological network and its predictions become more accurate. In this chapter we introduce model building, parameter estimation, model validation, and sensitivity analysis and present case studies in each section to demonstrate these concepts.

Systems Biology in Drug Discovery and Development, First Edition.
Edited by Daniel L. Young, Seth Michelson.
© 2012 John Wiley & Sons, Inc. Published 2012 by John Wiley & Sons, Inc.

2.2. MODEL BUILDING

2.2.1. Types of Models

Systems biologists use a variety of models to describe biological data. These models can be categorized into interaction-, constraint-, or mechanism-based models (Stelling, 2004). *Interaction-based models* represent network topology without consideration for reaction stoichiometry and kinetics. Topology maps reveal the modular organization of biological networks, a property that facilitates the study of biological organisms because it suggests that subnetworks can be studied in isolation. These maps also reveal the principles by which cellular networks are organized. Such principles provide insight into network behaviors.

Constraint-based approaches utilize information about interaction partners, stoichiometry, and reaction reversibility but contain no dynamic information. Due to the availability of such data, metabolic networks are frequently analyzed using constraint-based approaches. This approach can elucidate the range of phenotypes and behaviors that a system can achieve given the stoichiometry, interaction, and reversibility constraints. It has also been used to predict the optimal distribution of metabolic fluxes within a system from the range of possible solutions, where the optimal distribution is that which maximizes or minimizes some assumed objective, such as biomass production (Famili et al., 2003). Such analyses give insight into the behavior of an organism not only as it currently exists, but also its evolution; if the *in silico* predictions are in agreement with the experimental data, the assumption that the organism evolved to produce the optimized function is consistent with the data.

The most detailed models, the *mechanism-based models*, capture reaction stoichiometry and kinetics, providing quantitative insights into the dynamic behavior of biological networks. These models require substantial amounts of information about network connectivity and kinetic parameters. These requirements have limited the application of these models, although there are several systems for which this type of model has been constructed successfully. Such models are advantageous because they generate testable experimental hypotheses about dynamic cellular behavior. They also facilitate *in silico* experiments designed to elucidate biological design principles. For example, a model of the heat shock response in *Escherichia coli* was analyzed to determine the role of the feedback and feedforward loops that characterize this system (El-Samad et al., 2005). The *heat shock response* (HSR) is a mechanism that compensates for stress in the cytoplasm. Stress leads to the accumulation of unfolded and misfolded proteins and subsequently triggers the HSR, which induces the expression of genes that relieve the accumulation of these denatured proteins in the cytoplasm. Induced genes include those that encode chaperone proteins, which facilitate the folding of unfolded and misfolded proteins, and proteases to eliminate denatured proteins from the system. The HSR is a tightly controlled process governed by a complex regulatory architecture consisting of interconnected feedback and feedforward loops. Although simpler systems could in theory also prevent protein accumulation, evolution and natural selection led to this more complex design. *In silico* experiments in which the feedback and feedforward loops were removed from the system successively showed that this relatively complex design provides enhanced robustness compared to simpler systems (El-Samad et al., 2005). These insights would be difficult if not impossible to generate *in vivo*.

2.2.2. Specification of Model Granularity and Scope

One of the design challenges a modeler faces is that of determining the appropriate granularity and scope of a model. These choices are made based on the intended purpose of the model and the available data. When designed prudently, models will yield useful testable predictions and provide insights to pertinent mechanisms underlying an observed behavior. *Granularity* defines the level of scale that a model encompasses for a given biological network. In modeling biological systems, granularity from the level of molecules to cells to organ systems is considered. Usually, a model encompasses several levels based on the available data, the current understanding of the biological components, the model complexity, and the intended model applications. The appropriate level of granularity is also determined by considering the biological properties and behaviors of interest.

On the other hand, *scope* describes the extent of mechanistic details represented in a model. For example, at the molecular level, one has to decide which molecular components and reactions to include, and when modeling tissue behavior, one may have to decide what cell types to include. Mechanism-based models are typically very granular but reduced in scope compared to less detailed but larger-scoped topology networks. Constraint-based models are intermediate in scope and detail. Regardless of the modeling approach, the appropriate level of abstraction, taking into consideration granularity and scope, will yield consistent links between biological levels without including every detail (Stelling, 2004). The case study presented in Section 2.2.6 illustrates the impact of granularity and scope on model predictions.

2.2.3. Approaches to Model Construction

Model construction can be approached in a top-down or bottom-up manner. Top-down approaches are essentially a reverse-engineering exercise and are not to be confused with the traditional reductionist approach frequently taken by biologists. The top-down approach to *in silico* model building starts with genome-wide data, such as microarray data, and attempts to infer the underlying networks leading to the observed behavior from these data. This type of approach is facilitated by the availability of high-throughput data and is advantageous when mechanistic details and connectivity, or the wiring diagram for a system, are not well known (Kholodenko et al., 2002). The building of more empirical models in which the mechanistic details are "lumped" together is also considered a top-down approach; this results in a model that captures the relevant behavior although the mechanistic details are masked. Bottom-up approaches, on the other hand, combine connectivity and pathway information into a larger network. They start with the constitutive elements, such as genes or proteins, link them to their interaction partners, and identify the reaction-rate parameters associated with each interaction. Both top-down and bottom-up approaches can lead to detailed models able to predict dynamic response to perturbations.

A method that combines concepts from the top-down and bottom-up approaches has been proposed and applied with success to model protein folding (Hildebrandt et al., 2008). This top-down mechanistic modeling approach starts with the most basic mathematical model possible and successively expands the model scope. The impact of each model addition on the system's performance is evaluated, elucidating the structural requirements of the system (Hildebrandt et al., 2008). In essence, this top-down approach starts with a model that captures limited mechanistic detail of the system and elucidates the most critical network interactions as it progressively adds detail to the wiring diagram, ultimately resulting in a highly detailed mechanistic model. A case study employing this method to study protein folding of a single-chain antibody is described in Section 2.2.8.

2.2.4. Metabolic Network Analysis

Metabolic behavior is closely associated with phenotype, and the sequencing of the human genome enables the possibility of metabolic network analysis (Cornish-Bowden and Cardenas, 2000; Oliveira et al., 2005; Schwartz et al., 2007). Metabolic networks are highly complex, formed by hundreds of densely interconnected chemical reactions. Powerful computational tools are required to characterize such complex metabolic systems (Famili et al., 2003; Klamt and Stelling, 2003; Nielsen, 1998; Palsson et al., 2003; Reed and Palsson, 2003; Schilling et al., 2000; Wiback et al., 2004).

Two basic approaches are available for metabolic network analysis. First, the kinetic approach is based on fundamental reaction engineering principles, but this approach generally suffers from a lack of detailed kinetic information. The Palsson group (University of California–San Diego) has developed a dynamic model for a human red blood cell, a system for which detailed kinetic information is available. Second, structural approaches require only the stoichiometry of the metabolic network. For a structure-based metabolic network analysis, four approaches are available:

1. Metabolic flux analysis
2. Flux balance analysis
3. Extreme pathway analysis
4. Elementary mode analysis

The fundamental principle of metabolic flux analysis (MFA) and flux balance analysis (FBA) is the conservation of mass (Cornish-Bowden and Cardenas, 2000; Covert et al., 2001; Edwards et al., 2002; Follstad et al., 1999; Mahadevan and Palsson, 2005; Nielsen, 1998; Nissen et al., 1997; Oliveira et al., 2005; Pramanik and Keasling, 1997; Ramakrishna et al., 2001; Stelling et al., 2002; Stephanopoulos, 1999). Mathematically, MFA is applicable for a fully determined system (zero degrees of freedom) (Cornish-Bowden and Cardenas, 2000; Follstad et al., 1999; Stephanopoulos, 1999). However, biological systems are underdetermined, requiring, instead, FBA by imposing a linear optimization constraint (Edwards et al., 2002; Ramakrishna et al., 2001; Wiback et al., 2004). Recently, two other approaches, extreme pathway analysis (EPA) and elementary mode analysis (EMA), have become popular (Bell and Palsson, 2005; Edwards et al., 2001; Gayen and Venkatesh, 2006; Gayen et al., 2007; Kell, 2006; Price et al., 2002, 2003; Wiback and Palsson, 2002). EMA is the most promising, as it offers several advantages. Whereas EPA may neglect important routes connecting extracellular metabolites, EMA is capable of accounting for all possible routes (Klamt and Stelling, 2003). Another advantage of EMA is that the connecting routes between different extracellular metabolites can be traced out and the maximum theoretical yield can readily be computed. A number of tools are available for generating elementary modes, including ScrumPy and YANA (Poolman, 2006; Schwarz et al., 2005). Recently, EMA has been used to predict optimal growth and optimal phenotypic space of a specific target metabolite (Gayen and Venkatesh, 2006). It has also been used to analyze biochemical networks in mixed substrates and has biomedical applications (Edwards et al., 2001; Gayen and Venkatesh, 2006; Gayen et al., 2007; Kell, 2006; Schwartz et al., 2007; Stelling et al., 2002).

Quantifying the elementary modes of fluxes is possible, as accumulation rates of external metabolites can be represented as the fluxes of the elementary modes (Gayen and Venkatesh, 2006; Gayen et al., 2007). Mathematically, this can be represented as

$$S \cdot E = M \tag{2.1}$$

where S is a matrix representing the stiochiometry of the elementary modes, E the unknown vector of the fluxes of the elementary modes, and M a vector representing the accumulation rates of the external metabolites. Unfortunately, biological systems are underdetermined, as measurement of vector M is not sufficient for evaluating the elements of the vector E. In such scenarios, a linear optimization technique can be employed to evaluate the fluxes of the elementary modes. Mathematically, the linear optimization formulation for maximizing the accumulation rate of the ith metabolite, M_i, can be represented as

$$\max\left(\frac{dM_i}{dt}\right) \quad \text{such that} \quad M' = A'V' \quad \text{and} \quad 0 \le v_i \le \infty \quad \forall \text{ elements} \tag{2.2}$$

Elementary mode analysis enables an efficient comparison of the functional capacities of metabolic networks. In medicine, it can be used as an initial guide to evaluate the severity of enzyme deficiencies and to devise a more specific treatment of such conditions; for example, by stimulating alternative enzymatic activities that are easily overlooked without exact analysis or to better understand the metabolic routes adopted by various diseases, allowing microorganisms to survive in the host and to circumvent the host's defense mechanisms (Sauro and Ingalls, 2004). In this regard, the internal fluxes adopted by microorganisms could be traced out using EMA. Moreover, using this approach, one could identify key metabolic routes that are contributing to the survival of the microorganism in the host and point to potential drug targets. This application of elementary mode analysis makes it an attractive tool for *in silico* analysis.

2.2.5. Modeling Challenges

Building a realistic model of a biological network is challenging, due to the complexity of biological organisms and the relative sparsity of quantitative data to inform model construction. Establishing the granularity and scope of a model is the first obstacle to be overcome, although this is usually determined by the questions the systems biologist wishes to answer. More troublesome is the identification of the model structure, as knowledge about gene regulation and the proteome is incomplete and varies according to cell type, environmental conditions, genetic background, disease state, and stage of development. These issues also complicate the task of parameter identification and estimation and one must be wary about using kinetic data reported in the literature. For example, if a degradation rate for a species is determined from an *in vitro* experiment, that rate may be vastly different *in vivo*. Even if determined from an *in vivo* experiment, the conditions under which the experiment was conducted must be considered carefully. Usually, the parameters for a model cannot be derived solely from the literature but must be estimated to produce a model that behaves in the manner expected. When it is unclear which is the best of multiple competing models because all capture well the experimental data, tools such as the Akaike Information Criterion (AIC) can be used to facilitate model selection. Analyzing the model to identify conditions in which their behaviors diverge can also be useful if those conditions can be replicated experimentally. These types of validation experiments can rule out some competing models, providing insight into the nature of the biological system under study. As additional model-relevant data are generated, the predictive ability of these models and their value to the drug discovery process will increase.

Paradoxically, the advent of high-throughput genomic and proteomic technologies such as microarrays has presented new challenges because of the vast number of data points they provide. Visualizing and exploring such data sets is not straightforward; clustering and gene ontology classification have been employed heavily to facilitate data interpretation and generate hypotheses.

Much attention is devoted to data mining and the development of unsupervised, automated methods to infer the interaction networks and regulatory relationships underlying these data. Unfortunately, such efforts are complicated by the nature of experimental design for these high-throughput experiments, which usually generate extensive measurements with little replication and under a limited set of conditions. There is also no systematic means to integrate genome-wide data sets generated by disparate laboratories or to relate genomic information to proteomic data. These limitations restrict the ability to construct detailed, predictive models from genomic and proteomic data, but as technologies become cheaper and faster, analysis tools improve, and a systematic means of sharing data is developed, these limits will gradually be overcome.

2.2.6. Case Study: Synchronization and Phase Behavior of Mammalian Circadian Pacemaker

Living organisms have developed sustained oscillations to adapt to the light–dark cycles on Earth, dictating the presence and absence of light. These biological oscillations, called *circadian rhythms*, have a period around 24 hours and allow an organism to anticipate transitions in light–dark cycles. The rhythms stem from a regulatory network of clock genes in a negative feedback loop. Environmental stimuli such as light can change circadian rhythms, which in turn influence organism behavior. This phenomenon is what causes the sensation of jet lag in humans.

Effects of external stimuli on the circadian clock can be assessed by constructing a phase response curve (PRC). Typically, to construct a PRC, pulses of stimuli such as light or neuropeptides are given at different internal times of the clock. Once the rhythms have stabilized, the shift in phase is calculated. PRCs have been developed for animal and tissue behavior (Daan and Pittendrigh, 1976; Ding et al., 1994). PRCs can have regions of negligible phase shift, phase delays, and phase advances (Figure 2.1).

In mammals, the master pacemaker of the circadian clock resides in a population of neurons called the *suprachiasmatic nucleus* (SCN) located in the hypothalamus. To present a coherent rhythm to other parts of the body, the rhythms of the SCN neurons have to be synchronized. The nature of this synchronization is still unknown. First, to model the synchronization and phase responses of the SCN, one needs to determine the appropriate granularity and scope of the model. A model that captures events on the molecular and cellular levels is a logical choice for studying synchronization in the SCN. Specifically, a model of the gene regulatory network generating the rhythmic behavior in individual neurons must be integrated into a model of broader scope that describes how those neurons communicate. At the cellular level, one may hypothesize that intercellular coupling is responsible for synchronization. There are several different models of the gene regulator network with varying scope (Becker-Weimann et al., 2004; Forger and Peskin, 2003; Leloup and

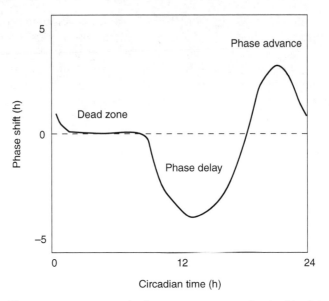

Figure 2.1   Phase response curves. A phase response curve is a tool to determine how a circadian clock is affected by a stimulus. A stimulus pulse (e.g., neuropeptides, or light) is applied to the circadian clock at some internal time. This internal time is represented by the circadian time (CT), which is real time normalized to a 24-hour period [CT = $t(24/\tau)$ where t is real time and τ is the period of the oscillator]. Once the oscillator has stabilized from the pulse, the phase shift from the reference rhythms (no stimulus applied) is calculated. PRCs can exhibit negligible phase shifts (dead zones), phase delays, and phase advances.

Goldbeter, 2003). In some models, certain multiprotein species have been modeled as one entity while phosphorylation, dephosphorylation, and translocation between the nucleus and cytosol have been omitted. Auxiliary feedback loops involving newly discovered genes are included in some models.

Different factors appear to couple SCN neurons and regulate synchrony (Aton and Herzog, 2005; Michel and Colwell, 2001). Synchronization could involve coupling via neuropeptides such as γ-aminobutyric acid (GABA) and vasoactive intestinal polypeptide (VIP). Electrical coupling such as gap junctions may also be involved. To et al. (2007) explored the effect of VIP signaling and its effect in synchronization. Previous models have also demonstrated synchronization of the SCN via coupling, but represented abstract states having no direct physiological correlates (Gonze et al., 2005). Increasing the scope of the model to include VIP signaling allows verification by comparing simulation results to experimental data.

The model developed by To et al. (2007) was extended to capture new experimental evidence. Given this evidence, the model was increased with the addition of changes in the VIP receptor (VPAC$_2$) density (Figure 2.2). VIP in the extracellular space binds with VPAC$_2$ and activates it. The activated VPAC$_2$

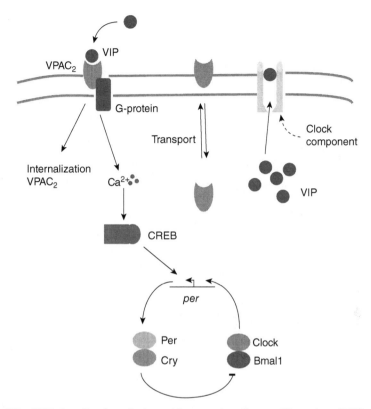

Figure 2.2 VIP signaling interfacing with core circadian oscillator in a SCN neuron. VIP from the extracellular milieu binds and activates VIP receptor, VPAC$_2$. Activated VPAC$_2$, in turn, activates G-proteins that initiate a sequence of events that lead to increases in intracellular calcium. This event is correlated with phosphorylation and activation of CREB, which serves as the link to the core oscillator by inducing *Per* transcription. The primary component of the core oscillator consists of negative feedback between the PER/CRY and CLK/BMAL1 dimers. This core oscillator is assumed to be the driving force behind release of VIP and increase of VPAC$_2$ density on the cell surface. VPAC$_2$, in both the VIP bound and unbound states, is also internalized from the cell surface.

receptor can then activate G-proteins, which eventually lead to increases in intracellular calcium. Increases in calcium lead to activation of a transcription factor, CREB, which induces the clock gene *per*. In addition, VPAC$_2$ receptors can be translocated into the cell with or without VIP bound. VPAC$_2$ and VIP transport to the cell surface is influenced by the clock gene *bmal1*.

Studies indicate that light acts on the molecular components of the circadian clock even though the neurons of the SCN do not have photoreceptors. This behavior implies that modeling of phase responses could be modeled at the single-cell level. The validity of this assumption was tested for the phase

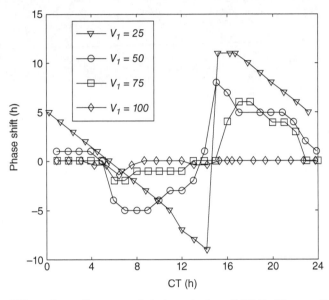

Figure 2.3 Effect of coupling strength (v_1) on single-cell PRCs. The coupling strength parameter, v_1, was set to 25, 50, 75, or 100 and the resulting single-cell PRC was calculated for a 1-hour pulse of 10 mM VIP.

behavior in response to VIP. PRCs in response to 1-hour pulses of 10 μM VIP in the single-cell and population-level model with varying degrees in coupling strength, v_1, were evaluated. For some values of v_1, the PRCs from the single-cell model agree qualitatively with the population model (Figures 2.3 and 2.4b). On the other hand, PRCs generated with v_1 set to 25 show the crossover from phase delays to phase advances from the population model to be quite different from that in the single-cell model. One piece of information lost in abstracting to the single-cell model is the synchronization property indicated by the Synchronization Index (SI). Varying coupling strength changes the SI of the population (Figure 2.4a). Hence, in this situation, a population model would be more appropriate in elucidating the phase behavior in response to VIP.

2.2.7. Case Study: Elementary Mode Analysis for the Ovarian Steroidogenesis Process of *Pimephales promelas*

Steroids play a vital role in reproduction, and their concentration varies significantly during different phases of the life cycle. Therefore, quantification of the steroidogenic process under diverse conditions can provide insight into the mechanisms controlling reproduction. We have applied elementary mode analysis to a steroidgenesis model of the *Pimephales promelas* shown in Figure 2.5. In this model, cholesterol is the precursor for all steroid hormones. It is

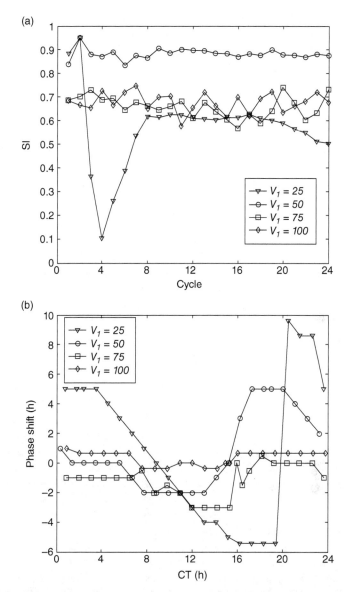

Figure 2.4 Effect of coupling strength on neuronal populations. The single-cell model was used to generate populations of neurons coupled via VIP with v_1 set to 25, 50, 75, or 100. (a) The SI was calculated after each cycle for each population. (b) Corresponding PRCs reveal that increasing v_1 reduces the magnitude of phase shifts.

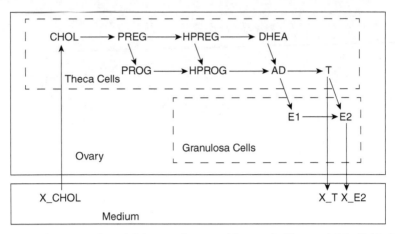

Figure 2.5 Conceptual model for ovarian steroidogenesis. The model is divided into two compartments: the medium and the ovary. X_prefixes denote the external metabolites present in the system. Steroids and their precursors are: cholesterol (CHOL), pregnenolone (PREG), 17-hydroxypregnenolone (HPREG), dehydroepiandrosterone (DHEA), progesterone (PROG), 17-hydroxyprogesterone (HPROG), androstenedione (AD), testosterone (T), estrone (E1), and estradiol (E2).

transferred to the inner mitochondrial membrane from the outer mitochondrial membrane by steroidogenic acute regulatory protein (STAR). Two steroids (testosterone, T and estradiol, E2) are excreted into the media.

Elementary modes for the ovarian steroidogenesis model are generated by attempting to optimize the production of T and E2 using YANA software. For this network, nine elementary modes are responsible for the production of both E2 and T (see Figure 2.6). Six elementary modes are available for conversion of cholesterol to E2, and three are responsible for T production. Figure 2.7 shows the relative flux distribution of enzyme activities. Cholesterol uptake and cholesterol side-chain cleavage enzymes have an activity of 1; this suggests that the steroidogenic process will cease completely if any steroidogenic disrupting elements fully inhibit either of these two enzymes.

In a drug development program, it is essential to discover suitable target enzymes. Elementary mode analysis facilitates the identification of the relative importance of various enzymes in a metabolic network. For example, the activity of cholesterol uptake and cholesterol side-chain cleavage enzymes should be prioritized, as these enzymes have the highest activity level for the ovarian steroidogenesis process. The activity of other enzymes is less important, as there are alternative routes to maintaining the steroidogenic process should the activity of these enzymes be disturbed. Moreover, this type of analysis provides insights that enable multitarget drugs or combination therapies that alter the activity of several enzymes simultaneously.

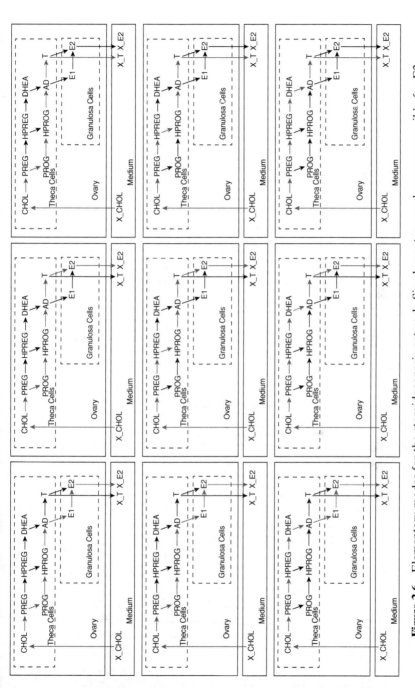

Figure 2.6 Elementary modes for the steroidogenesis network. Six elementary modes for E2 production, while three elementary modes are associated with T production. Red arrows indicate the active pathways, and black arrows indicate the inactive pathways in the network. (See insert for color representation.)

19

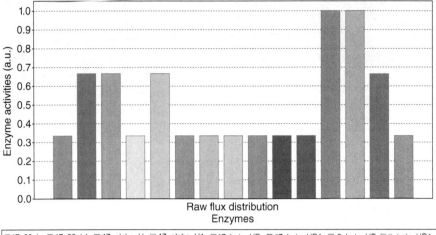

Figure 2.7 Enzyme activity diagram of the steroidogenesis process that can help guide drug development. Enzymes: cholesterol side-chain cleavage (Chol_SCCE); 17α-hydroxylase (17_alpha_H, 17_alpha_H1); 17, 20-lyase (17_20_L, 17_20_L1); 3β-hydroxysteroid dehydrogenase (3_beta_HD, 3_beta_HD1, 3_beta_HD2); 17β-hydroxysteroid dehydrogenase (17_beta_HD, 17_beta_HD1); and aromatase (Aromatase). Transport reactions: cholesterol uptake into inner mitochondrial membrane (Cholesterol_uptake); external E2 (Ex_E2); and external T (Ex_T). (See insert for color representation.)

2.2.8. Case Study: A Top-Down Approach to Bottom-Up Model Building

Understanding protein folding in the endoplasmic reticulum has important implications for the biotechnology industry. Protein therapeutics are expensive and relatively difficult to produce, so small increases in yield translate to large benefits. Elaborating the process by which proteins are folded could suggest perturbations to increase yields and maximize benefits in organisms that serve as platforms for recombinant protein production.

In the model organism baker's yeast, simultaneous overexpression of the chaperone binding protein BiP and the foldase PDI have been shown to increase the yield of recombinantly expressed single-chain antibody (scFv) over the amplification observed by overexpressing these proteins individually (Xu et al., 2005). Xu et al. hypothesized that BiP facilitates translocation of newly synthesized proteins into the endoplasmic reticulum (ER) and PDI aids in protein folding, and that these increases in complementary, serial functions account for the amplification effect observed during co-overexpression (Xu et al., 2005). To test this hypothesis and to clarify the mechanisms required for such behavior, Hildebrandt et al. (2008) employed top-down mechanistic modeling to protein folding in the ER.

Eight models of increasing complexity were developed and their analysis suggested three requirements for a system to reproduce the observed behavior. First, a two-state model was developed that captured BiP-dependent translocation and PDI dependent folding of scFv. Although this simple model was incapable of reproducing the desired behavior, enumeration of the assumptions under which it was constructed suggested the next modification—modeling the degradation of unfolded protein. Indeed, this modification created a model that captured the behavior during BiP and PDI overexpression. It was further shown that the competition between PDI-assisted folding and degradation was an important factor in determining the magnitude of PDI dependence. This analysis led the authors to conclude that the detailed model should include PDI-mediated folding and competition between degradation and folding.

Similar analyses of the remaining six models led to the formulation of an additional requirement and structural modification for the model. Using these requirements and insights, the authors developed a more detailed mechanistic model that captured the desired behaviors and was used for further analysis of the protein-folding system in the ER of *Saccharomyces cerevisiae*.

2.3. PARAMETER ESTIMATION

Numerical values must be assigned to parameters of mathematical models to analyze biological behavior. For example, these parameters include rate constants, equilibrium constants, diffusion constants, and initial conditions. Although these data may be available in the literature, more often they have not been measured, as obtaining the required data is typically difficult and costly. Even when data are available, they are often context specific, so the experimental model and conditions under which the data were gathered must be considered carefully.

Parameter estimation methods are used to determine the parameter values for which the model simulations most closely resemble the observed behavior of experimental systems. Three key elements make up the parameter estimation problem: decision variables, the objective function, and constraints. *Decision variables* are variables that are changed during the estimation process to obtain a model with the specified behaviors. The *objective function* is a measure of the performance of the solution and is sometimes referred to as a cost or fitness function. *Constraints* are bounds on the acceptable values of the decision variables or relationships between them.

Parameter estimation methods can be broadly classified as local or global. *Local methods* such as Newton's method and sequential quadratic programming methods are based on gradient-based searches that sample the parameter space around the current values and determines the direction in which the objective function is maximally decreasing until it reaches a minimum. Because they do not sample all of the parameter space and the solution depends on the initial guesses for the parameters, it is possible to get "stuck" in a trough or local minimum for multimodal objective functions. These approaches also require that the objective function always be continuous and differentiable.

Global methods sample the entire feasible region for parameters and find (nearly) optimal solutions. The simplest such method is the multistart method, in which a local method is used repeatedly to solve the optimization problem, starting with different initial guesses for the parameters. Evolutionary algorithms, which include evolutionary strategies, genetic algorithms, and evolutionary programming, are also popular and are based on principles of biological evolution: competition, reproduction, and selection (Fogel, 1994). Such methods are stochastic in nature and not gradient-based; they do not guarantee the global optimum and may generate different results from different starting conditions because of their stochastic nature. In the next section we focus on the implementation of evolutionary strategies.

2.3.1. Evolutionary Strategies

Evolutionary strategies (ESs) were introduced more than 40 years ago (Coello Coello, 2005). To implement an evolutionary strategy, offspring are generated from a population of parents and the fittest individuals are selected as parents for the next generation; this process is repeated many times. There are two general strategies for choosing offspring, the $(\mu + \lambda)$-ES and the (μ,λ)-ES strategies. For the former, new generations are established by choosing the fittest individuals from the total population of parents and their offspring, while the latter considers offspring only when choosing fit individuals to establish new generations. The $(\mu + \lambda)$-ES strategy is elitist, because the fittest individuals are never discarded. In contrast, the fittest individual may be discarded by the (μ,λ)-ES strategy if that individual is a member of the parent population μ and not the offspring population λ (Coello Coello, 2005).

Mathematically, individuals are represented by a vector containing the values of the decision variables, or parameters. Offspring are generated from individuals according to the equation

$$\overline{x}^{t+1} = \overline{x}^{t} + N\left(0,\sigma^{2}\right) \tag{2.3}$$

This equation states that an offspring is generated from the parent by adding normally distributed noise (N) with mean 0 and standard deviation σ^2. The fitness of the parents and offpsring are calculated and a new generation is selected from the fittest individuals from both populations, $(\mu + \lambda)$-ES, or from only the offspring population, (μ,λ)-ES. The process is repeated until convergence is achieved or the number of generations exceeds a preset threshold. A popular variation of the evolutionary strategy applies recombination to the parent vectors before Gaussian noise is added, where recombination can involve two or more parents.

Over the course of an optimization, both the decision variables and the standard deviations used to generate offspring may be modified. The standard deviations are adjusted according to the equation

$$\sigma'(i) = \sigma(i)\exp[\tau'N(0,1) + \tau N_i(0,1)] \tag{2.4}$$

where the proportionality constants τ' and τ depend on N. The following relationships are recommended (Beyer and Schwefel, 2002):

$$\tau' = \frac{c}{\sqrt{2n}} \quad \text{and} \quad \tau = \frac{c}{\sqrt{2\sqrt{n}}}$$

The number of decision variables is n. This feature, known as *self-adaption*, is a particularly advantageous characteristic of modern ES implementations that improves performance.

2.3.2. Parameter Estimation Challenges

A variety of considerations complicate the implementation of parameter estimation techniques. Biological optimization problems usually encompass a large search space and are of high dimension (i.e., many parameters must be estimated). These types of problems are computationally expensive. Constraining the search space based on experimental data and reducing dimensionality by specifying parameters for which experimental measurements have been taken will improve the performance and speed of the optimization.

In addition, the fitness function must be expressed mathematically. It is typical to formulate the fitness function as the sum of squared errors between the simulated and observed data:

$$f(x) = \sum (y_{obs} - y_{sim})^2 \tag{2.5}$$

This construction has several drawbacks. Namely, for objectives that vary over several orders of magnitude as parameters are adjusted, differences between the simulated and observed outputs are less pronounced when the outputs simulated are high compared to those observed. This scenario may result in a stalled optimization. Furthermore, this construction weights observations with high values greater than it weights those with low values. Therefore, the weighted sum of squared errors is a better option:

$$f(x) = \sum w_i \left(\frac{y_{obs} - y_{sim}}{y_{obs}} \right)^2 \tag{2.6}$$

For data known to have lognormally distributed errors, the objective function given

$$f(x) = \sum w_i (\log y_{obs} - \log y_{sim})^2 \qquad (2.7)$$

is preferred. The weighting factors, w_i, are used to emphasize or diminish the importance of each contribution to a multimodel objective function, and setting these factors can be problematic, although using the alternative functions given in Eqs. (2.6) and (2.7) make this process more intuitive, because it puts those objectives on the same scale.

Evolutionary algorithms have some unique implementation challenges. The size of the parent and offspring populations must be chosen as well as rates of mutation and recombination. Loss of diversity of the population of solutions may also be a problem, a phenomenon known as *premature convergence*. Diversity can be reintroduced slowly by mimicking genetic mutation, while premature convergence is less problematic with large parent and offspring populations.

2.3.3. Case Study: Use of Evolution Strategy to Create a Realistic Model of the Circadian Rhythm

Biological systems widely exhibit circadian behavior (Dunlap, 1999), as observed in, for example, the onset of sleep in higher vertebrates or flower opening in angiosperms. These organism-level patterns are mimicked and ultimately controlled by underlying intracellular molecular oscillations with about 24-hour periodicity (DeCoursey, 2004). Because the circadian system for the mouse at the cellular level has been relatively well characterized, it provides an excellent template for sound model development.

It is reasonable to suppose that a successful mathematical model of an intracellular system can be built if at least three conditions are met: (1) the molecular relationships must be largely known, including any genetic regulation and protein modifications, associations, and reactions; (2) the key attributes that define the system are known; and (3) sufficient experimental data are available for both model creation and validation.

In the mouse circadian system, the principal molecular relationships have been elucidated over the last decade. In brief, the core system is comprised of a set of clock genes. Some of the clock genes [the period genes (*per1* and *per2*) and the cryptochrome genes (*cry1* and *cry2*)] are activated constitutively by heterodimers of Clock/Bmal1. When levels of Per and Cry are low, repression is at a minimum and the *per* and *cry* genes are "on." Per and Cry protein concentrations therefore increase, ultimately repressing the production of their own mRNAs (Reppert and Weaver, 2002). This negative feedback loop is made more complex by the presence of additional activators and repressors, such as RorC and Rev-ErbA, respectively, that act at additional promoter elements on the clock genes (Liu et al., 2008) (see Figures 2.8 and 2.9).

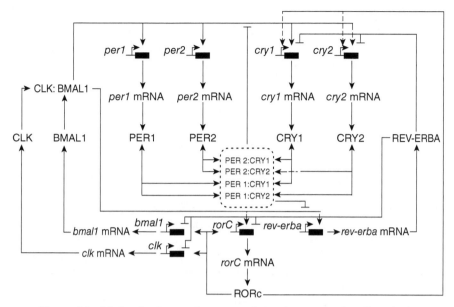

Figure 2.8 Molecular interaction network for the mouse circadian clock.

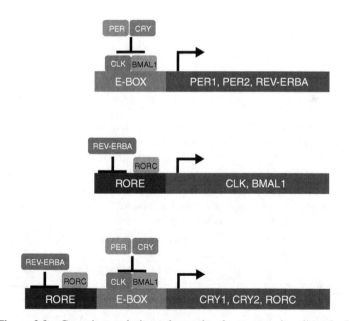

Figure 2.9 Genetic regulation scheme for the mouse circadian clock.

The importance of phase for the behavior of the circadian system has been recognized for some time. This is clearly true at the organ level (Pittendrigh and Daan, 1976) and is becoming increasingly apparent at the molecular level. As the feedback mechanisms act on the regulatory apparatus, the levels of clock components rise and fall, and their peaks arrive at repeatable times each day. Furthermore, sufficient experimental data exist to allow a "fit" to a model. Note that these data *must* be gathered at the level of individual cells, since our goal is to build a cell-level model, as neurons in communication with one another behave differently. Specifically, the peak of *rev-erba* mRNA precedes the peaks of *per1* and *per2* mRNA by 4 hours; the peaks of *per1* and *per2* mRNA precede the peaks of *cry1*, *cry2*, and *rorc* mRNA by 4 hours; the peaks of *cry1*, *cry2*, and *rorc* mRNA precede the peaks of *bmal1* and *clock* mRNA by 8 hours; and the peaks of *bmal1* and *clock* mRNA precede the peak of *rev-erba* mRNA by 8 hours (unpublished data). Additionally, mRNA peaks are known to precede their corresponding protein peaks (for most species in the system) by approximately 5 hours (Lee et al., 2001).

Given the molecular network and the corresponding genetic regulation, a mathematical representation was developed consisting of a set of ordinary differential equations (ODEs). Using an appropriate cost function, an evolutionary algorithm was employed to identify a set of parameters that resulted in oscillations with the correct phase relationships (Figure 2.10). Note that the cost function did not include a mandate for a 24-hour oscillation period. Rather, correct periodicity was obtained by multiplying by the identical factor all kinetic parameters obtained. For example, if the evolutionary strategy had produced a final parameter set resulting in a 12-hour period (a system that clearly is operating twice as fast as its desired speed), all kinetic parameters would have been multiplied by 0.5 to slow the system to once-daily operation.

A critical component of any model development effort is validation against retained data. For the mouse circadian system, the effect of numerous knockout mutations on rhythmicity is known (Liu et al., 2008). The fully parameterized model described here was evaluated with seven knockout mutations and two double-knockout mutations. In all nine cases, the model correctly predicts the experimental phenotypes (see Table 2.1). Furthermore, in 11 of 13 cases where knockout of a gene leads to changes in the expression level of the remaining components, the model predicts the change correctly. Finally, the model also predicts more subtle behaviors: for example, the continuance of rhythmicity when *bmal1* is produced constitutively (Liu et al., 2008).

In this case study, a highly predictive mathematical model was developed utilizing the wealth of data describing the interaction network and gene regulation of the system. Model parameters were estimated using an evolutionary strategy that used an objective function based on the system's principal attributes describing its phase relationships. This highly predictive tool can thus be employed with confidence to enhance scientific understanding and bolster drug discovery efforts.

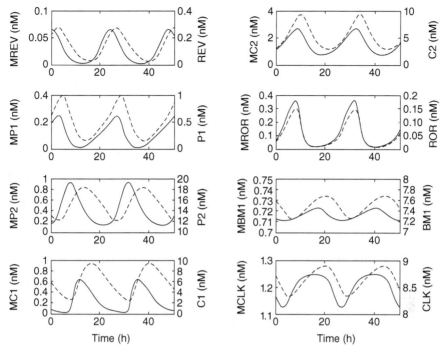

Figure 2.10 Simulated time courses for mRNAs and proteins in the mouse circadian clock. Solid lines represent mRNA time courses, and dashed lines represent protein time courses. REV, RevErbA; P1, Per1; P2, Per2; C1, Cry1; C2, Cry2; ROR, RorC; BM1, Bmal1; and CLK, Clock. An "M" prefix signifies mRNA.

TABLE 2.1 Experimental and Simulated Knockout Phenotypes for Intracellular Mouse Circadian Clock

Mutant	Experimental	Simulated
cry1 −/−, cry2 −/−	Arrhythmic	Arrhythmic
per1 −/−, per2 −/−	Arrhythmic	Arrhythmic
cry1 −/−	Arrhythmic	Arrhythmic
cry2 −/−	Rhythmic, long period	Rhythmic, 32.1-hour period
per1 −/−	Arrhythmic	Arrhythmic
per2 −/−	Arrhythmic	Arrhythmic
bmal1 −/−	Arrhythmic	Arrhythmic
rev-erbA −/−	Rhythmic, normal period	Rhythmic, 23.7-hour period
rorC −/−	Rhythmic, normal period	Rhythmic, 23.7-hour period

2.4. MODEL ANALYSIS

Once a suitable model has been constructed and its parameters estimated, analysis of that model can begin. Model simulations can generate testable hypotheses and predictions that would not have otherwise been evident and can elucidate the triggers leading to undesirable or pathological behavior. They can also uncover basic principles underlying a system. For example, feedback and feedforward loops are ubiquitous in biological networks. Analysis of models with and without these loops may suggest evolutionary reasons for systems to have developed such complex structures. To gain such insights, sensitivity analysis can be an important tool for the systems biologist. It identifies the strengths and vulnerabilities of a biological system, information that is useful in selecting drug targets. Such analyses can also be used to help design experiments and are discussed in detail in the next section.

2.4.1. Sensitivity Analysis

Because experiments in biological systems can be time consuming and/or costly, experimental design should be carefully considered. Sensitivity analysis of ODE models, which may be preliminary in nature or well established and validated, can help investigators design efficient, productive experiments. Using the methods described below, one can select a set of feasible system inputs, states (species of interest) to measure, and, potentially, time points that will give maximum information about the system—particularly the set of parameters for a model.

For a model of ordinary differential equations, a change in a parameter p_j from its nominal value may cause a change in state x_i, which is captured by a sensitivity coefficient, $s_{ij}(t_k)$ (where i ranges from 1 to the number of states that will be measured, j ranges from 1 to the number of parameters in the model that are of interest, and k ranges from 1 to the total number of time points). The sensitivity coefficient is given by

$$s_{ij}(t_k) = \frac{\partial x_i(t_k)}{\partial p_j} \tag{2.8}$$

Brute-force methods can be used to calculate s_{ij}, but it can be calculated more efficiently. For an ODE model $\dot{x} = f(x,t)$, application of the chain rule to Eq. (2.8) yields

$$\dot{s}_{ij} = \frac{\partial f}{\partial x_i} s_{ij} + \frac{\partial f}{\partial p_j} \tag{2.9}$$

Integration of Eq. (2.9) gives the sensitivity coefficients $s_{ij}(t_k)$. These coefficients are combined to form a sensitivity matrix, $S(t_k)$, for each time point.

Taking these "sensitivity matrices" and estimating the measurement error for each state, one can generate what is known as the Fisher information matrix (FIM). For a given experimental protocol, the FIM consolidates model information (i.e., the sensitivity matrices) and measurement error to estimate how many and how well model parameters can be identified from these data. For discrete-time-point measurements, the FIM is calculated as follows (Zak et al., 2003):

$$\text{FIM} = \sum_{k=1}^{N_k} S^T(t_k) V^{-1}(t_k) S(t_k) \tag{2.10}$$

N_k is the total number of time steps, and $V(t_k)$, which describes estimates of measurement covariance at time point t_k, is a diagonal matrix with elements:

$$V(t_k) = \begin{pmatrix} \sigma_1^2(t_k) & 0 & 0 \\ 0 & \ddots & 0 \\ 0 & 0 & \sigma_{N_x}^2(t_k) \end{pmatrix} \tag{2.11}$$

$$\sigma_i(t_k) = \text{RE}_i x_i(t_k) + \text{AE}_i$$

where RE_i is an estimated relative error in the measurement of state i, and AE_i (absolute error) is a small but nonzero number to eliminate numerical errors associated with inverting the matrices $V(t_k)$.

Once calculated, the FIM can be used to estimate lower bounds on how large the variance around the nominal model parameter ($\sigma_{p_j}^2$) would be if it were identified using data from the selected experimental protocol as follows [for a more rigorous treatment, refer to the article by Zak et al. (2003)]:

$$\sigma_{p_j}^2 \geq (\text{FIM}^{-1})_{jj} \tag{2.12}$$

These sizes of standard deviations for each parameter of interest can then be used to select between experimental protocols. In the case study that follows, if the 95% confidence interval, $[p_{\text{nominal}} - 1.96\sigma_p, p_{\text{nominal}} + 1.96\sigma_p]$, does not contain zero, a parameter is taken to be identifiable—the more parameters that can be identified from a protocol, the better. For equal numbers of identifiable parameters, one possible optimization is to choose the experimental protocol that minimizes the average normalized 95% confidence interval $[(1/N_j)\sum_j 1.96\sigma_{p_j}/p_j]$ over all identifiable parameters. Using these formulations of identifiability and optimality, one can design experiments to maximize the accuracy of parameter estimation by selecting a set of input profiles, measured states, and time points.

2.4.2. Case Study: Application of Sensitivity Analysis to Design of Experiments to Elucidate the Insulin Signaling Pathway

The optimal input profile and measurement selection approach outlined above were applied to a published model of the insulin signaling pathway (Sedaghat et al., 2002). Differential equations, largely mechanistic in nature, were used to describe the time-varying concentrations of 21 state variables, as illustrated in Figure 2.11.

The Sedaghat model, with a slight modification, was compiled in XPP and solved with numerical integration over a 60-minute "experiment" (Kwei et al., 2008). Following Sedaghat et al., the nominal insulin input concentration was a 15-minute pulse input, going from 0 M to 10^{-7} M and returning to 0 M.

Thirty parameters for the model were perturbed by 1% of their nominal values to calculate sensitivities for all states for each time step; the time steps were nearly continuous, but smaller numbers of time steps can also be consid-

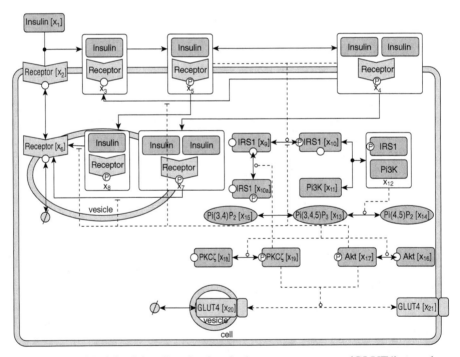

Figure 2.11 Model of insulin-stimulated glucose transporter (GLUT4) translocation with feedback mechanisms. Abbreviations used: insulin receptor substrate 1 (IRS1), phosphatidylinositol 3-kinase (PI3K), phosphatidylinositol 3,4-bisphosphate (PI(3,4)P$_2$), phosphatidylinositol 3,4,5-trisphosphate (PI(3,4)P$_2$), phosphatidylinositol 4,5-bisphosphate (PI(4,5)P$_2$), protein kinase B (Akt), atypical protein kinase C-ζ (PKCζ), and facilitated glucose transporter 4 (GLUT4). [Adapted from Sedaghat et al. (2002).]

ered with this method. This sensitivity analysis was conducted using the sensitivity analysis tool BioSens (Taylor et al., 2005).

When all 21 states were "measured," the relative error for each state (RE) was set to 1%, while absolute error (AE) was set to 10^{-7} to ensure that V could be inverted—these numbers can easily be changed to more realistic ones. To remove a state i from the set of measured states (see below), RE_i was set to 10^7% to simulate a highly noisy measurement.

2.4.2.1. Optimal Input Selection

Varying insulin input to the system is one method to maximize parameter estimation accuracy. Simple insulin input profiles were analyzed for maximum parameter identification in the model with feedback (Table 2.2). The inputs were ranked first by the number of identifiable parameters (out of 31) and then by the average normalized 95% confidence interval.

Of the insulin inputs tested, the best result was the 1-minute pulse with 21 identifiable parameters, while the worst was the step input, with 19 identifiable parameters (Table 2.2). Although the difference in the number of identifiable parameters is small, this example shows that the input profile dynamics can have quantifiable effects on the identifiability of model parameters.

2.4.2.2. Optimal Measurement Selection

For ease of calculation, measurement selection was carried out on the 1-minute pulse, which had 21 identifiable parameters, since insulin input dynamics did not seem to have a significant effect on parameter identifiability. As many states as possible were removed from the FIM while maintaining the same number of identified parameters. The FIM including all permutations of the remaining states were calculated, ranking the results by the number of identified parameters and by the average width of 95% confidence intervals. The

TABLE 2.2   Parameter Identification from Various Input Selections, Ranked by Number of Identifiable Parameters Followed by Average Width of 95% Confidence Interval for Identifiable Parameters

Input Description	Parameters	$\dfrac{1}{N_p}\sum_j 1.96\sigma_{p_j}/p_j$
1-min pulse	21	9.84%
5-min pulse	21	9.98%
0.5-min pulse	21	11.2%
15-min pulse	20	6.58%
Ramp up	20	7.61%
Ramp down	20	11.3%
Two 1-min pulses	19	7.37%
Step	19	15.1%

TABLE 2.3 Parameter Identification from Optimized Measurement Selection

State Measurement	Parameters	$\dfrac{1}{N_p}\sum\limits_j 1.96\sigma_{p_j}/p_j$
x2, x3, . . . , x21	21	9.84%
x15, x17, x19, x20, x21	21	11.7%
x15, x17, x19, x20	21	16.5%
x15, x17, x20	20	23.0%
x15, x17	14	25.1%
x17	9	46.3%

optimal measurement selection for each number of allowed measurements is given in Table 2.3.

Measurement of only five states, $x_{15}, x_{17}, x_{19}, x_{20}$, and x_{21}, provides 21 identifiable parameters; nearly all of the parameter information content available is included in these five states, all of which are near the end of the signaling pathway (see Kwei et al., 2008, for more information). The fact that such sparse measurement selection of the signaling cascade can yield high parameter information suggests that measurements of downstream signaling states can contain rich information about upstream reactions and their parameter values. In fact, measuring just one state (x_{17}) allows one to identify nine model parameters accurately.

2.5. CONCLUSIONS

The sequencing of the human genome was a revolutionary advance that provides a foundation for a better understanding of disease pathology and more effective identification of disease treatments. It has enabled the characterization of genes and their encoded proteins, the fundamental components of biological systems. Systems biology builds on this knowledge by focusing on the connections and interactions between those components and the influences of environment stimuli. This network-level understanding enables the prediction of behaviors in different conditions and in response to various perturbations. These predictions may suggest potential new drug targets, facilitate the discovery of off-target or unanticipated drug effects, and lead to the introduction of preventive, individualized medicine.

REFERENCES

Aton, S.J., and Herzog, E.D. (2005). Come together, right . . . now: synchronization of rhythms in a mammalian circadian clock. *Neuron 48*, 531–534.

Becker-Weimann, S., Wolf, J., Herzel, H., and Kramer, A. (2004). Modeling feedback loops of the mammalian circadian oscillator. *Biophys J 87*, 3023–3034.

Bell, S.L., and Palsson, B.O. (2005). expa: a program for calculating extreme pathways in biochemical reaction networks. *Bioinformatics 21*, 1739–1740.

Beyer, H.-G., and Schwefel, H.-P. (2002). Evolution strategies: a comprehensive introduction. *Nat Comput 1*, 3–52.

Coello Coello, C.A. (2005). An introduction to evolutionary algorithms and their applications. In: F. F. Ramos et al. (editors), International Symposium and School on Advanced Distributed Systems (ISSADS), pp. 425–442, *Springer-Verlag Lecture Notes in Computer Science* Vol. 3563, Guadalajara, Mexico.

Cornish-Bowden, A., and Cardenas, M.L. (2000). From genome to cellular phenotype: a role for metabolic flux analysis? *Nat Biotechnol 18*, 267–268.

Covert, M.W., Schilling, C.H., Famili, I., Edwards, J.S., Goryanin, II, Selkov, E., and Palsson, B.O. (2001). Metabolic modeling of microbial strains *in silico*. *Trends Biochem Sci 26*, 179–186.

Daan, S., and Pittendrigh, C.S. (1976). Functional-analysis of circadian pacemakers in nocturnal rodents: 2. Variability of phase response curves. *J. Comp Physiol 106*, 253–266.

DeCoursey, P. (2004). Overview of biological timing from unicells to humans. In: *Chronobiology: Biological Timekeeping* (Dunlap, J., Loros, J., and DeCoursey, P., eds.). Sinauer Associates, Sunderland, MA, pp. 3–24.

Ding, J.M., Chen, D., Weber, E.T., Faiman, L.E., Rea, M.A., and Gillette, M.U. (1994). Resetting the biological clock: mediation of nocturnal circadian shifts by glutamate and NO. *Science 266*, 1713–1717.

Dunlap, J.C. (1999). Molecular bases for circadian clocks. *Cell 96*, 271–290.

Edwards, J.S., Ibarra, R.U., and Palsson, B.O. (2001). *In silico* predictions of *Escherichia coli* metabolic capabilities are consistent with experimental data. *Nat Biotechnol 19*, 125–130.

Edwards, J.S., Covert, M., and Palsson, B. (2002). Metabolic modelling of microbes: the flux-balance approach. *Environ Microbiol 4*, 133–140.

El-Samad, H., Kurata, H., Doyle, J.C., Gross, C.A., and Khammash, M. (2005). Surviving heat shock: control strategies for robustness and performance. *Proc Natl Acad Sci USA 102*, 2736–2741.

Famili, I., Forster, J., Nielson, J., and Palsson, B.O. (2003). *Saccharomyces cerevisiae* phenotypes can be predicted by using constraint-based analysis of a genome-scale reconstructed metabolic network. *Proc Natl Acad Sci USA 100*, 13134–13139.

Fogel, D.B. (1994). An introduction to simulated evolutionary optimization. *IEEE Trans Neural Networks 5*, 3–14.

Follstad, B.D., Balcarcel, R.R., Stephanopoulos, G., and Wang, D.I.C. (1999). Metabolic flux analysis of hybridoma continuous culture steady state multiplicity. *Biotechnol Bioeng 63*, 675–683.

Forger, D.B., and Peskin, C.S. (2003). A detailed predictive model of the mammalian circadian clock. *Proc Natl Acad Sci USA 100*, 14806–14811.

Gayen, K., and Venkatesh, K.V. (2006). Analysis of optimal phenotypic space using elementary modes as applied to *Corynebacterium glutamicum*. *BMC Bioinf 7*, 445.

Gayen, K., Gupta, M., and Venkatesh, K.V. (2007). Elementary mode analysis to study the preculturing effect on the metabolic state of *Lactobacillus rhamnosus* during growth on mixed substrates. *In Silico Biol 7*, 12.

Gonze, D., Bernard, S., Waltermann, C., Kramer, A., and Herzel, H. (2005). Spontaneous synchronization of coupled circadian oscillators. *Biophys J 89*, 120–129.

Hildebrandt, S., Raden, D., Petzold, L.R., Robinson, A.R., and Doyle, F.J., III (2008). A top-down approach to mechanistic biological modeling: application to the single-chain antibody folding pathway. *Biophys J 95*, 3535–3558.

Kell, D.B. (2006). Systems biology, metabolic modelling and metabolomics in drug discovery and development. *Drug Discov Today 11*, 1085–1092.

Kholodenko, B.N., Kiyatkin, A., Bruggeman, F.J., Sontag, E., Westerhoff, H.V., and Hoek, J.B. (2002). Untangling the wires: a strategy to trace functional interactions in signaling and gene networks. *Proc Natl Acad Sci USA 99*, 12841–12846.

Klamt, S., and Stelling, J. (2003). Two approaches for metabolic pathway analysis? *Trends Biotechnol 21*, 64–69.

Kwei, F.C., Sanft, K.R., Petzold, L.R., and Doyle, F.J., III (2008). Systems analysis of the insulin signaling pathway. Presented at the 17th International Federation of Automatic Control World Congress, Seoul, Korea.

Lee, C., Etchegaray, J.P., Cagampang, F.R., Loudon, A.S., and Reppert, S.M. (2001). Posttranslational mechanisms regulate the mammalian circadian clock. *Cell 107*, 855–867.

Leloup, J.C., and Goldbeter, A. (2003). Toward a detailed computational model for the mammalian circadian clock. *Proc Natl Acad Sci USA 100*, 7051–7056.

Liu, A.C., Tran, H.G., Zhang, E.E., Priest, A.A., Welsh, D.K., and Kay, S.A. (2008). Redundant function of REV-ERBalpha and beta and non-essential role for Bmal1 cycling in transcriptional regulation of intracellular circadian rhythms. *PLoS Genet 4*, e1000023.

Mahadevan, R., and Palsson, B.O. (2005). Properties of metabolic networks: structure versus function. *Biophys J 88*, L7–L9.

Michel, S., and Colwell, C.S. (2001). Cellular communication and coupling within the suprachiasmatic nucleus. *Chronobiol Int 18*, 579–600.

Nielsen, J. (1998). Metabolic engineering: techniques for analysis of targets for genetic manipulations. *Biotechnol Bioeng 58*, 125–132.

Nissen, T.L., Schulze, U., Nielsen, J., and Villadsen, J. (1997). Flux distributions in anaerobic, glucose-limited continuous cultures of *Saccharomyces cerevisiae*. *Microbiology UK 143*, 203–218.

Oliveira, A.P., Nielsen, J., and Forster, J. (2005). Modeling *Lactococcus lactis* using a genome-scale flux model. *BMC Microbiol 5*.

Palsson, B.O., Price, N.D., and Papin, J.A. (2003). Development of network-based pathway definitions: the need to analyze real metabolic networks. *Trends Biotechnol 21*, 195–198.

Pittendrigh, C.S., and Daan, S. (1976). Functional-analysis of circadian pacemakers in nocturnal rodents: 1. Stability and lability of spontaneous frequency. *J Comp Physiol 106*, 223–252.

Poolman, M.G. (2006). ScrumPy: metabolic modelling with python. *Syst Biol (Stevenage) 153*, 375–378.

Pramanik, J., and Keasling, J.D. (1997). Stoichiometric model of *Escherichia coli* metabolism: incorporation of growth-rate dependent biomass composition and mechanistic energy requirements. *Biotechnol Bioeng 56*, 398–421.

Price, N.D., Famili, I., Beard, D.A., and Palsson, B.O. (2002). Extreme pathways and Kirchhoff's second law. *Biophys J 83*, 2879–2882.

Price, N.D., Reed, J.L., Papin, J.A., Famili, I., and Palsson, B.O. (2003). Analysis of metabolic capabilities using singular value decomposition of extreme pathway matrices. *Biophys J 84*, 794–804.

Ramakrishna, R., Edwards, J.S., McCulloch, A., and Palsson, B.O. (2001). Flux-balance analysis of mitochondrial energy metabolism: consequences of systemic stoichiometric constraints. *Am J Physiol Regul Integr Comp Physiol 280*, R695–R704.

Reed, J.L., and Palsson, B.O. (2003). Thirteen years of building constraint-based *in silico* models of *Escherichia coli*. *J Bacteriol 185*, 2692–2699.

Reppert, S.M., and Weaver, D.R. (2002). Coordination of circadian timing in mammals. *Nature 418*, 935–941.

Sauro, H.M., and Ingalls, B. (2004). Conservation analysis in biochemical networks: computational issues for software writers. *Biophys Chem 109*, 1–15.

Schilling, C.H., Edwards, J.S., Letscher, D., and Palsson, B.O. (2000). Combining pathway analysis with flux balance analysis for the comprehensive study of metabolic systems. *Biotechnol Bioeng 71*, 286–306.

Schwartz, J.M., Gaugain, C., Nacher, J.C., Daruvar, A.D., and Kanehisa, M. (2007). Observing metabolic function at the genome scale. *Gerome Biol 8*, R132.

Schwarz, R., Musch, P., von Kamp, A., Engels, B., Schirmer, H., Schuster, S., and Dandekar, T. (2005). YANA: a software tool for analyzing flux modes, gene-expression and enzyme activities. *BMC Bioinf 6*, 135.

Sedaghat, A.R., Sherman, A., and Quon, M.J. (2002). A mathematical model of metabolic insulin signaling pathways. *Am J Physiol Endocrinol Metab 283*, E1084–E1101.

Stelling, J. (2004). Mathematical models in microbial systems biology. *Curr Opin Microbiol 7*, 513–518.

Stelling, J., Klamt, S., Bettenbrock, K., Schuster, S., and Gilles, E.D. (2002). Metabolic network structure determines key aspects of functionality and regulation. *Nature 420*, 190–193.

Stephanopoulos, G. (1999). Metabolic fluxes and metabolic engineering. *Metab Eng 1*, 1–11.

Taylor, S.R., Gunawan, R., Gadkar, K., and Doyle, F.J., III (2005). *BioSens Sensitivity Analysis Toolkit* (UCSB's contribution to Bio-SPICE), v2beta.

To, T.L., Henson, M.A., Herzog, E.D., and Doyle, F.J., III (2007). A molecular model for intercellular synchronization in the mammalian circadian clock. *Biophys J 92*, 3792–3803.

Wiback, S.J., and Palsson, B.O. (2002). Extreme pathway analysis of human red blood cell metabolism. *Biophys J 83*, 808–818.

Wiback, S.J., Mahadevan, R., and Palsson, B.O. (2004). Using metabolic flux data to further constrain the metabolic solution space and predict internal flux patterns: the *Escherichia coli* spectrum. *Biotechnol Bioeng 86*, 317–331.

Xu, P., Raden, D., Doyle, F.J., III, and Robinson, A.S. (2005). Analysis of unfolded protein response during single-chain antibody expression in *Saccaromyces cerevisiae* reveals different roles for BiP and PDI in folding. *Metab Eng 7*, 269–279.

Zak, D.E., Gonye, G.E., Schwaber, J.S., and Doyle, F.J., III (2003). Importance of input perturbations and stochastic gene expression in the reverse engineering of genetic regulatory networks: insights from an identifiability analysis of an *in silico* network. *Genome Res 13*, 2396–2405.

CHAPTER 3

Methods in *In Silico* Biology: Modeling Feedback Dynamics in Pathways

PETER WELLSTEAD

The Hamilton Institute, NUIM, Maynooth, Republic of Ireland

OLAF WOLKENHAUER

Systems Biology and Bioinformatics, University of Rostock, Rostock, Germany

Summary

Statistical modeling has become an established tool in biology. Less well accepted is the role that is performed by mathematical modeling in the understanding of biochemical network dynamics. In this chapter we address this area, beginning with a discussion of general statistical modeling issues, and followed by a discussion of relevant issues in mathematical modeling of dynamical systems. It is the construction of mathematical models that will allow biologists to understand and interpret dynamic features of biological processes. The most important of these features is the role of model structure in modifying dynamics. Here we consider one class of structural modification—feedback and feedforward—and how it is used to achieve biological and metabolic functions.

3.1. INTRODUCTION

Statistical modeling and pattern recognition are established techniques in bioinformatics, drug discovery, and drug development. However, the mathematical modeling of dynamic processes, together with the corresponding analysis of their behavior, is not yet accepted in the life science community. If the goal is to identify a set of genes or proteins that *may* play a role in a particular

Systems Biology in Drug Discovery and Development, First Edition.
Edited by Daniel L. Young, Seth Michelson.
© 2012 John Wiley & Sons, Inc. Published 2012 by John Wiley & Sons, Inc.

experiment, simple experiments (e.g., Western blotting, microarrays, two-dimensional gel proteomics) will suffice to answer this question. To understand the role of a protein in processes such as apoptosis, cell differentiation, and the cell cycle, conventional models are not sufficient. In most subcellular processes related to cell signaling and metabolism, time matters. Nonlinear temporal interactions of genes and proteins can only be understood with concepts from systems theory—there is no alternative. This observation is slowly being accepted, and although many are quick to embrace the label *systems biology*, few understand the consequences that this approach will have on the design of experiments, related technologies, and the time and effort required. The complexity of nonlinear dynamics in subcellular processes is a source of surprises in experiments. However, understanding such surprises is crucial, as they contribute to nonspecific and unanticipated side effects of drugs and treatments.

It is not necessary to develop mathematical models for every question that arises in systems biology, but if nonlinearity and temporal changes in the quantity of components matter, a language other than qualitative textual and pictorial descriptions is required. In this spirit, it is imperative that biologists realize that mathematical modeling provides a quantitative basis for the analysis of molecular and cellular process dynamics. The immediate benefit is to provide both a means of organizing life science experimentation and a framework within which to explain the outcomes. This framework is objective (e.g., it is not driven by personal views) and thus offers a guide for experiment design when groups of researchers and laboratories are involved. The associated mathematical model forms a common repository of biological knowledge and a rational basis for the evaluation of hypotheses. Sasagawa's use of mathematical modeling to validate hypotheses on the ERK signaling network is an example of how a mathematical model might be used in this way (Sasagawa et al., 2005).

However, mathematical models have an additional significance; they reveal the crucial importance of system analytic properties such as *causality* and *feedback* in determining biological outcomes. The analysis of these system properties can guide wet laboratory experiments and also help verify proposed dynamic models of cellular processes, as well as showing how dynamic and structural features of models can determine biological behavior. This set of interacting processes is illustrated in Figure 3.1, in which *statistical modeling* enables and informs important decisions concerning data structure and information content. *Mathematical modeling*, on the other hand, allows us to embody our ideas concerning the temporal evolution of a process in quantitative form. On the other hand, *systems analysis* reveals features and properties of the dynamic performance (e.g., the sensitivity of the response to changes, the robustness of the system and its stability properties).

Thus, the systems approach fits into the overall biological investigation process as shown in Figure 3.1. The aim of this chapter is to clarify this approach by reviewing the importance of statistical modeling, mathematical

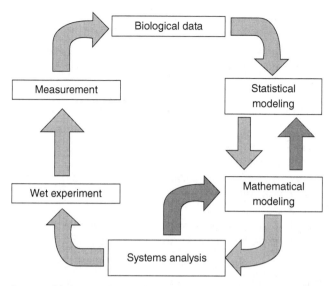

Figure 3.1 Systems biology cycle: placing statistical modeling, mathematical modeling, and systems analysis in the context of biological investigation. Note that the two darker arrows are used to emphasize that iterative feedback among analysis, mathematical modeling, and statistical modeling helps build our understanding of the biological process before we need to return to wet experiments.

modeling, and two crucial systems analysis areas: the role of feedback and feedforward in biological dynamic systems.

A particular theme of this chapter is to demonstrate (1) how mathematical methods are supported by statistical modeling and (2) how principles used to characterize the dynamics of physical systems can be (and are being) applied to biological systems in a quantitative and informative way. In this spirit, and following the pattern shown in Figure 3.1, this chapter is laid out as follows: In Section 3.2 we describe how *statistical modeling* helps us understand basic biological interactions. In Section 3.3 we review the *mathematical modeling* forms required to characterize dynamic system performance. Section 3.4 focuses selectively on *feedback* and *feedforward* and their role in determining a system's dynamic behavior.

3.2. STATISTICAL MODELING

Modeling of a network or pathway assumes a good understanding of the components whose interactions are described by dynamic models. Thus, the analysis of biological data proceeds by a sequence of modeling steps, starting with statistical modeling and proceeding toward a mathematical model, as described by kinetic rate equations—in other words, the state dynamics (Figure 3.2). Prior to the modeling of subcellular dynamic systems, one has to confirm the components (genes, metabolites, proteins) that should be represented in the dynamic model. In the present section we review key ideas in statistical modeling that are used in molecular and cell biology. We begin with the most basic task of testing for differences, followed by correlation and regression analyses. The latter is a first step toward an analysis of time-course data. From simple statistical significance tests to state-space representations, each method allows us to ask specific questions. The more informative the question is, the more demanding are the techniques required to collect the type and quality of data. Rate equation models are the most expressive description of the mechanisms that underlie cell function, but these models are also the most demanding with respect to the required accuracy and the effort required to produce them. Rich, quantitative time-course data remain a main bottleneck for applications of dynamic pathway modeling in drug design and discovery.

3.2.1. Testing Differences

The vast majority of experiments in molecular and cellular biology are directed at the detection of differences. In knockout experiments this approach is obvious, but in Western blotting and two-dimensional gel analysis, one typically attempts to detect the presence of a component or test for a change. Despite the advances in detection technology, we must handle uncertainty in data through replicate experiments. Repeating an experiment generates a sample from which we can establish a statistical model. The most frequently employed statistical model is that of a Gaussian (or normal) distribution:

$$p(x) = \frac{1}{\sigma\sqrt{2\pi}} e^{-(x-\mu)^2/2\sigma^2}$$

where μ is a measure of *central tendency*, determining a point around which the values of a sample will cluster (μ is also referred to as the *expected* or *mean value*). *Variance* σ^2 is a measure of how far the data are spread around the expected value. Both μ and σ^2 are parameters of the statistical model and must therefore be estimated from the data sampled. The density function above represents a *model*, that is, an abstraction from the sample of experimental data. Once the model is accepted (and in contrast to differential equation models, this type of model does not cause any concern among experimentalists), we can use it to make predictions.

Given two samples, how does one—with confidence—establish a difference between them? The mean value and variance can be estimated from data, but this means that their value will also vary, something quantified with the *standard error*:

$$\overline{SE} = \frac{s}{\sqrt{n}}, \quad \text{where} \quad s = \sqrt{\frac{n}{n-1}\sigma_n^2} \quad \text{and} \quad \sigma_n^2 = \frac{1}{n}\sum_{i=1}^{n}(x_i - \bar{X})^2$$

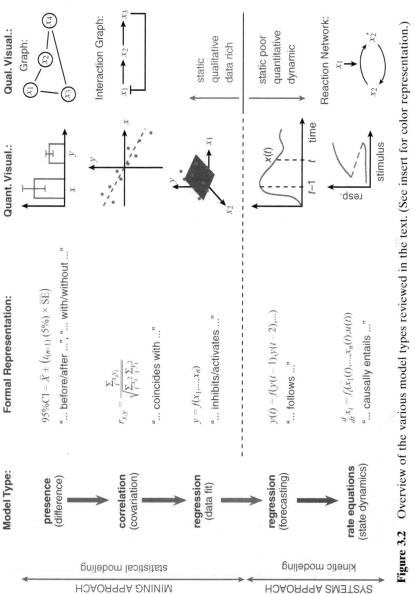

Figure 3.2 Overview of the various model types reviewed in the text. (See insert for color representation.)

Here n is the size of the sample and the subscript n to σ^2 indicates the sample variance as an estimate of the variance of the model above. The sample mean does not follow a Gaussian but rather a t-distribution, enabling one to calculate a 95% *confidence interval* (CI):

$$95\%\text{CI}(\text{mean}) = \bar{X} \pm \left[t_{n-1}(5\%) \times \overline{\text{SE}} \right]$$

Using a statistical table (or computer program), one can determine the *critical value* $t_{n-1}(5\%)$ as an interval defined by the number of standard errors ($\overline{\text{SE}}$) away from the mean value ($\bar{X}$) within which 95 out of 100 times the real mean value would be found (i.e., with a probability of 0.95).

The two-sample t-test is used to decide whether the means of two sets of measurements, sampled from two independent populations, are significantly different. The following steps are performed for this analysis:

1. The null hypothesis is that the mean of the differences is not different from zero. In other words, the two groups X and Y from which the samples were obtained have the same mean.

2. The test statistic t is given by

$$t = \frac{\text{mean difference}}{\text{SE of difference}} = \frac{\bar{X} - \bar{Y}}{\overline{\text{SE}}_d}$$

The standard error of the difference $\overline{\text{SE}}_d$ is more difficult to calculate because this would involve comparing each member of the first population with each member of the second. Assuming that the variance of both populations is the same, we can estimate $\overline{\text{SE}}_d$ using the equation

$$\overline{\text{SE}}_d = \sqrt{\left(\overline{\text{SE}}_x\right)^2 + \left(\overline{\text{SE}}_y\right)^2}$$

where $\overline{\text{SE}}_x$ and $\overline{\text{SE}}_y$ are the standard errors of the two populations.

3. Calculate the significance probability p that the absolute value of the test statistic would be equal to or greater than t if the null hypothesis were true. There are $n_x + n_y - 2$ degrees of freedom, where n_x and n_y are the sizes of samples X and Y.

4. Using a statistical software package, if $p < 0.05$, reject the null hypothesis; the sample means are significantly different from each other. If $p \geq 0.05$, there is no evidence to reject the null hypothesis; the two sample means are not significantly different from each other.

5. The 95% confidence interval for the mean difference is given by

$$95\% \text{ CI}(\text{difference}) = \bar{X} - \bar{Y} \pm \left[t_{n_x + n_y - 2}(5\%) \times \overline{\text{SE}}_d \right]$$

We summarize this illustration for the handling of uncertainty with statistical models as follows. Starting from a set of experimental data (our two samples), we adopted an abstract (statistical) model. Once the model is established it allows one to make predictions, which here is related to the significance of these sample differences. The primary purpose of a statistical model is to account for uncertainty, and there is no doubt that this type of modeling is well established and accepted by experimentalists. We have argued above that dynamical models are necessary for dealing with the complexity arising from nonlinear spatiotemporal interactions among cellular components. Nonetheless, the difference models described here are frequently used because they demand little with respect to sampling technology or experiment design. The downside is that these models allow us to consider only the presence of a protein, whether a gene is active or not, or more generally whether or not there is a change. If our technologies allow us to measure "levels" of concentrations or numbers of molecules, we require a different statistical concept, leading us to correlation and regression analysis.

3.2.2. Associations and Regression Modeling

If activity levels can be quantified in experiments, one can establish and test for *associations* using the (product-moment) correlation coefficient:

$$r_{x,y} = \frac{\sum_i x_i y_i}{\sqrt{\sum_i x_i^2 \sum_i y_i^2}}$$

The correlation coefficient is a value between -1 and 1 that describes whether the sizes of two variables are independent or whether they co-vary. A value of -1 means that if one variable is large, the other is small. The other extreme is when $r_{x,y} = +1$, meaning that if one variable is large, the value of the other is also large. A correlation coefficient near zero means that there is no association in the sizes of two variables. In other words, using correlation analysis we can test whether the size of one variable coincides with the level of another. As with the test for differences, the correlation coefficient is subject to variations that can be described with a confidence interval. We do not pursue this issue further, but we should comment on an error in the interpretation of correlation that is widespread and damaging. Namely, it is a common misconception that correlations imply causation. This notion may arise from correlation plots. If the values of two variables coincide, one being large or small as the values of the other are small or large, or large or small, this should not be interpreted to mean that "increasing one variable induces an increase or decrease in the other variable." It is, of course, the aim of most research to determine the causal effects of change; however, many technologies and experimental designs cannot deliver on this goal. Toward this end, dynamic models aim to represent and explain the causal relationships among variables. A step in this direction is regression modeling.

Let y denote a dependent variable that we wish to predict on the basis of independent variables $x_1, x_2, \ldots, x_m$. Note that we now refer to a *variable*, that is, a changeable quantity of the system. A variable is thus a concept: for example, the *expression level* of a gene or protein, and the sampling or measurement gives us a value (or sample of values) for this variable. Using small capital letters to denote variables as well as sample values can be confusing, which is why capital letters are often used in the statistical literature to denote variables. This notation is not, however, very common in systems theory, where Y is used to denote the space of possible values that the variable y can take. In this chapter the difference between a sample value and a variable should be clear from the context.

There are two main purposes of multiple regression analysis. The first is to establish a linear prediction equation that will enable a better prediction of y than is possible by any single independent variable x_j. The aim is to define a set of independent variables that predict a significant proportion of the variance in y. The second purpose is to estimate and fit a structural model to "explain" variation in the observations of the response variable y in terms of ("as a function of") the independent regressor variables x_j. Such a *functional relationship* is formally expressed by a mapping denoted by f, such that for given values of $x_1, \ldots, x_m$, these are "mapped into" a value y. The mathematical notation for this mapping is $x_1, \ldots, x_m \mapsto y$ and is equivalent to writing $y = f(x_1, \ldots, x_m)$. The relationship between the independent and dependent variables, indicated by f, can be linear or nonlinear in nature. A linear multiple regression model takes the form

$$\hat{y} = \theta_0 + \theta_{y_1} x_1 + \theta_{y_2} x_2 + \cdots + \theta_{y_m} x_m$$

where the value $\hat{y}$ of y predicted is a function of m independent variables $x_1, \ldots, x_m$. The partial regression coefficients θ_{y_i} are the parameters of this model. The key advance given by the multiple regression model compared to the previous statistical models is that the relationship between the variables $x_1, \ldots, x_m$ and y is now given structure (here, a weighted sum). In other words, the value of y predicted is specified in terms of the parameters θ_{y_i}, which specify the model performance precisely. The use of a parameterized model separates regression analysis from the parameter–free approach of correlation analysis. If the parameters of a model have a biochemical interpretation, these values may be extracted from the literature. In most cases the parameters must be determined ("estimated") from experimental data. However, with the current state of the art in experimental design and instrumentation, this determination is usually impractical. Nonetheless, regression techniques are a huge step forward toward dynamic models that are described subsequently in this chapter and reviewed in Jaqaman and Danuser (2006).

3.2.3. Time-Series Analysis

Thus far we have assumed that gene and protein expression levels do not depend on the point in time at which they are measured. Many experiments are, however, of a stimulus–response nature in which a change in one variable is induced and the subsequent changes in one or more other variables are observed. For example, a cell signaling pathway may be stimulated by adding ligands to a culture, the response to stress, including changes in pH levels, assessed by inducing changes in temperature, oxygen supply, or modifying levels of small-molecule concentrations. To use the statistical tools described above, one assumes that in these before-and-after experiments the system is initially at rest (in a steady state), and following the stimulus (perturbation, stress), the system will eventually settle into another steady state. In other words, one must demonstrate that the before-and-after measurements are independent of time. This can only be done by a series of subsequent measurements to test whether there are no further changes. Measurements at only two time points would therefore rarely suffice. There are, however, many situations, arising from Western blots, microarrays, and more recently, from two-dimensional gel technologies, that have a small number of time points (say, less than 12) for which we want to test whether there is a basic trend (up/down) in the data. Regression modeling allows this analysis by considering time as the independent variable:

$$\hat{y}(t) = \theta_0 + \theta_1 t$$

where θ_1 is the regression coefficient and θ_0 determines the intercept of the trend line with the y-axis. Given that the experiments are expensive and time consuming, this type of analysis is often sufficient. However, for cell functions, including apoptosis and cell differentiation, we find that the behavior of the system is more complex and such analyses will not suffice. Observing quantitative changes in protein concentrations in these processes reveals characteristic patterns, including cyclic changes or transient dynamics that could not be captured with a simple trend line. Autoregressive models intuitively appear to offer a solution in these cases, but since the prediction of y is only a function of its past values, such a model would not provide any insight into the mechanisms that have generated the observed data. Although very successful in econometrics and the engineering sciences, conventional time-series analysis is not very useful in systems biology. Hopefully, this situation will change as measurement technologies are developed that allow temporal measurements of the correct variables and at a sufficiently high sampling rate [see the article by Crampin et al. (2004) for another perspective on this issue].

The main point of the present section is thus to illustrate a class of statistical models, each model requiring different experiments or technologies and providing answers to different questions. This model class is shown diagrammatically in the top part of Figure 3.2 (the "mining approach"). In the next two sections the systems approach is employed, as illustrated in the lower part of Figure 3.2. The aim of the systems approach is to extract as much information as possible from the data and from the theoretical consideration of biochemical reactions that occur in an experiment. The more informative the models, the more demanding are the experiments. An apoptotic process is an example in which statistical models of the type described in this section provide a starting point with which one can then establish the system components that could compose a kinetic model. Apoptotic pathways are nonlinear dynamic processes, requiring systems-theoretic tools of the type described above. Cellular decisions in apoptosis are not made on the basis of whether a gene is present or a protein is expressed, but rather, it is the history of changes in concentration that determines the outcome. Not even a steady-state analysis will suffice, and sophisticated tools are required to develop and analyze such models. The behavior of such subcellular processes is characterized by mathematical modeling, discussed in Section 3.3, and feedback and feedforward mechanisms, discussed in Section 3.4.

3.3. MATHEMATICAL MODELING

The replacement of qualitative, case-by-case explanations of dynamic phenomena by explanations based on mathematical models was central to the development of manufacturing industries and the physical sciences over the past two centuries. Now at the beginning of the twenty-first century it is necessary to repeat this advancement for living systems. Mathematical modeling will again be the basis for this analysis, although in this case applied to the kinetics of biochemical processes rather than purely physical components. Mathematical models instantiate our understanding of a living system's dynamical characteristics in a way that extends the understanding given by the statistical modeling tools outlined in Section 3.2.

3.3.1. System Memory and Dynamics

Mathematical modeling of most physical systems[1] can be unified in terms of energy storage, that is, by the corresponding fluxes and potentials of physical systems (MacFarlane, 1970; Paynter, 1961; Wellstead, 1979). In this paradigm, energy is transformed, generated, stored, and dissipated in isolated (or lumped) components. In such systems, the dynamic behavior exhibited by a system's time-course behavior is an outward expression of energy transactions within the system and the patterns of interconnection of system components. Storage gives a system memory and the capacity to modify future behavior based on historical performance. In the same spirit, energy transactions imbue a system

---

[1] In general, we should mention partial differential equation models as well as stochastic and hybrid models.

with temporal precedence—the phenomenon of causality. The interconnection pattern between energy storage elements is crucial in determining the causality in a system.

For biochemical networks it is critical to model material fluxes and corresponding concentrations (Boogerd et al., 2007; Cornish-Bowden, 2004; Fell, 1997). The corresponding stored variables are the concentrations of the various biochemical species that are active in the reaction sets. It is these variables, along with the interconnection patterns that link them, that determine the dynamical response of the kinetic model.

3.3.2. State-Space Models

Newton's laws of motion provide the basis for the concept of system state—one for each storage quantity. Over time the concept of a set of states that quantify the dynamical behavior of a system has come to dominate mathematical modeling of dynamic systems. In a lumped-parameter system, the temporal evolution of the state vector is described completely by a set of initial conditions $\underline{x}(0)$, and a set of first-order ordinary differential equations:

$$\dot{\underline{x}} = f(\underline{x}, u, t)$$

where $\dot{\underline{x}}$ denotes the time derivative of the state vector and u represents external signals that influence the states in some way. Note that a minimum number of independent state variables $\underline{x}(t)$ are required for a complete and unique description of the performance of the system, an observation that explains the need to reduce the number of equations associated with biochemical differential equations to a set that describes the key biochemical concentrations.

The nature of biochemical reaction systems is such that they have specific structures (Feinberg, 1979) and performance properties (Sontag, 2007). These characteristics impose special forms on the object $f(\underline{x}, u, t)$ and the associated dynamic behavior. Such properties are important to an analysis of the complex nonlinear dynamics found in living systems, although they are not the focus of this chapter. Instead, we discuss how feedback and feedforward interconnections can contribute to dynamic responses. As a precursor to this topic, we informally discuss the role of causality and memory in mathematical modeling using linear forms of the state-space equations.

3.3.3. Linear Forms

Cell signaling and metabolic processes give rise to mathematical models that are frequently highly nonlinear. It is, however, often informative to linearize locally about specific operating points. The linear form can give valuable information about the stability of a process and its time-course behavior within the linearized region. Even in nonlinear form it is instructive (where possible) to

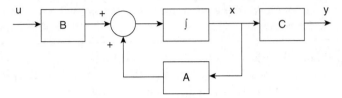

Figure 3.3   Linear state-space description showing the system memory in the forward path integrator block.

reformulate a model to show the states explicitly. The states are important because they are a biochemical system's memory bank—they determine the future behavior of a process and are the variables that a systems analyst seeks to understand. This formalism is seen graphically in a sketch of a linearized state space model (Figure 3.3), in which the block of integrators represents the memory mechanism within the system. Integration is the mechanism that makes the behavior of biochemical systems dependent on past behavior. This dependence on the past imparts dynamic characteristics to the concentrations of biochemical species represented in the state vector.

The state-space form is represented by the equations

$$\dot{x} = A\underline{x} + Bu$$
$$y = C\underline{x}$$

where y is an output variable that is a function of the states. The integrator memory bank shown in Figure 3.3 illuminates the way in which past behavior can influence future outcomes. For example, Figure 3.4 shows two time-course histories of the same model for a hypothetical biochemical signaling process (actually, an idealized biological switch for apoptotic triggering). In each of the two time courses shown, the only difference in the systems is a small difference in their histories (as quantified by the system initial values). However, the measured biological outcomes over time are very different even though only the initial conditions differ. This example gives a mathematical rationale for the problem, whereby differences in handling of samples and laboratory conditions leads to different experimental outcomes.

The model used to generate the results shown in Figure 3.4 is a relatively simple example. It was chosen to show how small changes in initial conditions typically found in signaling processes can lead to large differences in dynamic performance. When dynamic models become more complex and have more interacting components, the differences caused by very small differences in initial conditions can be huge. This insight into the importance of initial conditions was the essence of Edward Lorenz's work with models of climate systems (Gleick, 1988). The same applies in biological systems. For example, as illustrated by Wolkenhauer et al. (2007), there is a comparably dramatic potential for conditions prior to an experiment to influence biological outcomes. Such

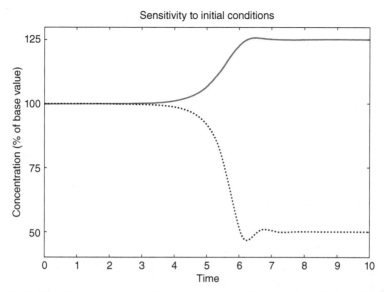

Figure 3.4 Two time courses for the same system, showing the relative differences from basal conditions for transient and steady-state behavior caused by very small changes in the prior history (as reflected in the initial states) of a mathematical model.

issues are, in part, responsible for problems with repeatability in experimental biology.

3.4. FEEDBACK AND FEEDFORWARD

The theories and analyses of dynamical systems are central to the field of control systems engineering, and the ideas of feedback and feedforward described here are core concepts in control theory. The need for such concepts emerged from the industrial revolution and the urgent need to understand the behavior of the automatic machines that replaced handcrafts [see Bennett's (1979) historical account of this transition]. A result of this history is that the approaches applied to biological feedback and feedforward are strongly influenced by experts in technological control.

3.4.1. Feedback

To quote Arnold Tustin, a twentieth-century pioneer of control systems analysis (Tustin, 1952): "It [feedback] is the fundamental principle that underlies all self-regulating systems, not only machines but also the processes of life and the tides of human affairs." While the realization that feedback is crucial to understanding living systems was not unique to Tustin,[2] his words are highly relevant as our understanding of biochemical reactions and network dynamics increases. In this section some basic insights are given into the roles of feedback and its partner, feedforward. First, we give a basic definition of *feedback*: Feedback occurs when a continuous path of signaling steps exists in which a downstream step influences an upstream step in the sequence, thus forming a feedback loop. There are two forms of feedback, negative and positive. *Negative feedback*, for which the desired effect is usually to reduce activity, is generally stabilizing. *Positive feedback*, on the other hand, increases activity and is generally destabilizing (except when used to switch variables from one state to another).

3.4.1.1. Negative Feedback Loops

In technological systems, the purpose of negative feedback is to hold key variables within desired ranges and to isolate a system against external changes; that is, it provides resistance to unwanted changes. The same is true in signaling and metabolic pathways, where negative feedback is used to maintain production levels within biologically acceptable limits. Negative regulatory loops are best known in physiological and metabolic systems by Cannon's principle of *homeostasis* (Cannon, 1932). Homeostasis is characterized by the ability of negative feedback to return key physiological variables to desired values in the face of external disturbances. The recently coined term *allostasis* is used to designate that physiological loops are not constant but adapt to particular disturbances triggered by the brain (Schulkin, 2004). In either case, negative feedback is present to manage the process dynamics.

There are multiple ways in which feedback is achieved in biochemical systems. One of the simplest forms is an unbranched biochemical pathway (Figure 3.5) in which the concentration $X_f(t)$ of the final stage exercises an inhibitory action on the first stage.

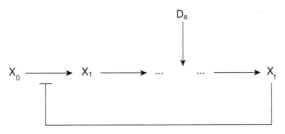

Figure 3.5   Unbranched pathway with inhibitory feedback from the final stage to the first, and a disturbance at some intermediate point.

---

[2] In his seminal book *Gaia*, James Lovelock (Lovelock, 2000) makes similar remarks about the fundamental role of control theory (of which feedback as the core element) in explaining complexity in living things.

Thus, if X_f tends to increase due to some variation in the pathway, inhibition of the first stage of the loop X_1 will tend to restore X_f toward its desired value. The negative nature of the feedback can be seen by considering the inhibitory action of the final stage on the production of the first stage as given by

$$v_1 = \frac{X_1 k_1}{1 + X_f k_f}$$

where k_1 and k_f are, respectively, kinetic coefficients associated with the initial and final stages of the pathway. Linearizing this system about small deviations, ΔX_1 and ΔX_f, from the equilibrium values of the pathway state leads to an expression for the corresponding small variations of flux in the first stage of Δv_1:

$$\Delta v_1 = \Delta X_1 \frac{k_1}{1 + X_f k_f} - \Delta X_f \frac{k_1 k_f X_1}{(1 + X_f k_f)^2}$$

In this expression changes in the flux are clearly show to be driven by the difference between the first-stage and final-stage concentrations. This differencing mechanism is at the heart of all negative feedback setups.

In addition to the illustrations of negative feedback in physiology and metabolism in Cannon (1932), many other examples have appeared in the literature. For example, Thomas and D'Ari (1990) quote an early account of negative feedback control by inhibition (Umbarger, 1961). More recently, Barkai and Leibler (1997) showed that a negative feedback loop in the chemotaxis network maintains the concentration of active enzymes constant despite variations in external (ligand) signals.

3.4.1.2. Dynamics of Negative Feedback

The usual function of negative feedback is to introduce a corrective adjustment to maintain concentrations and fluxes within biologically and metabolically acceptable limits. The time course—the dynamic response—during a correction will, however, vary depending on the dynamics of the mathematical model. For example, with a pulselike disturbance, D_e, to the pathway in Figure 3.5, the response X_f at the final stage can vary between the simple recovery shown in Figure 3.6a and the oscillatory type of response shown in Figure 3.6b. In biological processes a range of such recovery responses are observed. Whereas oscillatory response modes are rare in homeostatic loops, they are observed more frequently elsewhere in living systems. In particular, with appropriate parameter values, negative feedback can cause self-sustaining oscillations of the type that are widespread in biological processes (see, e.g., Pomerening et al., 2003). However, as emphasized below, reliable biological oscillations often involve two coupled feedback loops (see the article by Tsai

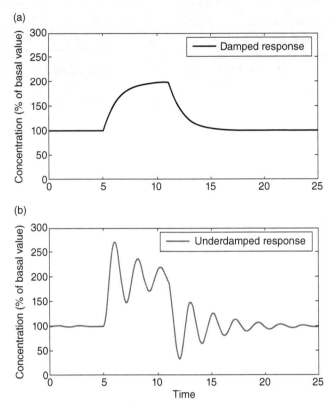

Figure 3.6 Variations in dynamic response during recovery from a pulselike disturbance from basal state. The disturbance (D_e in Figure 3.5) lasted from 5 to 10 seconds and with the same intensity in both cases. (a) Damped response of X_f with rapid inhibitory feedback from the final stage of Figure 3.5. (b) A more usual response when there is a time delay in the inhibitory feedback.

et al., 2008). When discussing negative feedback and oscillatory behavior, it is also important to distinguish coupled feedback oscillators from cases in which a well-behaved negative feedback mechanism is used to control the timing of an intrinsically oscillatory process. Hirata and colleagues present such an example in which the Notch effector Hes1 oscillations are regulated by negative feedback (Hirata et al., 2002).

3.4.1.3. Positive Feedback Loops
A positive feedback loop is formed when the feedback from one reaction to a previous reaction is excitatory. Positive feedback is inherently unstable and usually leads to a response that switches rapidly from one state to another or is persistently oscillating [see, e.g., the oscillatory mechanism described by Hirata et al. (2002) and Li and Qian (2003) and the previous remark concern-

ing negative feedback oscillators]. In the physical sciences, positive feedback is the basis of binary switching circuits in electronic computers. In the life science analog, positive feedback is the biological basis for binary switching between two stable states and reliably (i.e., robustly) maintaining those states even in the face of external disturbances (Ferrell and Xiong, 2001). The reliability of the holding mechanism can be modulated by varying the gain of the positive feedback, where usually the stronger the level of excitatory feedback, the faster the change from one state to the other. However, strong positive feedback can come with increased susceptibility to false switching under disturbances. Biological systems use this property to fine-tune the level of positive feedback, trading-off the speed of the switching state with the resistance to erroneous switching. Brandman et al. (2005) showed elegantly that combining two positive feedback loops (one fast and one slow) can create more reliable, yet fast, cell decisions. Zhang et al. (2007) have provided a theoretical explanation for this process.

3.4.2. Feedforward

After feedback, feedforward is the next most important generic interconnection pattern found in dynamical systems. It is used in technological systems when there is a need to achieve a specific performance goal, or to provide some form of redundancy within a system. Even when redundant pathways are not vital, living systems frequently use feedforward paths to speed responses to input stimuli when rapid responses to transient demands are required before the main path can respond adequately. This combination of a fast and a slow feedforward path in biological processes parallels the corresponding fast–slow feedback mentioned earlier.

At the cellular level, an example of fast–slow feedforward to achieve perfect adaptation during cell signaling has been provided by Tyson et al. (2003). At the metabolic level, an example is mitochondrial ATP production in response to a stimulus triggering energy demand.

As shown in Figure 3.7, in addition to the slow feedfoward glycolytic pathway for stimulating ATP production, there is a second direct feedforward activation pathway. The direct activation of mitochondria allows the mitochondrial reaction rate to increase as soon as there is energy demand. This mechanism is limited, as the directly activated mitochondria could consume pyruvate faster than it is produced by the glycolytic reactions. Fortunately, this fast feedforward activation combines with the slower response of the feedback control of the HK–PFK complex in the glycolysis process. The glycolysis path therefore constitutes the main pathway and the main response to energetic demands.

Figure 3.8 shows that these two control mechanisms interact to achieve rapid, stable control of the ATP level. For example, a pulse of 10% of the baseline value was imposed on the ATPase reaction for 20 units of time. The resulting ATP concentration profiles are presented for three distinct cases:

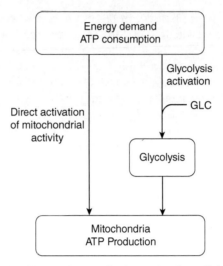

Figure 3.7   Fast–slow feedforward control scheme for the cellular response to energy requirements.

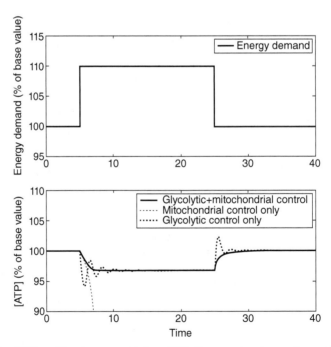

Figure 3.8   ATP profiles in response to a 10% increase in energy demand. Note the increased quality of regulation when glycolytic and mitochondrial control are combined.

glycolytic control, mitochondrial control, and a combination of both (which is the normal, physiological case).

Interestingly, taken separately, the two mechanisms perform poorly. The activation of glycolysis (without mitochondrial feedforward control) induces oscillations, while the direct mitochondrial activation (without glycolysis activation) cannot sustain prolonged demand in ATP. In the latter case, ATP levels drop below 5% of the baseline value (not shown on the graph). Thus, it is clear that the two control mechanisms, even though they might appear redundant, are actually part of a composite control structure that allows the energy level within a cell to respond robustly to varying energetic requirements. This idea that a set of interdependent control mechanisms may be used to achieve a required objective is basic to technological control theory, so it is not surprising that similar composite control structures have evolved in life. We elaborate on this below.

3.4.3. Connections of Modules in Biological Networks

Because feedback is so widely and (because of its intrinsic nonlinearity) variously used in cell signaling, there have been many attempts to categorize the basic forms and their coupling. In this context, Tyson et al. (2003) built upon analogies with electronic subsystems to classify molecular circuits according to their function and use of feedback. Other researchers have extended these ideas to describe additional biological building blocks and subsystems that can be used to form larger networks. An important problem is how to identify the modules and separate them in such large networks. The challenge is that the strong (spatial and temporal) coupling in biology makes it hard to unscramble the interconnective patterns in realistic networks. Kholodenko's (2007) commentary (including the numerous references) on Santos' study of the RAF-MEK-ERK cascade (Santos et al., 2007) presents a method of determining structure by perturbing different connection points within a network. As in all biological processes, however, the key problem is the practical one of obtaining appropriate time-course data for key network components in massively coupled and complex systems.

3.4.4. Robustness and Sensitivity

In this section we have shown that feedback can reduce the sensitivity to external disturbances in negative feedback systems (homeostatic control) and make biological decisions resistant to noise by positive feedback by means of bistable biological switches that drive the biochemical states between the maximum and minimum concentrations. These are the two basic mechanisms with which feedback introduces robustness: the first by some dynamical stability mechanism, and the second by a binary switching mechanism. However, the idea of robustness has existed in biology for many years in connection with evolutionary capabilities, and thus there is a need to reconcile the biological and the control theoretic interpretations. In the context of control theory, the idea of robustness has a long history (Bode, 1945) and has acquired specialized meaning (Dorato and Vlack, 1987). It is natural, therefore, that the control and biological interpretations should be linked and used to explain biological function. In this spirit, El-Samad's interpretation of heat shock (El-Samad et al., 2005) is an example of work that utilizes the control engineering meaning of a dynamic stabilizing principle. More generally, Kitano (2004) interprets robustness in a more subtle way and suggests an overarching theory of robustness (Kitano, 2007). However, in these various interpretations and robustness examples, a set of feedback loops—often interacting—are involved, and feedforward paths are not far away.

3.5. CONCLUSIONS

Statistical modeling is an established element of computational biology, but as illustrated in Figures 3.1 and 3.2 and Section 3.2, it is only part of a much richer systems approach involving mathematical modeling, understanding dynamic responses, and analyzing their behavior. Thus, mathematical modeling is the first step in applying a systems approach to living systems by understanding dynamics and architectural structure. We illustrated these concepts using the themes of feedback and feedforward in terms of relatively simple examples and showed that distinguishing features of feedback in biochemical reaction networks include (1) a high degree of intrinsic nonlinearity, (2) pervasiveness in living systems, and (3) a range of subtle feedback methods to achieve specific control objectives. Advanced methods and skills need to be developed to account properly for these issues and to understand the central role played by feedback and feedforward in living systems. In this spirit, the ideas outlined here introduce threads needed for work on a richer tapestry—this work in progress we call systems biology.

Acknowledgments

The apoptosis example (Figure 3.4) showing the impact of small changes in initial conditions was prepared by Mark Readman. The feedforward example for ATP control (Figure 3.7) was supplied by Mathieu Cloutier and is part of his work on brain energy metabolism. Fernando Lopez Caamal helped with the graphics. O.W. acknowledges support by the Helmholtz-Alliance on Systems Biology and through the EU FP6 project AMKIN. P.W. acknowledges support from Science Foundation Ireland under grant 03/RP1/I382.

REFERENCES

Barkai, N., and Leibler, S. (1997). Robustness in simple biochemical networks. *Nature* *387*, 913–917.

Bennett, S. (1979). *A History of Control Engineering, 1800-1930*. Peter Peregrinus, London.

Bode, H.W. (1945). *Network Analysis and Feedback Amplifier Design*. Van Nostrand, Princeton, NJ.

Boogerd, F.C., Westerhoff, H.V., and Hofmeyr, H.S. (2007). *Systems Biology: Philosophical Foundations*. Elsevier Science, New York.

Brandman, O., Ferrell, J.E., Li, R., and Meyer, T. (2005). Interlinked fast and slow positive feedback loops drive reliable cell decisions. *Science 310*, 496–498.

Cannon, W. (1932). *The Wisdom of the Body*. Norton Press, New York.

Cornish-Bowden, A. (2004). *Fundamentals of Enzyme Kinetics*. Portland Press, London.

Crampin, E.J., Schnell, S., and McSharry, P.E. (2004). Mathematical and computational techniques to deduce complex biochemical reaction mechanisms. *Prog Biophys Mol Biol 86*, 77–112.

Dorato, P., and Vlack, D. (1987). *Robust Control*. IEEE Press, Piscataway, NJ.

El Samad, H., Kurata, H., Doyle, J.C., Gross, C.A., and Khammash, M. (2005). Surviving heat shock: control strategies for robustness and performance. *Proc Natl Acad Sci USA 102*(8), 2736–2741.

Feinberg, M. (1979). *Lectures on Chemical Reaction Networks*. Notes on lectures given at the Mathematics Research Center, University of Wisconsin, Madison, WI.

Fell, D.A. (1997). *Understanding the Control of Metabolism*. Portland Press, London.

Ferrell, J.E., and Xiong, W. (2001). Bistability in cell signalling: how to make continuous processes discontinuous, and reversible processes irreversible. *Chaos 11*, 227–235.

Gleick, J. (1988). *Chaos*. Penguin Books, London.

Hirata, H., Yoshiura, S., Ohtsuka, T., Bessho, Y., Harada, T. and Yoshikawa, K. (2002). Oscillatory expression of the bHLH factor Hes1 regulated by a negative feedback loop. *Science 298*, 840–843.

Jaqaman, K., and Danuser, G. (2006). Linking data to models: data regression. *Nat Rev Mol Cell Biol 7*, 813–819.

Kholodenko, B.N. (2007). Untangling the signalling wires. *Nat Cell Biol 9*, 247–249.

Kitano, H. (2004). Biological robustness. *Nat Rev 5*, 826–837.

Kitano, H. (2007). Toward a theory of biological robustness. *Mol Syst Biol 3*(137), 1–7.

Li, G., and Qian, H. (2003). Sensitivity and specificity amplification in signal transduction. *Cell Biochem Biophy 39*, 39–49.

Lovelock, J. (2000). *Gaia: A New Look at Life on Earth*, 3rd ed. Oxford University Press, Oxford, UK.

MacFarlane, A.G.J. (1970). *Dynamical System Models*. George Harrap and Co., London.

Paynter, H.M. (1961). *Analysis and Design of Engineering Systems*. MIT Press, Cambridge, MA.

Pomerening J.R., Sontag E.D., and Ferrell J.E. (2003). Building a cell cycle oscillator: hysteresis and bistability in the activation of Cdc2. *Nat Cell Biol 5*(4), 346–351.

Santos, S.D.M., Verveer, P.J., and Bastiaens, P.I.H. (2007). Growth factor-induced MAPK network topology shapes ERK response determining PC-12 cell fate. *Nat Cell Biol 9*, 329–330.

Sasagawa, S., Ozaki, Y., Fujita, K., and Kuroda, S. (2005). Prediction and validation of the distinct dynamics of transient and sustained ERK activation. *Nat Cell Biol 7*(4), 366–373.

Schulkin, J. (2004). *Allostasis, Homeostasis, and the Costs of Physiological Adaption.* Cambridge University Press, Cambridge, MA.

Sontag, E.D. (2007). Monotone and near-monotone biochemical networks. *Syst Synth Biol 1*, 59–87.

Thomas, R., and D'Ari, R. (1990). *Biological Feedback.* CRC Press, Boca Raton, FL.

Tustin, E. (1952). Feedback. *Sci Am* Sept. pp. 48–55.

Tyson, J.J., Chen, K.C., and Novak, B. (2003). Sniffers, buzzers, toggles and blinkers: dynamics of regulatory and signalling pathways in the cell. *Curr Opin Cell Biol 15*, 221–321.

Tsai, T.Y.-C., Choi, Y.S., Ma, W., Pomerening, J.R., Tang, C., and Ferrell, J.E. (2008). Robust, tunable biological oscillations from interlinked positive and negative feedback loops. *Science 321*(5885), 126–129.

Umbarger, II.E. (1961). Feedback control by end product inhibition. *Cold Spring Harbour Symp Quant Biol 23*, 301.

Wellstead, P.E. (1979). *Introduction to Physical System Modelling.* Academic Press, London.

Wolkenhauer, O., Mesarovic, M., and Wellstead, P. (2007). A plea for more theory in molecular biology. In *Systems Biology: Applications and Perspectives*, Bringmann, P., Butcher, E.C., Parry, G., Weiss, B., (eds.). Springer-Verlag, Berlin.

Zhang, X.P., Cheng, Z., Liu, F., and Wang, W. (2007). Linking fast and slow positive feedback loops creates an optimal bistable switch in cell signaling. *Phys Rev E 76*, 031924-1 to 031924-7.

CHAPTER 4

Simulation of Population Variability in Pharmacokinetics

JIANSONG YANG

Simcyp Ltd., Sheffield, UK

Summary

Interindividual variability in pharmacokinetics can have direct consequences for therapeutic reliability. Physiologically based pharmacokinetic modeling provides a mechanistic framework for predicting interindividual variability in human pharmacokinetics based on *in vitro* data. This chapter identifies the determinants of variability in drug absorption, distribution, metabolism, and excretion and provides algorithms for predicting interindividual variability in pharmacokinetics.

4.1. INTRODUCTION

Differences in drug response among patients may affect drug safety and effectiveness (Wilkinson, 2005), leading to challenges in optimizing the dosage regimen for individual patients. It has long been recognized that such differences in drug response may be due to pharmacokinetic and/or pharmacodymanic variability (Wood, 1999). Interindividual variability in pharmacokinetics is multifactorial, including environmental, genetic, physiological, and disease factors that affect the absorption, distribution, metabolism, and excretion of a given drug. The interplay of these factors determines the profile of the plasma concentration over time for a drug and therefore its elicited pharmacologic effect at the site of action (Wilkinson, 2005).

Over the past few decades, several approaches have been developed for predicting pharmacokinetic behavior in humans, including quantitative

Systems Biology in Drug Discovery and Development, First Edition.
Edited by Daniel L. Young, Seth Michelson.

structure–activity relationship (QSAR), allometry and physiologically based pharmacokinetic (PBPK) modeling. These approaches have been integrated increasingly into all stages of the drug discovery and development process. However, reports on predicting pharmacokinetics are usually based on mean data that give no estimate of interindividual variability and therefore have a limited ability to address the extremes of risk in real patients. It is increasingly recognized that predicting pharmacokinetics in the "virtual patient population" as opposed to the "virtual reference man" is particularly relevant and desirable (Rostami-Hodjegan and Tucker, 2007).

Of the aforementioned approaches for predicting pharmacokinetic behavior in humans, the PBPK approach has advantages over the other approaches in terms of predicting interindividual variability. With the advances in our understanding of key determinants in pharmacokinetics and the development of *in vitro* assays over the past decade, the task of predicting overall pharmacokinetic behavior *in vivo* is becoming more feasible by integrating PBPK modeling and *in vitro* data. Such data integration also provides a mechanistic framework for predicting interindividual variability in pharmacokinetics. The purpose of this chapter is twofold: to identify sources of variability that contribute to interindividual variability in pharmacokinetics, and to provide a strategy for predicting population variability in pharmacokinetics.

4.2. PBPK MODELING

PBPK modeling represents an evolution from classical compartmental models toward more realistic biological descriptions of the determinants that regulate the disposition of drugs in the body (Andersen et al., 2005). A PBPK model is composed of mathematical representations of the tissues and organs of the body (e.g., adipose, bone, brain, gut, heart, kidney, liver, lung, muscle, skin, spleen), which are perfused by and connected via the vascular system. Drug distribution into a tissue can be rate limited by either perfusion or permeability. *Perfusion-rate-limited kinetics* applies when the tissue membrane presents no barrier to distribution. As expected, this condition is likely to be met by small lipophilic drugs. In contrast, *permeability-rate-limited kinetics* applies when drug distribution into a tissue is rate limited by the drug's permeability across the tissue membrane, and this condition is more likely to happen to polar compounds with large molecular structures. Accordingly, PBPK models may exhibit different degrees of complexity. In the simplest and most commonly applied form (Figure 4.1), each tissue is regarded as a well-stirred system, and drug distribution into a tissue is rate limited by perfusion (i.e., tissue blood flow rate). However, more complex models that take the permeability barriers into account are often needed.

A PBPK model comprises three components: the system, which consists of a body of independent physiological, anatomical, and biochemical data; drug-specific data, which are overlaid onto the system; and the model structure,

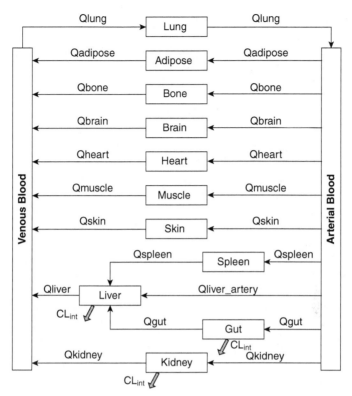

Figure 4.1 Typical PBPK model. The tissues and organs of the body are arranged anatomically and are connected via the vascular system. Q represents blood flow; CL_{int} represents intrinsic clearance.

which refers to the tissues and organs included in the model and their arrangement (Rowland et al., 2004). In a sense, PBPK modeling is an integrated systems approach to both understanding the pharmacokinetic behavior of compounds and predicting concentration–time profiles in plasma and tissues. More details on PBPK modeling are presented elsewhere (Gerlowski and Jain, 1983; Nestorov, 2003; Reddy et al., 2005; Rowland et al., 2004).

4.3. SIMULATION OF PHARMACOKINETIC VARIABILITY

Interindividual variability in pharmacokinetics can have direct consequences for therapeutic reliability and the likelihood of toxicity, especially for compounds with narrow therapeutic windows. Therefore, simulation of interindividual variability should be an integral part of the prediction of pharmacokinetics in humans. An attractive feature of PBPK modeling is that its mechanistic framework provides a capacity for predicting interindividual variability in pharmacokinetics when coupled with Monte Carlo methods.

Early attempts to use Monte Carlo methods to simulate pharmacokinetic behavior in virtual populations date back to the mid-1980s. Jackson et al. assessed the robustness of different experimental *in vivo* indices to detect and display genetic polymorphisms in human drug-metabolizing activity (Jackson and Tucker, 1990; Jackson et al., 1986). These simulations were later expanded to show the effect of variability in absorption, distribution, metabolism, and excretion (ADME) parameters on the power of single-time-point estimates for the assessment of metabolic activity (Jackson et al., 1991), the differentiation of parent drug and metabolite data in bioequivalence assessment (Rostami-Hodjegan et al., 1994), the discriminatory power of different indices of *in vivo* enzyme activity, and the optimization of sampling to assess such activity (Rostami-Hodjegan et al., 1996). Coupled with Monte Carlo methods, PBPK modeling has been used by others to assess the quantitative impact of physiological and environmental factors on human variability in toxicokinetics and pharmacokinetics, Bogaards et al., 2000; Clewell and Andersen, 1996; Jamei et al., 2009a; Nestorov, 2001; Sato, 1991; Sato et al., 1991.

The overall interindividual variability in pharmacokinetics can be simulated by considering the variability in key system parameters in PBPK modeling (Figure 4.2). Details that follow on the prediction of interindividual variability

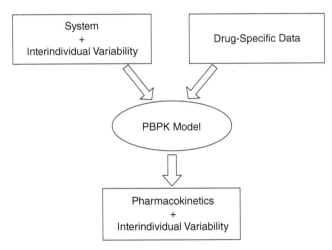

Figure 4.2 Schematic for predicting population variability in pharmacokinetics. A PBPK model comprises three components: the system, which composes a body of independent physiological, anatomical, and biochemical data; drug-specific data overlaid on the system; and the model structure, which refers to the tissues and organs included in the model and their arrangement. By incorporating variability into system parameters, interindividual variability in pharmacokinetics can be mechanistically simulated. [From Rowland et al. (2004).]

in pharmacokinetics are divided into four sections: absorption, distribution, metabolism, and excretion.

4.3.1. Absorption

Oral administration remains the most popular and convenient route of drug administration because of its advantages of convenience and cost over the other routes. Nevertheless, it is often associated with low bioavailability and high interindividual variability. After oral administration, the drug is first released from its formulation, then gets dissolved in the gastrointestinal fluid and passes sequentially through the intestinal wall and the liver before entering the systemic circulation. Thus, *oral bioavailability* (F_{oral}) is defined as

$$F_{oral} = F_a F_G F_H \qquad (4.1)$$

where F_a is the net fraction of dose absorbed from the intestinal tract, F_G the fraction of dose that escapes intestinal first-pass metabolism in the enterocytes, and F_H the fraction of dose that escapes hepatic first-pass metabolism. In this section we focus on the prediction of F_a and its interindividual variability. F_G and F_H are discussed in Section 4.3.3.

Drug absorption from the gastrointestinal tract is a prerequisite for drugs that are administered orally and are intended to act systemically. The majority of drug absorption occurs at the small intestine because of its large absorptive surface area and high blood perfusion rate. The large intestine has a considerably smaller absorptive surface area than the small intestine, but it may still serve as a site of drug absorption for compounds that are not completely absorbed from the small intestine. Various factors that can affect oral drug absorption (Mayersohn, 2002) are listed in Table 4.1. Generally, these determinants can be divided into two categories: system (physiological and biological)-related factors and drug (physicochemical and pharmaceutical)-related factors. These factors can all contribute to the overall rate and extent

TABLE 4.1 Determinants of Oral Drug Absorption

System Factors	Drug-Related Factors
Gastric emptying time	Disintegration
Intestinal residence time	Deaggregation
Gastrointestinal pH	Dissolution
Intestinal transporters	Chemical stability
Intestinal blood flow	Solubility
Food effects	Permeability
Gastrointestinal fluid dynamics	Precipitation
Gut surface area	Affinity to transporters
Disease states	

of absorption, but only the system factors determine the interindividual variability in absorption.

4.3.1.1. Prediction of Drug Absorption

Key physiochemical properties, such as solubility and permeability, are used in empirical methods to estimate the absorption potential of a drug (Artursson and Karlsson, 1991; Dressman et al., 1985). The Biopharmaceutical Classification System (Amidon et al., 1995), which classifies compounds based on their solubility and permeability, is widely used in lead optimization during drug discovery and has been expanded to regulatory practices in determining whether an *in vivo* bioequivalence study may be waived for immediate-release solid oral dosage forms (FDA, 2000).

Physiological models such as the compartmental absorption and transit (CAT) model have also been developed to simulate drug absorption mechanistically (Yu and Amidon, 1999). The CAT model has been developed further into the advanced compartmental absorption and transit (ACAT) model (Agoram et al., 2001) and the advanced dissolution, absorption, and metabolism (ADAM) model (Jamei et al., 2009b), which are implemented in the software Gastroplus (Simulation Plus Inc., California, http://www.simulationsplus.com) and Simcyp population-based ADME simulator (Simcyp Ltd., Sheffield, UK, http://www.simcyp.com), respectively. In brief, these absorption models consist of physiologically based compartments corresponding to different segments of the gastrointestinal tract. A series of differential equations are used to describe drug release, dissolution, degradation, metabolism, and absorption within each compartment and drug transit from one compartment to the next.

4.3.1.2. Sources of Variability in Drug Absorption

Gastric Emptying Time The residence time of a drug in the stomach is an important factor determining the initiation of oral drug absorption. Variability in gastric emptying rates would probably result in variable absorption rates and sometimes even variable absorption extents. As expected, the rate of gastric emptying is influenced by both volume and composition of gastric contents. Several factors influence the residence time of a drug in the stomach, including the nature of the dosage form, the volume of water coadministered, the particle size if the drug is in solid dosage form, and the presence of food (Dressman, 1986). Although the process of gastric emptying is complex, it is generally described as a first-order process (Jamei et al., 2009b; Rebecca and Gordon, 1987). The associated rate constant varies for solids and liquids (Davis et al., 1986) and is reported to be age- and gender-dependent (Brogna et al., 1999; Graff et al., 2001; Gryback et al., 2000).

Intestinal Residence Time Intestinal residence time can greatly affect oral drug absorption, particularly to those drugs with low permeability (Jamei

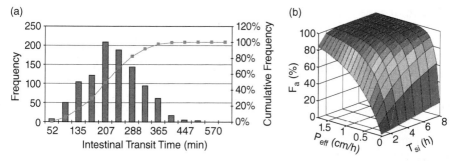

Figure 4.3 Small intestinal residence time: interindividual variability (A) and its impact on F_a (B). P_{eff} refers to effective intestinal permeability and T_{si} refers to the intestinal transit time shown in (A). [Adapted from Jamei et al. (2009b).] (See insert for color representation.)

et al., 2004). Yu and co-workers collected and analyzed published data for small intestinal residence time for over 400 subjects, and reported a mean value of 199 minutes with ranges of about 1 and 6 hours (Yu et al., 1996). Intestinal residence time appears to be relatively less dependent than gastric residence time on the nature of the dosage form (liquid vs. solid) (Davis et al., 1986). The presence of food appears not to influence intestinal transit (Davis et al., 1986; Fadda et al., 2009). The large variation in small intestinal residence time may affect F_a and its variability, particular for compounds with low permeability, as illustrated by Figure 4.3. Transit along the colon is characterized by abrupt movement and long periods of stasis (Metcalf et al., 1987). Colonic residence time is considerably longer than in the small intestine and is also more variable. The transit time can range from several hours to 60 hours (Mayersohn, 2002).

Gastrointestinal pH As most drugs are weak acids or weak bases, regional pH in the gastrointestinal tract can influence drug solubility and hence the dissolution of solid dosage forms. Gastrointestinal pH may also affect drug permeability by influencing the balance between ionized and nonionized moieties. Fallingborg et al. (1989) measured pH profiles along the gastrointestinal tract in 39 healthy volunteers and observed a range of values up to two pH units at the same site in different subjects.

The presence of food in the gastrointestinal tract can raise the pH in the stomach and the proximal part of the small intestine, due to the buffering capacity of proteins. Following a meal, gastric pH gradually returns to its basal value, corresponding to the fasted state (Dressman et al., 1990). The return rate is considerably slower in elderly subjects than in young subjects (Russell et al., 1993). Gastrointestinal pH is affected by many other factors, including pathological states such as achlorhydria and hypergastrinemia (Feldman and Barnett, 1991), diseases such as acquired immunodeficiency syndrome (AIDS)

(Lake-Bakaar et al., 1988), and medicines such as H_2 receptor antagonists (Lin, 1991) and proton pump inhibitors (Shi and Klotz, 2008).

Transporters on the Gastrointestinal Wall   Various transporters are expressed in the apical and basolateral membranes of intestinal epithelial cells (Hilgendorf et al., 2007; Koepsell, 1998; Koepsell et al., 2007; Kunta and Sinko, 2004; Murakami and Takano, 2008; Su and Sinko, 2007; Tsuji and Tamai, 1996; Zhang et al., 1998). Much attention has been given to the efflux transporters [e.g., P-glycoprotein (P-gp, MDR1, *ABCB1*), MRP2 (*ABCC2*), and BCRP (*ABCG2*)] at the apical (brush border) membrane of the intestine, as they can limit the intestinal absorption of drugs administered orally.

Von Richter et al. (2004) measured P-gp in the human small intestine obtained from 15 patients, and reported a marked interindividual variation in intestinal P-gp expression. Additional data were reported in several later publications (Canaparo et al., 2007; Dietrich et al., 2004; Mouly and Paine, 2003). Available data demonstrate that the expression levels of transporters vary along the gastrointestinal tract. Mouly and Paine (2003) determined P-gp expression by Western blotting along the entire length of the human small intestine and found that relative P-gp levels increased progressively from the proximal to the distal region. Other intestinal transporters may or may not follow the same pattern, and further studies are warranted to determine their regional distribution along the human small intestine.

4.3.2. Distribution

Distribution refers to the reversible transfer of drug from one location to another within the body. Distribution of drugs to and from the blood and other tissues occurs at various rates and extents (Rowland and Tozer, 1995). Factors that determine the distribution pattern of a drug with time include delivery of drug to tissue by blood, ability to cross tissue membranes, binding within blood and tissues, partitioning into fat, and tissue uptake (Rowland and Tozer, 1995). The traditional description of the volume of distribution at steady state (V_{ss}) corresponds to the sum of the products of each tissue:plasma partition coefficient ($K_{p,t}$) and the respective tissue volume in addition to the plasma volume (Sawada et al., 1984), as described by

$$V_{ss} = V_p + V_e \times (E:P) + \sum V_t \times K_{p,t} \qquad (4.2)$$

where V_p, V_e, and V_t are the volumes of plasma, erythrocyte, and tissue, respectively, and E:P is a erythrocyte-to-plasma coefficient.

The volume of distribution of a specific drug can vary widely among individuals. Several factors are responsible for the distribution pattern of a drug within the body over time, as noted in Table 4.2. System factors affecting drug distribution include tissue volumes, tissue composition, blood perfusion rates to the tissues, plasma protein concentrations, hematocrit, and the expression

TABLE 4.2   Determinants of Oral Drug Distribution

System Factors	Drug-Related Factors
Tissue volumes	Lipophilicity
Tissue composition	Ionization
Tissue blood flows	Protein-binding affinity
Plasma protein levels	Erythrocyte-to-plasma partition
Hematocrit	Affinity to transporters
Transporters	
Disease states	

of transporter proteins. Drug-specific factors determining the distribution behavior of a drug include its ability to cross membranes, to bind to plasma proteins, and to partition into red blood cells and fat, as well as its specific affinity to influx or efflux transporter proteins.

4.3.2.1. Prediction of Drug Distribution

Tissue-to-plasma partition coefficients [$K_{p,t}$; see Eq. (4.2)] form an essential component of mechanistic prediction of drug distribution and PBPK modeling. Direct determination of $K_{p,t}$ involves intravenous constant infusions to animals followed by an extraction and quantification of drugs from tissue homogenates (Lin et al., 1982; Sawada et al., 1984), which is costly and time consuming. It is, therefore, of interest to predict $K_{p,t}$ values without conducting *in vivo* animal studies.

Poulin and co-workers first developed mechanistic equations to predict the affinity of drugs for various tissues and organs (Poulin and Theil, 2000; Poulin et al., 2001) and subsequently, V_{ss} predictions (Poulin and Theil, 2002) using Eq. (4.2). The mechanistic basis of these equations is that each tissue and plasma is a mixture of lipids, water, and plasma proteins in which the drug can be distributed homogeneously. The assumption is that the drug distributes homogeneously into each tissue (and plasma) by passive diffusion. Consequently, the drug would partition between lipids and water as well as bind reversibly to common proteins present in plasma and tissue interstitial space. The main compound-specific input parameters are *in vitro* data describing drug lipophilicity and plasma protein binding. The species-specific tissue composition parameters can be found in the literature and have been summarized by Poulin and Theil (2002). Later, corrections were introduced to these equations by Berezhkovskiy (2004).

More recently, Rodgers and co-workers extended and improved these equations by considering drug ionization and incorporating more details on drug distribution inside tissues (Rodgers and Rowland, 2006; Rodgers et al., 2005). Briefly, the equations developed by Rodgers et al. are based on the assumption that all drugs will dissolve in intra- and extracellular tissue water and partition into the neutral lipids and neutral phospholipids located within tissue cells. An additional mechanism incorporated for compounds with at least one basic $pK_a \geq 7$ (ionized bases and corresponding zwitterions) is electrostatic interaction with tissue acidic phospholipids. For other drug classes, association with extracellular proteins are an essential component where acids and weakly basic compounds are assumed to bind primarily to albumin, and neutral drugs to lipoproteins (Rodgers and Rowland, 2006; Rodgers et al., 2005).

As mentioned earlier, drug distribution into a tissue can be rate limited by either perfusion or permeability. If drug distribution into a tissue is perfusion limited, the tissue can be regarded as a well-stirred system; if drug distribution into a tissue is permeability limited, a more realistic, yet more complex model is needed and the tissue is often divided into two or more compartments to take the permeability barriers into account. Examples of permeability-limited models can be found in the literature (Kawai et al., 1998; Meno-Tetang et al., 2006; Nasu et al., 2005; Sato et al., 1987; von Kleist and Huisinga, 2007).

Traditionally, drug distribution in the body is described using classical compartmental models. However, these models are descriptive and cannot be used in prediction. In comparison, PBPK models provide a mechanistic and more realistic description of the behavior of a substance in various tissues. It also provides the possibility of predicting interindividual variability in drug distribution. An increasing body of physiological and biological data has become available over the years to inform PBPK modeling. Moreover, these aforementioned mechanistic methods for predicting $K_{p,t}$ values have greatly extended the application of PBPK modeling in drug discovery.

4.3.2.2. Sources of Variability in Distribution

Tissue Volumes and Tissue Blood Flows   Tissue volumes and tissue blood flows are essential components of a PBPK model. Early publications reported representative physiological parameters values but did not indicate the biological variability associated with those data (Arms and Travis, 1988; Davies and Morris, 1993; Snyder et al., 1975; Williams and Leggett, 1989). Interindividual variability on tissue volumes and tissue blood flows have been reported in later publications (Brown et al., 1997; de la Grandmaison et al., 2001; Price et al., 2003; Valentin, 2002). It should be emphasized that the possible correlations between tissue volumes and tissue blood flows should be considered when modeling interindividual variability in drug distribution using PBPK models.

Tissue Composition   As mentioned earlier, a tissue-to-plasma partition coefficient ($K_{p,t}$) is determined by drug partitioning between lipids and water as well as binding to common proteins present in the tissue interstitial space. Most studies on tissue composition (water, neutral lipids, phospholipids, etc.) were carried out between the late 1960s and mid-1980s (Diagne et al., 1984; Gray and Yardley, 1975; Hof and Simon, 1970; Rouser et al., 1969; Simon and

Rouser, 1969). Overall, data on human tissue composition and related variability are very limited.

Hematocrit and Plasma Proteins   *Hematocrit* refers to the percentage of total blood volume composed of red blood cells. It is influenced by such factors as age, gender, seasonal influence, and habits of physical activity (Morse et al., 1947; Thirup, 2003; Wennesland et al., 1959). Women on average have lower hematocrits than those of men. Hematocrit ranges between 40 and 54% in males and between 38 and 47% in females.

Drug protein binding is the reversible interaction of drugs with plasma proteins. The extent of protein binding is a function of drug and protein concentrations, the affinity constant for the drug–protein binding, and the number of protein-binding sites (Grandison and Boudinot, 2000). The major drug-binding proteins in plasma are albumin, α_1-acid glycoprotein (AAG), and lipoproteins. Albumin levels generally decrease with age, whereas AAG levels are not affected significantly by age. Many pathophysiological, pharmacological, and environmental factors, such as renal disease, hepatic disease, obesity, trauma, stress, surgery, pregnancy, concomitant drug therapy, and smoking can alter the concentration of albumin and/or AAG (Benedek et al., 1984a,b; Blain et al., 1985; Blaschke, 1977; Edwards et al., 1982; Jackson et al., 1982; Pacifici et al., 1986; Piafsky, 1980; Routledge, 1986; Veering et al., 1990; Viani et al., 1992).

Transporters   Numerous drug transporters are found on the membranes of various tissues. These transporters can influence drug distribution into the tissues, particularly for drugs with low passive permeability. There is now increasing evidence to suggest that transporters may affect the volumes of distribution of certain drugs (Grover and Benet, 2009). For most drugs, however, transporters may not influence the volume of distribution significantly, but may still influence the local kinetics in certain tissues (e.g., brain, liver) and cause pharmacological or toxicological consequences. Numerous polymorphisms have been identified in transporters, as reviewed by Ho and Kim (2005).

4.3.3. Metabolism

Metabolism is the conversion of one chemical species to another and is the major mechanism for the elimination of most drugs. Drug metabolism reactions are generally grouped into two phases, I and II. Phase I metabolism includes oxidation, reduction, hydrolysis, and hydration reactions. Phase II reactions use an endogenous compound, such as glucuronic acid, glutathione, or sulfate, for conjugation to the drug or its phase I–derived metabolite to produce a more polar end product that can be excreted more readily in bile or urine.

Although drug metabolism can take place in many organs, the liver has long been recognized as the major site of metabolism for most drugs. Various phase I and II enzymes are expressed in the liver. More recently, the role of gut metabolism in first-pass metabolism has been recognized increasingly. The intestinal tissue is also endowed with phase I and II enzymes, although at lower levels than those for the liver (Ilett et al., 1990; Pang, 2003). Several CYP enzymes have been detected in the human small intestine, including CYP1A2, CYP2D6, CYP2E1, CYP2C8, CYP2C9, CYP2C19, CYP3A4, and CYP3A5 (Kaminsky and Fasco, 1992; Kolars et al., 1992; Lindell, 2003; Paine et al., 2006; Zhang et al., 1999). Among them, CYP3A4 is the most prominent enzyme present in the human intestine (Kolars et al., 1992; Paine et al., 1997, 2006; Watkins et al., 1987; Zhang et al., 1999), contributing significantly to the first-pass metabolism of drugs such as cyclosporine (Hebert et al., 1992; Kolars et al., 1991; Wu et al., 1995), midazolam (Gorski et al., 1998; Paine et al., 1996; Thummel et al., 1996; Tsunoda et al., 1999), tacrolimus (Floren et al., 1997; Tuteja et al., 2001), nifedipine (Holtbecker et al., 1996; Rashid et al., 1995), felodipine (Lown et al., 1997), and verapamil (Fromm et al., 1996; von Richter et al., 2001). Although the total content of CYP3A in the entire human small intestine is only 1% of that in the liver (Paine et al., 1997; Yang et al., 2004), intestinal extraction of CYP3A substrates is often similar to or even exceeds hepatic extraction (Floren et al., 1997; Masica et al., 2004; Thummel et al., 1996; Wu et al., 1995).

4.3.3.1. Prediction of Hepatic Metabolism

Rane et al. (1977) successfully predicted *in vivo* hepatic metabolic clearance in rats based on *in vitro* data obtained from rat liver microsomes, taking into consideration the hepatic blood flow rate and the unbound fraction in blood. Since then, significant progress has been achieved in predicting human hepatic metabolic clearance from a variety of *in vitro* systems, such as human liver microsomes, recombinant enzymes, and hepatocytes (Galetin et al., 2004; Houston, 1994; Houston and Carlile, 1997; Howgate et al., 2006; Iwatsubo et al., 1997; McGinnity et al., 2004; Obach, 1999; Riley et al., 2005).

The unbound total hepatic intrinsic clearance ($CLu_{int,H}$) can be extrapolated from *in vitro* clearance determined in a variety of *in vitro* systems using scaling factors as described by Barter et al. (2007) and according to the procedure described by Rostami-Hodjegan and Tucker (2007):

Recombinantly expressed enzymes:

$$CLu_{int,H} = \left[\sum_{j=1}^{n} \left(\sum_{i=1}^{n} ISEF_{ji} \times \frac{V_{max_i}(rhEnz_i) \times Enz_i abundance}{K_{m_i}(rhEnZ_i)} \right) \right] \times \tag{4.3}$$
$$MPPGL \times liver\ weight$$

where there are i metabolic pathways for each of j enzymes, "rh" indicates recombinantly expressed enzyme, V_{max} is the maximum rate of metabolism by an individual enzyme, K_m is the Michaelis constant, MPPGL is the amount of microsomal protein per gram of liver, and ISEF is a scaling factor that compensates for any difference in the activity per unit of enzyme between recombinant systems and hepatic enzymes.

Human liver microsomes:

$$CLu_{int,H} = CLu_{int}(\text{per mg microsomes}) \times MPPGL \times \text{liver weight} \qquad (4.4)$$

Human hepatocytes:

$$CLu_{int,H} = CLu_{int}(\text{per million hepatocytes}) \times HPGL \times \text{liver weight} \qquad (4.5)$$

where HPGL refers to hepatocellularity (millions of hepatocytes per gram of liver).

$CLu_{int,H}$ is then combined with other determinants to obtain total hepatic intrinsic clearance, using a liver model. Several hepatic clearance models have been developed to quantify the effects of hepatic blood flow, fraction unbound in blood, and hepatic intrinsic clearance on hepatic clearance (Wilkinson, 1987). Among these models the well-stirred model has been widely used for its mathematical simplicity and practicality:

$$CL_{H,B} = \frac{Q_{H,B} \cdot fu_B \cdot CLu_{int,H}}{Q_{H,B} + fu_B \cdot CLu_{int,H}} \qquad (4.6)$$

$$F_H = \frac{Q_{H,B}}{Q_{H,B} + fu_B \cdot CLu_{int,H}} \qquad (4.7)$$

where $CL_{H,B}$ is hepatic drug clearance based on whole-blood drug concentration, $Q_{H,B}$ is hepatic blood flow, fu_B is the free fraction of drug in blood. The well-stirred model assumes (1) that drug distribution into the liver is perfusion limited with no diffusion delay and that no active transport systems are involved, and (2) that the drug is distributed instantly and homogenously throughout liver water and that the unbound concentrations in plasma and liver water are identical.

4.3.3.2. Sources of Variability in Hepatic Metabolism

Determinants of hepatic metabolism are summarized in Table 4.3. As indicated by Eq. (4.6), interindividual variability in $CL_{H,B}$ is influenced by the variability in three key parameters: $Q_{H,B}$, fu_B, and $CLu_{int,H}$. When drug distribution into liver is permeability limited, $CL_{H,B}$ is also influenced by hepatic transporters.

Q_H Hepatic blood flow (Q_H) is the sum of hepatic arterial and hepatic portal vein blood flows, representing 6.5 and 19% of cardiac output in male adults, respectively; and 6.5 and 20.5% of cardiac output in female adults, respectively

TABLE 4.3   Determinants of Hepatic Metabolism

System Factors	Drug-Related Factors
Liver blood flow	Intrinsic metabolic clearance
Liver weight	Protein-binding affinity
Plasma protein levels	Erythrocyte-to-plasma partition
Hematocrit	Affinity to transporters
Liver enzyme abundances	
Enzyme polymorphism	
MPPGL/HPGL	
Hepatic transporters	
Disease states	

(Valentin, 2002). Cardiac output is dependent on body surface area as well as age (de Simone et al., 1997; Katori, 1979).

fu$_B$ fu_B is determined by the equation

$$fu_B = \frac{fu}{C_B : C_P} \tag{4.8}$$

where *fu* refers to unbound fraction in plasma, as defined by

$$fu = \frac{1}{1+[P]/K_D} \tag{4.9}$$

where [P] refers to the concentration of drug-binding protein in plasma, and K_D refers to the drug–protein dissociation constant; and $C_B:C_P$ refers to blood-to-plasma concentration ratio, as defined by (Tozer, 1981)

$$C_B : C_P = (E:P) \times \text{hematocrit} + (1-\text{hematocrit}) \tag{4.10}$$

Substituting Eqs. (4.9) and (4.10) into Eq. (4.8) yields the following relationship:

$$fu_B = \frac{1}{1+[P]/K_D} \times \frac{1}{(E:P) \times \text{hematocrit} + (1-\text{hematocrit})} \tag{4.11}$$

As K_D and E:P are drug-specific parameters, Eq. (4.11) indicates that inter-individual variability in fu_B is determined by variations in drug-binding protein concentration and hematocrit, which were discussed earlier (Section 4.3.2.2).

CLu$_{int,H}$ As shown in Eqs. (4.3) to (4.5), the unbound total hepatic intrinsic metabolic clearance ($CLu_{int,H}$) is dependent on MPPGL, HPGL, liver weight, and most important, enzyme abundances in the liver. Recently, Barter et al.

(2007) surveyed the available information on MPPGL and HPGL and on their variability in humans. They estimated 95% confidence intervals for the geometric mean of 27 to 32 mg per gram for MPPGL and 74 to 131 × 10^6 cells per gram for HPGL. A modest decrease in MPPGL with age was also detected. Johnson et al. (2005) have analyzed published data from more than 6000 people (aged from birth to 28 years) to provide a comprehensive, predictive model for liver weight based on body surface area and ethnic differences. The authors then used this model to predict successfully the clearance of 11 drugs in populations of neonates, infants, and children from *in vitro* data (Johnson et al., 2006).

Interindividual differences in the expressions and catalytic activities of various drug-metabolizing enzymes are often the major causes of the large interindividual variability observed in *in vivo* drug metabolism. The majority of the metabolism of drugs occurs via the cytochrome P450s (CYPs), which comprise a superfamily of hemoprotein enzymes involved in the metabolism of a variety of chemically diverse substances (Gonzalez, 1988; Nelson et al., 1993). In humans, about 15 different CYPs have been identified as being involved in drug metabolism in the liver (Guengerich, 2004). These P450s have been characterized to varying degrees with respect to their regulation of expression and catalytic activities (Shimada et al., 1994; Snawder and Lipscomb, 2000). Yeo et al. (2003) have reported a metaanalysis of data on CYP abundances in Caucasians and their variances from a large number of sources. A similar analysis of Japanese and Chinese livers was published later (Inoue et al., 2006). Recently, Izukawa and co-workers determined the abundances of UDP-glucuronosyltransferases (UGTs) in the human liver and their interindividual variability (Izukawa et al., 2009).

Differences in metabolism that result from functional genetic polymorphisms can be accommodated by knowing the frequency of various genotypes, and by modifying either the enzyme abundance (null alleles; e.g., in the case of CYP2D6, poor metabolizers) or the intrinsic enzyme activity (e.g., CYP2C9 variants). Pharmacokinetic differences between phenotypes are most relevant for drugs with low therapeutic indices (Tucker, 1999). Inherited defects in several drug-metabolizing enzymes, such as CYP2D6, CYP2C19, and CYP2C9, have long been recognized to be critical to the therapeutic efficacy or toxicities observed for certain drugs (Kirchheiner et al., 2005; Meyer, 2000). The content and activity of CYP enzymes can decline in patients with liver diseases (Villeneuve and Pichette, 2004). It is worth noting that some of the CYPs are regulated by common promoters; thus, their expression and activity can be related.

Hepatic Transporters   Numerous drug transporters are expressed on liver sinusoidal and canalicular membranes. These transporters are involved in hepatic uptake, sinusoidal efflux, and biliary excretion of some drugs (Giacomini and Sugiyama, 2005; Meier et al., 1997; van Montfoort et al., 2003). Hepatic transporters can affect the drug concentration in the liver, thereby influencing hepatic metabolism. For example, the net hepatic clearance of atorvastatin, which is highly taken up into hepatocytes by transporters, is affected by both metabolism and hepatic uptake (Lau et al., 2006).

Polymorphisms have been identified in many drug transporters (Ho and Kim, 2005). Several publications have reported the interindividual variability of sinusoidal transporter expressions, such as OATP1B1 (Seithel et al., 2008), OATP1B3 (Ho et al., 2006), and OCT1 (Bleasby et al., 2006). However, studies relating the role of genetic polymorphisms of hepatic transporters to pharmacokinetics are just emerging in the literature (e.g., Kivisto and Niemi, 2007; Nishizato et al., 2003).

4.3.3.3. Prediction of Gut Metabolism
We have developed an operational model to predict first-pass metabolism in the gut. The Q_{gut} model [Eq. (4.12)] (Rostami-Hodjegan and Tucker, 2002; Yang et al., 2001, 2007) retains the form of the well-stirred model, but the flow term (Q_{gut}) is a hybrid of both permeability through the enterocyte membrane and villous blood flow:

$$F_G = \frac{Q_{gut}}{Q_{gut} + fu_G \cdot CLu_{int,G}} \tag{4.12}$$

where F_G is intestinal availability (fraction of dose that escapes intestinal first-pass metabolism in the enterocytes), fu_G is the fraction of drug unbound in the enterocyte, whose value is close to 1 in most cases (Yang et al., 2007), $CLu_{int,G}$ is the unbound total gut intrinsic clearance, and Q_{gut} is a hybrid of permeability through the enterocyte membrane and villous blood flow:

$$Q_{gut} = \frac{Q_{villi} \cdot CL_{perm}}{Q_{villi} + CL_{perm}} \tag{4.13}$$

where CL_{perm} is a clearance term defining permeability through the enterocyte and Q_{villi} is villous blood flow.

Substituting Eq. (4.13) into Eq. (4.12) gives the full model:

$$F_G = \frac{Q_{villi}}{Q_{villi} + fu_G \cdot CLu_{int,G} \cdot (1 + Q_{villi}/CL_{perm})} \tag{4.14}$$

$CLu_{int,G}$ can be extrapolated from *in vitro* clearance determined in a variety of *in vitro* systems, similar to the extrapolation of $CLu_{int,H}$. For recombinantly expressed enzymes, we have

$$CLu_{int,G} = \left[\sum_{j=1}^{n} \left(\sum_{i=1}^{n} ISEF_{ji} \times \frac{V_{max_i}(rhEnz_i) \times Enz_i abundance}{K_{m_i}(rhEnZ_i)} \right) \right] \times$$

$$MPPGI \times intestine\ weight \tag{4.15}$$

where there are i metabolic pathways for each of j enzymes, MPPGI is the amount of microsomal protein per gram of intestine, and ISEF is a scaling factor that compensates for any difference in the activity per unit of enzyme between recombinant systems and intestinal enzymes. For human intestinal microsomes,

$$CLu_{int,G} = CLu_{int}(\text{per mg microsomes}) \times MPPGI \times \text{intestine weight} \quad (4.16)$$

The Q_{gut} model is an operational model and is not a fully physiological model. The most sophisticated physiologically based models of first-pass intestinal drug metabolism are those elaborated in a series of articles by Pang and co-workers, culminating in their segmental segregated flow model (Pang, 2003; Tam et al., 2003). The latter incorporates route-dependent intestinal metabolism and the zonal distributions of intestinal enzymes and transporters, and provides unique insight into the likely interplay between lumenal transit, metabolism and active efflux.

4.3.3.4. Sources of Variability in Gut Metabolism

Determinants of gut metabolism are summarized in Table 4.4. Key parameters that determine variability in gut metabolism include Q_{villi}, $CLu_{int,G}$, and CL_{perm}.

Q_{villi} The blood supply to the small intestine is provided by the superior mesenteric artery, and constitutes about 10% of the cardiac output in an average adult (Valentin, 2002). In the unfed state, mucosal blood flow represents about 80% of the total mesenteric flow (Matheson et al., 2000), and, in turn, about 60% of mucosal blood flow supplies the epithelial cells of the villi (Dregelid et al., 1986; Granger et al., 1980; Matheson et al., 2000). Hence, villous blood flow (Q_{villi}) is about 4.8% of cardiac output (Yang et al., 2007). Q_{villi} is increased in the presence of food (Madsen et al., 2006; Muller et al., 1992).

TABLE 4.4   Determinants of Gut Metabolism

System Factors	Drug-Related Factors
Villous blood flow	Intrinsic metabolic clearance
Drug-binding proteins within enterocytes	Protein-binding affinity
Gut enzyme abundances	Permeability
Enzyme polymorphism	Affinity to transporters
MPPGI	
Gut weight	
Gut surface area	
Gut transporters	
Disease states	

*CL*_{uint,G}   The unbound total gut intrinsic clearance ($CLu_{int,G}$), as shown by Eqs. (4.15) and (4.16), is dependent on enzyme abundance, MPPGI, and intestine weight. Paine et al. (2006) analyzed the microsomes prepared from mucosal scrapings from the duodenal and jejunal portions of 31 human donor small intestines by Western blot. Total CYP3A content for the 31 donors averaged 50 pmol/mg and ranged from 18 to 151 pmol/mg. Along with CYP3A4, CYP2C9 and CYP2C19 were detected readily in all donor intestines and varied among individuals at least fivefold.

*CL*_{perm}   Permeability clearance (CL_{perm}) is the product of effective intestinal permeability (P_{eff}) and intestinal cylindrical surface area (Yang et al., 2007):

$$CL_{perm} = P_{eff} \times A \qquad (4.17)$$

where A is the intestinal cylindrical surface area and is variable from person to person. P_{eff} is related to drug permeability but can be affected by the abundance of intestinal transporters and pH in the gut lumen, as discussed in Section 4.3.1.2.

4.3.4. Excretion

Excretion is the irreversible loss of the chemically unchanged drug. For most drugs, excretion occurs predominantly via the kidneys. However, some drugs and their metabolites are excreted extensively via the bile. Drug excretion can also happen via saliva, sweat, breast milk, and lungs, although their contributions to overall drug elimination are often small.

The kidney is the major site of drug excretion. Net renal drug excretion is a combination of three processes: glomerular filtration, tubular secretion, and tubular reabsorption:

$$\text{rate of excretion} = (\text{rate of filtration} + \text{rate of active secretion})(1 - F_R) \quad (4.18)$$

The glomerular filtration of a drug is a passive process that is dependent on the unbound fraction of a drug in plasma (*fu*) and renal blood flow available for filtration:

$$\text{rate of filtration} = fu \times \text{GFR} \times C \qquad (4.19)$$

where F_R is the fraction of drug reabsorbed from tubule lumen, *fu* is the fraction unbound in plasma, GFR is the glomerular filtration rate, and C is the drug concentration in plasma.

Tubular secretion occurs predominantly in the proximal tubule and is mediated by several families of transporters, including the organic anion transporters (OATs) and organic cation transporters (OCTs) (Anzai and Endou, 2007).

Tubular reabsorption of a drug can be a passive or an active transport process. Passive reabsorption may occur throughout the nephron. The driving force is supplied largely by reabsorption of water, which concentrates the urine with respect to plasma. Drugs that have low molecular weights, are lipophilic, and nonionized are likely to be reabsorbed from the tubule into the circulation. For weak acids and weak bases, urine pH can affect their ionization degrees and therefore influence their reabsorption. Active reabsorption occurs in the proximal tubule and, similar to tubular secretion, is energy dependent, saturable, stereospecific, and also likely to be associated with competitive drug interactions (Tett et al., 2003).

Biliary excretion is one of the primary elimination routes for xenobiotics and their conjugate metabolites (Arias et al., 1993). Biliary excretion requires active secretory transport because drugs are transported across the biliary epithelium against a concentration gradient. Often, drugs excreted into the bile undergo some degree of reabsorption along the intestine (enterohepatic recirculation). If the entire biliary excreted drug is totally reabsorbed from the intestine, biliary secretion is a component of drug distribution rather than a route of elimination. Only when there is no or incomplete reabsorption from the intestine does biliary secretion become a route of elimination.

4.3.4.1. Prediction of Renal Clearance

According to Eqs. (4.18) and (4.19), it is apparent that renal clearance can be predicted from GFR and fu for drugs that are not subject to active secretion and tubular reabsorption. Current *in vitro* models to investigate the complex parallel processes for renal clearance are limited, and the prediction of renal clearance of drugs in humans is normally based on preclinical animal data.

4.3.4.2. Sources of Variability in Renal Excretion

Parameters influencing the renal clearance are summarized in Table 4.5. The primary determinants of renal excretion include renal blood flow, plasma protein binding, urine flow, urine pH, and renal transporters (Garrett, 1978; Tucker, 1981). The extent of sensitivity to these parameters depends on

TABLE 4.5   Determinants of Renal Excretion

System Factors	Drug-Related Factors
Renal function	Protein-binding affinity
Renal blood flow	Ionization
Plasma protein levels	Affinity to transporters
Urine flow	
Urine pH	
Renal transporters	
Disease states	

the nature of the compound and the mechanisms involved in its renal elimination (e.g., glumerular filtration, active secretion, passive reabsorption). Thus, interindividual variation in these parameters, together with renal function, determines the overall renal clearance. Urine flow is sensitive to individual fluid intake and the administration of diuretic drugs. Interindividual differences in urine pH are related primarily to differences in diet and physical activity.

Renal transporters play key roles in the secretion and reabsorption of many drugs and can contribute significantly to the variability in renal excretion of these compounds (Lee and Kim, 2004). Organic anion and organic cation transport systems are two major drug transport systems in the human kidney (Dresser et al., 2001), and the effects of genetic variations in transporters on renal clearance have been investigated recently (Erdman et al., 2006; Song et al., 2008; Urban et al., 2008; Wang et al., 2008).

A range of pathophysiological states influence the efficiency of individual renal elimination pathways (Tett et al., 2003; Tucker, 1981). It is well recognized that renal diseases alter the renal clearance and therefore the elimination of drugs. For a drug eliminated primarily via renal excretion, impaired renal function may alter its pharmacokinetics and pharmacodynamics to the extent that the dosage regimen needs to be changed from that used in patients with normal renal function (FDA, 1998). Although it is obvious that renal impairment is associated with a decrease in renal excretion of a drug and its metabolites, renal impairment has also been shown to be associated with other changes, such as changes in absorption, hepatic metabolism, plasma protein binding, and drug distribution (FDA, 1998). Accumulating evidence indicates that renal impairment can affect the pharmacokinetics of drugs that are eliminated predominantly by nonrenal processes such as metabolism and/or active transport (Nolin et al., 2008; Zhang et al., 2009). The underlying mechanisms of these effects are not fully understood in humans.

4.3.4.3. Prediction of Biliary Clearance

Biliary excretion of drugs can be investigated using *in vitro* systems with varying degrees of complexity, ranging from the entire hepatocyte to membrane vesicles prepared from cell lines transfected with specific transport proteins (Ghibellini et al., 2006). Nevertheless, the predictive accuracy of these methods in humans is largely unknown, owing to the lack of clinical data on biliary excretion of drugs. Ghibellini and co-workers used *in vitro* data obtained from sandwich-cultured human hepatocytes to predict the biliary clearance for three drugs, and the values predicted were significantly lower than those for *in vivo* data (Ghibellini et al., 2007). Alternatively, human biliary clearance can be estimated from animal data using interspecies scaling (Mahmood, 2005). However, the accuracy of interspecies scaling is hampered by the remarkable interspecies differences in biliary excretion of drugs and metabolites (Ishizuka et al., 1999; Li et al., 2008, 2009; Shilling et al., 2006).

TABLE 4.6   Determinants of Biliary Excretion

System Factors	Drug-Related Factors
Bile flow	Protein-binding affinity
Drug-binding proteins within hepatocytes	Ionization
Hepatic transporters	Affinity to transporters
Disease states	

4.3.4.4. Sources of Variability in Biliary Excretion

Determinants of biliary excretion are summarized in Table 4.6. Biliary excretion is mediated by transporters in the canilacular membrane. Therefore, genetic variation in these transporters contributes to the interindividual variability in biliary excretion. Several recent reviews have summarized the key transporters involved in hepatobiliary disposition of drugs (Chandra and Brouwer, 2004; Faber et al., 2003; Ghibellini et al., 2006; Kullak-Ublick and Becker, 2003). The absolute abundances of efflux transporters that are responsible for the hepatobiliary elimination of drugs have not been determined until very recently (Li et al., 2009). However, several publications have reported the variability of canalicular transporter expressions, such as P-gp (Meier et al., 2006), MRP2 (Li et al., 2009; Meier et al., 2006), and BCRP (Merino et al., 2005).

4.4. CONCLUSIONS AND FUTURE DIRECTIONS

Prediction of pharmacokinetics in humans plays an increasingly important role in drug discovery and development. PBPK modeling provides a mechanistic framework for predicting pharmacokinetic behavior of compounds in humans by integrating physiochemical and *in vitro* data available in drug discovery and early developmental stages. To provide meaningful predictions, system variables should be incorporated within PBPK modeling, allowing the prediction of pharmacokinetics in relevant patient populations rather than in an "average" person. As more information becomes available, it will be possible to predict the effects of certain diseases (e.g., liver cirrhosis and renal impairment) and environmental factors (e.g., smoking, alcohol consumption) on pharmacokinetics.

Over the years an increasing body of physiological and biological data needed in PBPK modeling has become available, and our understanding of how drugs interact with the components of the system has improved significantly. However, there are certain areas that still require further investigation. In particular, the roles of transporters and their genetic polymorphisms in the processes of drug absorption, distribution, metabolism, and excretion remain to be fully understood.

REFERENCES

Agoram, B., Woltosz, W.S., and Bolger, M.B. (2001). Predicting the impact of physiological and biochemical processes on oral drug bioavailability. *Adv Drug Deliv Rev 50*, S41–S67.

Amidon, G.L., Lennernas, H., Shah, V.P., and Crison, J.R. (1995). A theoretical basis for a biopharmaceutic drug classification: the correlation of *in-vitro* drug product dissolution and *in vivo* bioavailability. *Pharm Res 12*, 413–420.

Andersen, M.E., Reddy, M.B., Clewell, H.J., and Yang, R.S. (2005). Conclusions and future directions. In: *Physiologically Based Pharmacokinetic Modeling: Science and Applications* (Reddy, M.B., Yang, R.S.H., Andersen, M.E., and Clewell, H.J., eds.). Wiley, Hoboken, NJ, pp. 389–399.

Anzai, N., and Endou, H. (2007). Drug transport in the kidney. In: *Drug Transporters: Molecular Characterization and Role in Drug Disposition* (You, G., and Morris, M.E., eds.). Wiley, Hoboken, NJ, pp. 411–461.

Arias, I.M., Che, M., Gatmaitan, Z., Leveille, C., Nishida, T., and St. Pierre, M. (1993). The biology of the bile canaliculus. *Hepatology 17*, 318–329.

Arms, A.D., and Travis, C.C. (1988). *Reference Physiological Parameters in Pharmacokinetic Modelling*. Washington, DC: U.S. Environmental Protection Agency.

Artursson, P., and Karlsson, J. (1991). Correlation between oral drug absorption in humans and apparent drug permeability coefficients in human intestinal epithelial (Caco-2) cells. *Biochem Biophys Res Commun 175*, 880–885.

Barter, Z.E., Bayliss, M.K., Beaune, P.H., Boobis, A.R., Carlile, D.J., Edwards, R.J., Brian Houston, J., Lake, B.G., Lipscomb, J.C., Pelkonen, O.R., et al. (2007). Scaling factors for the extrapolation of *in vivo* metabolic drug clearance from *in vitro* data: reaching a consensus on values of human microsomal protein and hepatocellularity per gram of liver. *Curr Drug Metab 8*, 33–45.

Benedek, I.H., Blouin, R.A., and McNamara, P.J. (1984a). Influence of smoking on serum protein composition and the protein binding of drugs. *J Pharm Pharmacol 36*, 214–216.

Benedek, I.H., Blouin, R.A., and McNamara, P.J. (1984b). Serum protein binding and the role of increased alpha 1-acid glycoprotein in moderately obese male subjects. *Br J Clin Pharmacol 18*, 941–946.

Berezhkovskiy, L.M. (2004). Volume of distribution at steady state for a linear pharmacokinetic system with peripheral elimination. *J Pharm Sci 93*, 1628–1640.

Blain, P.G., Mucklow, J.C., Rawlins, M.D., Roberts, D.F., Routledge, P.A., and Shand, D.G. (1985). Determinants of plasma alpha 1-acid glycoprotein (AAG) concentrations in health. *Br J Clin Pharmacol 20*, 500–502.

Blaschke, T.F. (1977). Protein binding and kinetics of drugs in liver diseases. *Clin Pharmacokinet 2*, 32–44.

Bleasby, K., Castle, J.C., Roberts, C.J., Cheng, C., Bailey, W.J., Sina, J.F., Kulkarni, A.V., Hafey, M.J., Evers, R., Johnson, J.M., et al. (2006). Expression profiles of 50 xenobiotic transporter genes in humans and pre-clinical species: a resource for investigations into drug disposition. *Xenobiotica 36*, 963–988.

Bogaards, J.J.P., Hissink, E.M., Briggs, M., Weaver, R., Jochemsen, R., Jackson, P., Bertrand, M., and van Bladeren, P.J. (2000). Prediction of inter-individual variation in drug plasma levels *in vivo* from individual enzyme kinetic data and physiologically based pharmacokinetic modeling. *Eur J Pharm Sci 12*, 117–124.

Brogna, A., Ferrara, R., Bucceri, A.M., Lanteri, E., and Catalano, F. (1999). Influence of aging on gastrointestinal transit time: an ultrasonographic and radiologic study. *Invest Radiol 34*, 357–359.

Brown, R.P., Delp, M.D., Lindstedt, S.L., Rhomberg, L.R., and Beliles, R.P. (1997). Physiological parameter values for physiologically based pharmacokinetic models. *Toxicol Ind Health 13*, 407–484.

Canaparo, R., Finnstrom, N., Serpe, L., Nordmark, A., Muntoni, E., Eandi, M., Rane, A., and Zara, G.P. (2007). Expression of CYP3A isoforms and P-glycoprotein in human stomach, jejunum and ileum. *Clin Exp Pharmacol Physiol 34*, 1138–1144.

Chandra, P., and Brouwer, K.L. (2004). The complexities of hepatic drug transport: current knowledge and emerging concepts. *Pharm Res 21*, 719–735.

Clewell, H.J., and Andersen, M.E. (1996). Use of physiologically based pharmacokinetic modeling to investigate individual versus population risk. *Toxicology 111*, 315–329.

Davies, B., and Morris, T. (1993). Physiological parameters in laboratory animals and humans. *Pharm Res 10*, 1093–1095.

Davis, S.S., Hardy, J.G., and Fara, J.W. (1986). Transit of pharmaceutical dosage forms through the small intestine. *Gut 27*, 886–892.

de la Grandmaison, G.L., Clairand, I., and Durigon, M. (2001). Organ weight in 684 adult autopsies: new tables for a Caucasoid population. *Forensic Sci Int 119*, 149–154.

de Simone, G., Devereux, R.B., Daniels, S.R., Mureddu, G., Roman, M.J., Kimball, T.R., Greco, R., Witt, S., and Contaldo, F. (1997). Stroke volume and cardiac output in normotensive children and adults: assessment of relations with body size and impact of overweight. *Circulation 95*, 1837–1843.

Diagne, A., Fauvel, J., Record, M., Chap, H., and Douste-Blazy, L. (1984). Studies on ether phospholipids: II. Comparative composition of various tissues from human, rat and guinea pig. *Biochim Biophys Acta 793*, 221–231.

Dietrich, C.G., Geier, A., Salein, N., Lammert, F., Roeb, E., Oude Elferink, R.P., Matern, S., and Gartung, C. (2004). Consequences of bile duct obstruction on intestinal expression and function of multidrug resistance-associated protein 2. *Gastroenterology 126*, 1044–1053.

Dregelid, E., Haukaas, S., Amundsen, S., Eide, G.E., Soreide, O., Lekven, J., and Svanes, K. (1986). Microsphere method in measurement of blood flow to wall layers of small intestine. *Am J Physiol Gastrointest Liver Physiol 250*, G670–G678.

Dresser, M.J., Leabman, M.K., and Giacomini, K.M. (2001). Transporters involved in the elimination of drugs in the kidney: organic anion transporters and organic cation transporters. *J Pharm Sci 90*, 397–421.

Dressman, J.B. (1986). Comparison of canine and human gastrointestinal physiology. *Pharm Res 3*, 123–131.

Dressman, J.B., Amidon, G.L., and Fleisher, D. (1985). Absorption potential: estimating the fraction absorbed for orally administered compounds. *J Pharm Sci 74*, 588–589.

Dressman, J.B., Berardi, R.R., Dermentzoglou, L.C., Russell, T.L., Schmaltz, S.P., Barnett, J.L., and Jarvenpaa, K.M. (1990). Upper gastrointestinal (GI) pH in young, healthy men and women. *Pharm Res 7*, 756–761.

Edwards, D.J., Lalka, D., Cerra, F., and Slaughter, R.L. (1982). Alpha1-acid glycoprotein concentration and protein binding in trauma. *Clin Pharmacol Ther 31*, 62–67.

Erdman, A.R., Mangravite, L.M., Urban, T.J., Lagpacan, L.L., Castro, R.A., de la Cruz, M., Chan, W., Huang, C.C., Johns, S.J., Kawamoto, M., et al. (2006). The human organic anion transporter 3 (OAT3; SLC22A8): genetic variation and functional genomics. *Am J Physiol Renal Physiol 290*, F905–F912.

Faber, K.N., Muller, M., and Jansen, P.L. (2003). Drug transport proteins in the liver. *Adv Drug Deliv Rev 55*, 107–124.

Fadda, H.M., McConnell, E.L., Short, M.D., and Basit, A.W. (2009). Meal-induced acceleration of tablet transit through the human small intestine. *Pharm Res 26*, 356–360.

Fallingborg, J., Christensen, L.A., Ingeman-Nielsen, M., Jacobsen, B.A., Abildgaard, K., and Rasmussen, H.H. (1989). pH-profile and regional transit times of the normal gut measured by a radiotelemetry device. *Aliment Pharmacol Ther 3*, 605–613.

FDA (1998). Guidance for Industry. Pharmacokinetics in patients with impaired renal function: study design, data analysis, and impact on dosing and labeling. http://www.fda.gov/CBER/gdlns/renal.pdf.

FDA (2000). Guidance for Industry. Waiver of *in vivo* bioavailability and bioequivalence studies for immediate-release solid oral dosage forms based on a biopharmaceutics classification system. http://www.fda.gov/CDER/GUIDANCE/3618fnl.htm.

Feldman, M., and Barnett, C. (1991). Fasting gastric pH and its relationship to true hypochlorhydria in humans. *Dig Dis Sci 36*, 866–869.

Floren, L.C., Bekersky, I., Benet, L.Z., Mekki, Q., Dressler, D., Lee, J.W., Roberts, J.P., and Hebert, M.F. (1997). Tacrolimus oral bioavailability doubles with coadministration of ketoconazole. *Clin Pharmacol Ther 62*, 41–49.

Fromm, M.F., Busse, D., Kroemer, H.K., and Eichelbaum, M. (1996). Differential induction of prehepatic and hepatic metabolism of verapamil by rifampin. *Hepatology 24*, 796–801.

Galetin, A., Brown, C., Hallifax, D., Ito, K., and Houston, J.B. (2004). Utility of recombinant enzyme kinetics in prediction of human clearance: impact of variability, CYP3A5 and CYP2C19 on CYP3A4 probe substrates. *Drug Metab Dispos 32*, 1411–1420.

Garrett, E.R. (1978). Pharmacokinetics and clearances related to renal processes. *Int J Clin Pharmacol Biopharm 16*, 155–172.

Gerlowski, L.E., and Jain, R.K. (1983). Physiologically based pharmacokinetic modeling: principles and applications. *J Pharm Sci 72*, 1103–1127.

Ghibellini, G., Leslie, E.M., and Brouwer, K.L. (2006). Methods to evaluate biliary excretion of drugs in humans: an updated review. *Mol Pharm 3*, 198–211.

Ghibellini, G., Vasist, L.S., Leslie, E.M., Heizer, W.D., Kowalsky, R.J., Calvo, B.F., and Brouwer, K.L.R. (2007). *In vitro–in vivo* correlation of hepatobiliary drug clearance in humans. *Clin Pharmacol Ther 81*, 406–413.

Giacomini, K.M., and Sugiyama, Y. (2005). Membrane transporters and drug response. In: *Goodman & Gilman's The Pharmacological Basis of Therapeutics* (Brunton, L.L., Lazo, J.S., and Parker, K.L. eds.). McGraw-Hill, New York, pp. 41–70.

Gonzalez, F.J. (1988). The molecular biology of cytochrome P450s. *Pharmacol Rev 40*, 243–288.

Gorski, J.C., Jones, D.R., Haehner-Daniels, B.D., Hamman, M.A., O'Mara, E.M., and Hall, S.D. (1998). The contribution of intestinal and hepatic CYP3A to the interaction between midazolam and clarithromycin. *Clin Pharmacol Ther 64*, 133–143.

Graff, J., Brinch, K., and Madsen, J.L. (2001). Gastrointestinal mean transit times in young and middle-aged healthy subjects. *Clin Physiol 21*, 253–259.

Grandison, M.K., and Boudinot, F.D. (2000). Age-related changes in protein binding of drugs: implications for therapy. *Clin Pharmacokinet 38*, 271–290.

Granger, D.N., Richardson, P.D., Kvietys, P.R., and Mortillaro, N.A. (1980). Intestinal blood flow. *Gastroenterology 78*, 837–863.

Gray, G.M., and Yardley, H.J. (1975). Lipid compositions of cells isolated from pig, human, and rat epidermis. *J Lipid Res 16*, 434–440.

Grover, A., and Benet, L.Z. (2009). Effects of drug transporters on volume of distribution. *AAPS J 11*, 250–261.

Gryback, P., Hermansson, G., Lyrenas, E., Beckman, K.W., Jacobsson, H., and Hellstrom, P.M. (2000). Nationwide standardisation and evaluation of scintigraphic gastric emptying: reference values and comparisons between subgroups in a multicentre trial. *Eur J Nucl Med 27*, 647–655.

Guengerich, F.P. (2004). Human cytochrome P450 enzymes. In: *Cytochrome P450: Structure, Mechanism, and Biochemistry* (Ortiz de Montellano, P.R., ed.). KluwerAcademic/Plenum, New York, pp. 377–530.

Hebert, M.F., Roberts, J.P., Prueksaritanont, T., and Benet, L.Z. (1992). Bioavailability of cyclosporine with concomitant rifampin administration is markedly less than predicted by hepatic enzyme induction. *Clin Pharmacol Ther 52*, 453–457.

Hilgendorf, C., Ahlin, G., Seithel, A., Artursson, P., Ungell, A.-L., and Karlsson, J. (2007). Expression of thirty-six drug transporter genes in human intestine, liver, kidney, and organotypic cell lines. *Drug Metab Dispos 35*, 1333–1340.

Ho, R.H., and Kim, R.B. (2005). Transporters and drug therapy: implications for drug disposition and disease. *Clin Pharmacol Ther 78*, 260.

Ho, R.H., Tirona, R.G., Leake, B.F., Glaeser, H., Lee, W., Lemke, C.J., Wang, Y., and Kim, R.B. (2006). Drug and bile acid transporters in rosuvastatin hepatic uptake: function, expression, and pharmacogenetics. *Gastroenterology 130*, 1793–1806.

Hof, H., and Simon, R.G. (1970). Phospholipid content of human and guinea pig muscle: post-mortem changes and variations with muscle composition. *Lipids 5*, 485–487.

Holtbecker, N., Fromm, M.F., Kroemer, H.K., Ohnhaus, E.E., and Heidemann, H. (1996). The nifedipine–rifampin interaction: evidence for induction of gut wall metabolism. *Drug Metab Dispos 24*, 1121–1123.

Houston, J.B. (1994). Utility of *in-vitro* drug metabolism data in predicting *in-vivo* metabolic clearance. *Biochem Pharmacol 47*, 1469–1479.

Houston, J.B., and Carlile, D.J. (1997). Prediction of hepatic clearance from microsomes, hepatocytes, and liver slices. *Drug Metab Rev 29*, 891–922.

Howgate, E.M., Yeo, K.R., Proctor, N.J., Tucker, G.T., and Rostami-Hodjegan, A. (2006). Prediction of *in vivo* drug clearance from *in vitro* data: I. Impact of interindividual variability. *Xenobiotica 36*, 473–497.

Ilett, K.F., Tee, L.B.G., Reeves, P.T., and Minchin, R.F. (1990). Metabolism of drugs and other xenobiotics in the gut lumen and wall. *Pharmacol Ther 46*, 67–93.

Inoue, S., Howgate, E.M., Rowland-Yeo, K., Shimada, T., Yamazaki, H., Tucker, G.T., and Rostami-Hodjegan, A. (2006). Prediction of *in vivo* drug clearance from *in vitro* data: II. Potential inter-ethnic differences. *Xenobiotica 36*, 499–513.

Ishizuka, H., Konno, K., Shiina, T., Naganuma, H., Nishimura, K., Ito, K., Suzuki, H., and Sugiyama, Y. (1999). Species differences in the transport activity for organic anions across the bile canalicular membrane. *J Pharmacol Exp Ther 290*, 1324–1330.

Iwatsubo, T., Hirota, N., Ooie, T., Suzuki, H., Shimada, N., Chiba, K., Ishizaki, T., Green, C.E., Tyson, C.A., and Sugiyama, Y. (1997). Prediction of *in vivo* drug metabolism in the human liver from *in vitro* metabolism data. *Pharmacol Ther 73*, 147–171.

Izukawa, T., Nakajima, M., Fujiwara, R., Yamanaka, H., Fukami, T., Takamiya, M., Aoki, Y., Ikushiro, S.-I., Sakaki, T., and Yokoi, T. (2009). Quantitative analysis of UGT1A and UGT2B expression levels in human livers. *Drug Metab Dispos 37*, 1759–1768.

Jackson, P.R., and Tucker, G.T. (1990). Pharmacokinetic pharmacogenetic modeling in the detection of polymorphisms in xenobiotic metabolism. *Ann Occup Hyg 34*, 653–662.

Jackson, P.R., Tucker, G.T., and Woods, H.F. (1982). Altered plasma drug binding in cancer: role of alpha 1-acid glycoprotein and albumin. *Clin Pharmacol Ther 32*, 295–302.

Jackson, P.R., Tucker, G.T., Lennard, M.S., and Woods, H.F. (1986). Polymorphic drug oxidation: pharmacokinetic basis and comparison of experimental indices. *Br J Clin Pharmacol 22*, 541–550.

Jackson, P.R., Tucker, G.T., and Woods, H.F. (1991). Backtracking booze with Bayes: the retrospective interpretation of blood alcohol data. *Br J Clin Pharmacol 31*, 55–63.

Jamei, M., Yang, J., and Rostami-Hodjegan, A. (2004). Inter- and intra-individual variability in physiological parameters of gastro-intestinal tract has significant effects on the predicted fraction of dose absorbed. Presented at LogP 2004, The 3rd Lipophilicity Symposium, Physicochemical and Biological Profiling in Drug Research, Zurich, Switzerland.

Jamei, M., Dickinson, G.L., and Rostami-Hodjegan, A. (2009a). A framework for assessing inter-individual variability in pharmacokinetics using virtual human populations and integrating general knowledge of physical chemistry, biology, anatomy, physiology and genetics: a tale of "bottom-up" vs "top-down" recognition of covariates. *Drug Metab Pharmacokinet 24*, 53–75.

Jamei, M., Turner, D., Yang, J., Neuhoff, S., Polak, S., Rostami-Hodjegan, A., and Tucker, G.T. (2009b). Population-based mechanistic prediction of oral drug absorption. *AAPS J. 11*, 225–237.

Johnson, T.N., Tucker, G.T., Tanner, M.S., and Rostami-Hodjegan, A. (2005). Changes in liver volume from birth to adulthood: a meta-analysis. *Liver Transpl 11*, 1481–1493.

Johnson, T.N., Rostami-Hodjegan, A., and Tucker, G.T. (2006). Prediction of the clearance of eleven drugs and associated variability in neonates, infants and children. *Clin Pharmacokinet 45*, 931–956.

Kaminsky, L.S., and Fasco, M.J. (1992). Small intestinal cytochromes-P450. *Crit Rev Toxicol 21*, 407–422.

Katori, R. (1979). Normal cardiac output in relation to age and body size. *Tohoku J Exp Med 128*, 377–387.

Kawai, R., Mathew, D., Tanaka, C., and Rowland, M. (1998). Physiologically based pharmacokinetics of cyclosporine A: extension to tissue distribution kinetics in rats and scale-up to human. *J Pharmacol Exp Ther 287*, 457–468.

Kirchheiner, J., Roots, I., Goldammer, M., Rosenkranz, B., and Brockmoller, J. (2005). Effect of genetic polymorphisms in cytochrome P450 (CYP) 2C9 and CYP2C8 on the pharmacokinetics of oral antidiabetic drugs: clinical relevance. *Clin Pharmacokinet 44*, 1209–1225.

Kivisto, K.T., and Niemi, M. (2007). Influence of drug transporter polymorphisms on pravastatin pharmacokinetics in humans. *Pharm Res 24*, 239–247.

Koepsell, H. (1998). Organic cation transporters in intestine, kidney, liver, and brain. *Annu Rev Physiol 60*, 243–266.

Koepsell, H., Lips, K., and Volk, C. (2007). Polyspecific organic cation transporters: structure, function, physiological roles, and biopharmaceutical implications. *Pharm Res 24*, 1227–1251.

Kolars, J.C., Awni, W.M., Merion, R.M., and Watkins, P.B. (1991). First-pass metabolism of cyclosporine by the gut. *Lancet 338*, 1488–1490.

Kolars, J.C., Schmiedlinren, P., Schuetz, J.D., Fang, C., and Watkins, P.B. (1992). Identification of rifampin-inducible P450IIIA4 (CYP3A4) in human small bowel enterocytes. *J Clin Invest 90*, 1871–1878.

Kullak-Ublick, G.A., and Becker, M.-B. (2003). Regulation of drug and bile salt transporters in liver and intestine. *Drug Metab Rev 35*, 305–317.

Kunta, J.R., and Sinko, P.J. (2004). Intestinal drug transporters: *in vivo* function and clinical importance. *Curr Drug Metab 5*, 109–124.

Lake-Bakaar, G., Quadros, E., Beidas, S., Elsakr, M., Tom, W., Wilson, D.E., Dincsoy, H.P., Cohen, P., and Straus, E.W. (1988). Gastric secretory failure in patients with the acquired immunodeficiency syndrome (AIDS). *Ann Intern Med 109*, 502–504.

Lau, Y.Y., Okochi, H., Huang, Y., and Benet, L.Z. (2006). Multiple transporters affect the disposition of atorvastatin and its two active hydroxy metabolites: application of *in vitro* and ex situ systems. *J Pharmacol Exp Ther 316*, 762–771.

Lee, W., and Kim, R.B. (2004). Transporters and renal drug elimination. *Annu Rev Pharmacol Toxicol 44*, 137–166.

Li, M., Yuan, H., Li, N., Song, G., Zheng, Y., Baratta, M., Hua, F., Thurston, A., Wang, J., and Lai, Y. (2008). Identification of interspecies difference in efflux transporters of hepatocytes from dog, rat, monkey and human. *Eur J Pharm Sci 35*, 114–126.

Li, N., Zhang, Y., Hua, F., and Lai, Y. (2009). Absolute difference of hepatobiliary Transporter MRP2/Mrp2 in liver tissues and isolated hepatocytes from rat, dog, monkey and human. *Drug Metab Dispos 37*, 66–73.

Lin, J.H. (1991). Pharmacokinetic and pharmacodynamic properties of histamine H2-receptor antagonists: relationship between intrinsic potency and effective plasma concentrations. *Clin Pharmacokinet 20*, 218–236.

Lin, J.H., Sugiyama, Y., Awazu, S., and Hanano, M. (1982). *In vitro* and *in vivo* evaluation of the tissue-to-blood partition coefficient for physiological pharmacokinetic models. *J Pharmacokinet Pharmacodyn 10*, 637–647.

Lindell, M. (2003). Expression of genes encoding for drug metabolism in the small intestine. Department of Pharmaceutical Biosciences, Uppsala University, Uppsala, Sweden.

Lown, K.S., Bailey, D.G., Fontana, R.J., Janardan, S.K., Adair, C.H., Fortlage, L.A., Brown, M.B., Guo, W.S., and Watkins, P.B. (1997). Grapefruit juice increases felodipine oral availability in humans by decreasing intestinal CYP3A protein expression. *J Clin Invest 99*, 2545–2553.

Madsen, J.L., Sondergaard, S.B., and Moller, S. (2006). Meal-induced changes in splanchnic blood flow and oxygen uptake in middle-aged healthy humans. *Scand J Gastroenterol 41*, 87–92.

Mahmood, I. (2005). Interspecies scaling of biliary excreted drugs: a comparison of several methods. *J Pharm Sci 94*, 883–892.

Masica, A.L., Mayo, G., and Wilkinson, G.R. (2004). *In vivo* comparisons of constitutive cytochrome P450 3A activity assessed by alprazolam, triazolam, and midazolam. *Clin Pharmacol Ther 76*, 341–349.

Matheson, P.J., Wilson, M.A., and Garrison, R.N. (2000). Regulation of intestinal blood flow. *J Surg Res 93*, 182–196.

Mayersohn, M. (2002). Principles of drug absorption. In: *Modern Pharmaceutics* (Banker, G.S., and Rohodes, C.T. eds.). Marcel Dekker, New York, pp. 23–66.

McGinnity, D.F., Soars, M.G., Urbanowicz, R.A., and Riley, R.J. (2004). Evaluation of fresh and cryopreserved hepatocytes as *in vitro* drug metabolism tools for the prediction of metabolic clearance. *Drug Metab Dispos 32*, 1247–1253.

Meier, P.J., Eckhardt, U., Schroeder, A., Hagenbuch, B., and Stieger, B. (1997). Substrate specificity of sinusoidal bile acid and organic anion uptake systems in rat and human liver. *Hepatology 26*, 1667–1677.

Meier, Y., Pauli-Magnus, C., Zanger, U.M., Klein, K., Schaeffeler, E., Nussler, A.K., Nussler, N., Eichelbaum, M., Meier, P.J., and Stieger, B. (2006). Interindividual variability of canalicular ATP-binding-cassette (ABC)-transporter expression in human liver. *Hepatology 44*, 62–74.

Meno-Tetang, G.M.L., Li, H., Mis, S., Pyszczynski, N., Heining, P., Lowe, P., and Jusko, W.J. (2006). Physiologically based pharmacokinetic modeling of FTY720 (2-amino-2[2-(-4-octylphenyl)ethyl]propane-1,3-diol hydrochloride) in rats after oral and intravenous doses. *Drug Metab Dispos 34*, 1480–1487.

Merino, G., van Herwaarden, A.E., Wagenaar, E., Jonker, J.W., and Schinkel, A.H. (2005). Sex-dependent expression and activity of the ATP-binding cassette transporter breast cancer resistance protein (BCRP/ABCG2) in liver. *Mol Pharmacol 67*, 1765–1771.

Metcalf, A.M., Phillips, S.F., Zinsmeister, A.R., MacCarty, R.L., Beart, R.W., and Wolff, B.G. (1987). Simplified assessment of segmental colonic transit. *Gastroenterology 92*, 40–47.

Meyer, U.A. (2000). Pharmacogenetics and adverse drug reactions. *Lancet 356*, 1667–1671.

Morse, M., Cassels, D.E., and Schlutz, F.W. (1947). Blood volumes of normal children. *Am J Physiol 151*, 448–458.

Mouly, S., and Paine, M.F. (2003). P-glycoprotein increases from proximal to distal regions of human small intestine. *Pharm Res 20*, 1595–1599.

Muller, A.F., Fullwood, L., Hawkins, M., and Cowley, A.J. (1992). The integrated response of the cardiovascular system to food. *Digestion 52*, 184–193.

Murakami, T., and Takano, M. (2008). Intestinal efflux transporters and drug absorption. *Expert Opin Drug Metab Toxicol 4*, 923–939.

Nasu, R., Kumagai, Y., Kogetsu, H., Tsujimoto, M., Ohtani, H., and Sawada, Y. (2005). Physiologically based pharmacokinetic model for pralmorelin hydrochloride in rats. *Drug Metab Dispos 33*, 1488–1494.

Nelson, D.R., Kamataki, T., Waxman, D.J., Guengerich, F.P., Estabrook, R.W., Feyereisen, R., Gonzalez, F.J., Coon, M.J., Gunsalus, I.C., Gotoh, O., et al. (1993). The P450 superfamily: update on new sequences, gene mapping, accession numbers, early trivial names of enzymes, and nomenclature. *DNA Cell Biol 12*, 1–51.

Nestorov, I. (2001). Modeling and simulation of variability and uncertainty in toxicokinetics and pharmacokinetics. *Toxicol Lett 120*, 411–420.

Nestorov, I. (2003). Whole body pharmacokinetic models. *Clin Pharmacokinet 42*, 883–908.

Nishizato, Y., Ieiri, I., Suzuki, H., Kimura, M., Kawabata, K., Hirota, T., Takane, H., Irie, S., Kusuhara, H., Urasaki, Y., et al. (2003). Polymorphisms of *OATP-C* (*SLC21A6*) and *OAT3* (*SLC22A8*) genes: consequences for pravastatin pharmacokinetics. *Clin Pharmacol Ther 73*, 554–565.

Nolin, T.D., Naud, J., Leblond, F.A., and Pichette, V. (2008). Emerging evidence of the impact of kidney disease on drug metabolism and transport. *Clin Pharmacol Ther 83*, 898–903.

Obach, R.S. (1999). Prediction of human clearance of twenty-nine drugs from hepatic microsomal intrinsic clearance data: an examination of *in vitro* half-life approach and nonspecific binding to microsomes. *Drug Metab Dispos 27*, 1350–1359.

Pacifici, G.M., Viani, A., Taddeucci-Brunelli, G., Rizzo, G., Carrai, M., and Schulz, H.U. (1986). Effects of development, aging, and renal and hepatic insufficiency as well as hemodialysis on the plasma concentrations of albumin and alpha 1-acid glycoprotein: implications for binding of drugs. *Ther Drug Monit 8*, 259–263.

Paine, M.F., Shen, D.D., Kunze, K.L., Perkins, J.D., Marsh, C.L., McVicar, J.P., Barr, D.M., Gillies, B.S., and Thummel, K.E. (1996). First-pass metabolism of midazolam by the human intestine. *Clin Pharmacol Ther 60*, 14–24.

Paine, M.F., Khalighi, M., Fisher, J.M., Shen, D.D., Kunze, K.L., Marsh, C.L., Perkins, J.D., and Thummel, K.E. (1997). Characterization of interintestinal and intraintestinal variations in human CYP3A-dependent metabolism. *J Pharmacol Exp Ther 283*, 1552–1562.

Paine, M.F., Hart, H.L., Ludington, S.S., Haining, R., Rettie, A.E., and Zeldin, D.C. (2006). The human intestinal cytochrome P450 "pie." *Drug Metab Dispos 34*, 880–886.

Pang, K.S. (2003). Modeling of intestinal drug absorption: roles of transporters and metabolic enzymes (for the Gillette Review Series). *Drug Metab Dispos 31*, 1507–1519.

Piafsky, K.M. (1980). Disease-induced changes in the plasma binding of basic drugs. *Clin Pharmacokinet 5*, 246–262.

Poulin, P., and Theil, F.P. (2000). A Priori prediction of tissue:plasma partition coefficients of drugs to facilitate the use of physiologically-based pharmacokinetic models in drug discovery. *J Pharm Sci 89*, 16–35.

Poulin, P., and Theil, F.P. (2002). Prediction of pharmacokinetics prior to *in vivo* studies: 1. Mechanism-based prediction of volume of distribution. *J Pharm Sci 91*, 129–156.

Poulin, P., Schoenlein, K., and Theil, F.P. (2001). Prediction of adipose tissue: plasma partition coefficients for structurally unrelated drugs. *J Pharm Sci 90*, 436–447.

Price, P.S., Conolly, R.B., Chaisson, C.F., Gross, E.A., Young, J.S., Mathis, E.T., and Tedder, D.R. (2003). Modeling inter-individual variation in physiological factors used in PBPK models of humans. *Crit Rev Toxicol 33*, 469–503.

Rane, A., Wilkinson, G.R., and Shand, D.G. (1977). Prediction of hepatic extraction ratio from *in vitro* measurement of intrinsic clearance. *J Pharmacol Exp Ther 200*, 420–424.

Rashid, T.J., Martin, U., Clarke, H., Waller, D.G., Renwick, A.G., and George, C.F. (1995). Factors affecting the absolute bioavailability of nifedipine. *Br J Clin Pharmacol 40*, 51–58.

Rebecca, L.O., and Gordon, L.A. (1987). The influence of variable gastric emptying and intestinal transit rates on the plasma level curve of cimetidine; an explanation for the double peak phenomenon. *J Pharmacokinet Pharmacodyn 15*, 529–544.

Reddy, M.B., Yang, R.S.H., Andersen, M.E., and Clewell, H.J. (2005). *Physiologically Based Pharmacokinetic Modeling: Science and Applications.* Wiley, Hoboken, NJ.

Riley, R.J., McGinnity, D.F., and Austin, R.P. (2005). A unified model for predicting human hepatic, metabolic clearance from *in vitro* intrinsic clearance data in hepatocytes and microsomes. *Drug Metab Dispos 33*, 1304–1311.

Rodgers, T., and Rowland, M. (2006). Physiologically based pharmacokinetic modeling: 2. Predicting the tissue distribution of acids, very weak bases, neutrals and zwitterions. *J Pharm Sci 95*, 1238–1257.

Rodgers, T., Leahy, D., and Rowland, M. (2005). Physiologically based pharmacokinetic modeling: 1. Predicting the tissue distribution of moderate-to-strong bases. *J Pharm Sci 94*, 1259–1276.

Rostami-Hodjegan, A., and Tucker, G.T. (2002). The effects of portal shunts on intestinal cytochrome P450 3A activity. *Hepatology 35*, 1549–1550.

Rostami-Hodjegan, A., and Tucker, G.T. (2007). Simulation and prediction of *in vivo* drug metabolism in human populations from *in vitro* data. *Nat Rev Drug Discov 6*, 140–148.

Rostami-Hodjegan, A., Jackson, P.R., and Tucker, G.T. (1994). Sensitivity of indirect metrics for assessing "rate" in bioequivalence studies: moving the "goalposts" or changing the "game". *J Pharm Sci 83*, 1554–1557.

Rostami-Hodjegan, A., Nurminen, S., Jackson, P.R., and Tucker, G.T. (1996). Caffeine urinary metabolite ratios as markers of enzyme activity: a theoretical assessment. *Pharmacogenetics 6*, 121–149.

Rouser, G., Simon, G., and Kritchevsky, G. (1969). Species variations in phospholipid class distribution of organs: I. Kidney, liver and spleen. *Lipids 4*, 599–606.

Routledge, P.A. (1986). The plasma protein binding of basic drugs. *Br J Clin Pharmacol 22*, 499–506.

Rowland, M., and Tozer, T.N. (1995). *Clinical Pharmacokinetics: Concept and Applications.* Lea & Febiger, Philadelphia.

Rowland, M., Balant, L., and Peck, C. (2004). Physiologically based pharmacokinetics in drug development and regulatory science: a workshop report (Georgetown University, Washington, DC, May 29–30, 2002). *AAPS J 6*, 1–12.

Russell, T.L., Berardi, R.R., Barnett, J.L., Dermentzoglou, L.C., Jarvenpaa, K.M., Schmaltz, S.P., and Dressman, J.B. (1993). Upper gastrointestinal pH in seventy-nine healthy, elderly, North American men and women. *Pharm Res 10*, 187–196.

Sato, A. (1991). The effect of environmental factors on the pharmacokinetic behavior of organic solvent vapours. *Ann Occup Hyg 35*, 525–541.

Sato, A., Endoh, K., Kaneko, T., and Johanson, G. (1991). A simulation study of physiological factors affecting pharmacokinetic behavior of organic solvent vapours. *Br J Ind Med 48*, 342–347.

Sato, H., Sugiyama, Y., Sawada, Y., Iga, T., and Hanano, M. (1987). Physiologically based pharmacokinetics of radioiodinated human beta-endorphin in rats: an application of the capillary membrane-limited model. *Drug Metab Dispos 15*, 540–550.

Sawada, Y., Hanano, M., Sugiyama, Y., Harashima, H., and Iga, T. (1984). Prediction of the volumes of distribution of basic drugs in humans based on data from animals. *J Pharmacokinet Biopharm 12*, 587–596.

Seithel, A., Klein, K., Zanger, U.M., Fromm, M.F., and Konig, J. (2008). Non-synonymous polymorphisms in the human SLCO1B1 gene: an *in vitro* analysis of SNP c.1929A>C. *Mol Genet Genom 279*, 149–157.

Shi, S., and Klotz, U. (2008). Proton pump inhibitors: an update of their clinical use and pharmacokinetics. *Eur J Clin Pharmacol 64*, 935–951.

Shilling, A.D., Azam, F., Kao, J., and Leung, L. (2006). Use of canalicular membrane vesicles (CMVs) from rats, dogs, monkeys and humans to assess drug transport across the canalicular membrane. *J Pharmacol Toxicol Methods 53*, 186–197.

Shimada, T., Yamazaki, H., Mimura, M., Inui, Y., and Guengerich, F.P. (1994). Interindividual variations in human liver cytochrome P-450 enzymes involved in the oxidation of drugs, carcinogens and toxic chemicals: studies with liver microsomes of 30 Japanese and 30 Caucasians. *J Pharmacol Exp Ther 270*, 414–423.

Simon, G., and Rouser, G. (1969). Species variations in phospholipid class distribution of organs: II. Heart and skeletal muscle. *Lipids 4*, 607–614.

Snawder, J.E., and Lipscomb, J.C. (2000). Interindividual variance of cytochrome P450 forms in human hepatic microsomes: correlation of individual forms with xenobiotic metabolism and implications in risk assessment. *Regul Toxicol Pharmacol 32*, 200–209.

Snyder, W.S., Cook, M.J., Masset, E.S., Karhausen, L.R., Howells, G.P., and Tipton, I.H. (1975). *Report of the Task Group on Reference Man*. Pergamon Press, Oxford, UK.

Song, I.S., Shin, H.J., Shim, E.J., Jung, I.S., Kim, W.Y., Shon, J.H., and Shin, J.G. (2008). Genetic variants of the organic cation transporter 2 influence the disposition of metformin. *Clin Pharmacol Ther 84*, 559–562.

Su, Y., and Sinko, P.J. (2007). Drug transporters in the intestine. In: *Drug Transporters: Molecular Characterization and Role in Drug Disposition* (You, G., and Morris, M.E., eds.). Wiley, Hoboken, NJ, pp. 495–516.

Tam, D., Tirona, R.G., and Pang, K.S. (2003). Segmental intestinal transporters and metabolic enzymes on intestinal drug absorption. *Drug Metab Dispos 31*, 373–383.

Tett, S.E., Kirkpatrick, C.M.J., Gross, A.S., and McLachlan, A.J. (2003). Principles and clinical application of assessing alterations in renal elimination pathways. *Clin Pharmacokinet 42*, 1193–1211.

Thirup, P. (2003). Haematocrit: within-subject and seasonal variation. *Sports Med 33*, 231–243.

Thummel, K.E., Oshea, D., Paine, M.F., Shen, D.D., Kunze, K.L., Perkins, J.D., and Wilkinson, G.R. (1996). Oral first-pass elimination of midazolam involves both gastrointestinal and hepatic CYP3A-mediated metabolism. *Clin Pharmacol Ther 59*, 491–502.

Tozer, T.N. (1981). Concepts basic to pharmacokinetics. *Pharmacol Ther 12*, 109–131.

Tsuji, A., and Tamai, I. (1996). Carrier-mediated intestinal transport of drugs. *Pharm Res 13*, 963–977.

Tsunoda, S.M., Velez, R.L., von Moltke, L.L., and Greenblatt, D.J. (1999). Differentiation of intestinal and hepatic cytochrome P450 3A activity with use of midazolam as an *in vivo* probe: Effect of ketoconazole. *Clin Pharmacol Ther 66*, 461–471.

Tucker, G.T. (1981). Measurement of the renal clearance of drugs. *Br J Clin Pharmacol 12*, 761–770.

Tucker, G.T. (1999). Clinical aspects of polymorphic drug metabolism. In: *Variability in Human Drug Response* (Tucker, G.T., ed.). Excerpta Medica, Amsterdam, pp. 11–22.

Tuteja, S., Alloway, R.R., Johnson, J.A., and Gaber, A.O. (2001). The effect of gut metabolism on tacrolimus bioavailability in renal transplant recipients. *Transplantation 71*, 1303–1307.

Urban, T.J., Brown, C., Castro, R.A., Shah, N., Mercer, R., Huang, Y., Brett, C.M., Burchard, E.G., and Giacomini, K.M. (2008). Effects of genetic variation in the novel organic cation transporter, OCTN1, on the renal clearance of gabapentin. *Clin Pharmacol Ther 83*, 416–421.

Valentin, J. (2002). *Basic Anatomical and Physiological Data for Use in Radiological Protection: Reference Values*. Pergamon Press, Oxford, UK.

van Montfoort, J.E., Hagenbuch, B., Groothuis, G.M.M., Koepsell, H., Meier, P.J., and Meijer, D.K.F. (2003). Drug uptake systems in liver and kidney. *Curr Drug Metab 4*, 185–211.

Veering, B.T., Burm, A.G.L., Souverijn, J.H.M., Serree, J.M.P., and Spierdijk, J. (1990). The effect of age on serum concentrations of albumin and alpha 1-acid glycoprotein. *Br J Clin Pharmacol 29*, 201–206.

Viani, A., Rizzo, G., Carrai, M., and Pacifici, G.M. (1992). Interindividual variability in the concentrations of albumin and alpha-1-acid glycoprotein in patients with renal or liver disease, newborns and healthy subjects: implications for binding of drugs. *Int J Clin Pharmacol Ther Toxicol 30*, 128–133.

Villeneuve, J.P., and Pichette, V. (2004). Cytochrome P450 and liver diseases. *Curr Drug Metab 5*, 273–282.

von Kleist, M., and Huisinga, W. (2007). Physiologically based pharmacokinetic modeling: a sub-compartmentalized model of tissue distribution. *J Pharmacokinet Pharmacodyn 34*, 789–806.

von Richter, O., Greiner, B., Fromm, M.F., Fraser, R., Omari, T., Barclay, M.L., Dent, J., Somogyi, A.A., and Eichelbaum, M. (2001). Determination of *in vivo* absorption, metabolism, and transport of drugs by the human intestinal wall and liver with a novel perfusion technique. *Clin Pharmacol Ther 70*, 217–227.

von Richter, O., Burk, O., Fromm, M.F., Thon, K.P., Eichelbaum, M., and Kivisto, K.T. (2004). Cytochrome P450 3A4 and P-glycoprotein expression in human small intestinal enterocytes and hepatocytes: a comparative analysis in paired tissue specimens. *Clin Pharmacol Ther 75*, 172–183.

Wang, Z.J., Yin, O.Q., Tomlinson, B., and Chow, M.S. (2008). OCT2 polymorphisms and *in-vivo* renal functional consequence: studies with metformin and cimetidine. *Pharmacogenet Genom 18*, 637–645.

Watkins, P.B., Wrighton, S.A., Schuetz, E.G., Molowa, D.T., and Guzelian, P.S. (1987). Identification of glucocorticoid-inducible cytochromes P-450 in the intestinal mucosa of rats and man. *J Clin Invest 80*, 1029–1036.

Wennesland, R., Brown, E., Hopper, J., Jr., Hodges, J.L., Jr., Guttentag, O.E., Scott, K.G., Tucker, I.N., and Bradley, B. (1959). Red cell, plasma and blood volume in healthy men measured by radiochromium (Cr51) cell tagging and hematocrit: influence of age, somatotype and habits of physical activity on the variance after regression of volumes to height and weight combined. *J Clin Invest 38*, 1065–1077.

Wilkinson, G.R. (1987). Clearance approaches in pharmacology. *Pharmacol Rev 39*, 1–47.

Wilkinson, G.R. (2005). Drug metabolism and variability among patients in drug response. *N Engl J Med 352*, 2211–2221.

Williams, L.R., and Leggett, R.W. (1989). Reference values for resting blood flow to organs of man. *Clin Phys Physiol Meas 10*, 187–217.

Wood, A.J.J. (1999). Ethnic differences in drug response: a model for understanding inter-individual variability. In: *Variability in Human Drug Response* (Tucker, G.T., ed.). Excerpta Medica, Amsterdam, pp. 133–139.

Wu, C.Y., Benet, L.Z., Hebert, M.F., Gupta, S.K., Rowland, M., Gomez, D.Y., and Wacher, V.J. (1995). Differentiation of absorption and first-pass gut and hepatic metabolism in humans: studies with cyclosporine. *Clin Pharmacol Ther 58*, 492–497.

Yang, J., Rostami-Hodjegan, A., and Tucker, G.T. (2001). Prediction of ketoconazole interaction with midazolam, alprazolam and triazolam: incorporating population variability. *Br J Clin Pharmacol 52*, 472P–473P.

Yang, J., Tucker, G.T., and Rostami-Hodjegan, A. (2004). CYP3A expression and activity in the human small intestine. *Clin Pharmacol Ther 76*, 391–391.

Yang, J., Jamei, M., Yeo, K.R., Tucker, G.T., and Rostami-Hodjegan, A. (2007). Prediction of intestinal first-pass drug metabolism. *Curr Drug Metab 8*, 676–684.

Yeo, K.R., Rostami-Hodjegan, A., and Tucker, G.T. (2003). Abundance of cytochrome P450 in human liver: a meta-analysis. *Br J Clin Pharmacol 57*, 687–688.

Yu, L.X., and Amidon, G.L. (1999). A compartmental absorption and transit model for estimating oral drug absorption. *Int J Pharm 186*, 119–125.

Yu, L.X., Crison, J.R., and Amidon, G.L. (1996). Compartmental transit and dispersion model analysis of small intestinal transit flow in humans. *Int J Pharm 140*, 111–118.

Zhang, L., Brett, C.M., and Giacomini, K.M. (1998). Role of organic cation transporters in drug absorption and elimination. *Annu Rev Pharmacol Toxicol 38*, 431–460.

Zhang, Q.Y., Dunbar, D., Ostrowska, A., Zeisloft, S., Yang, J., and Kaminsky, L.S. (1999). Characterization of human small intestinal cytochromes P-450. *Drug Metab Dispos* *27*, 804–809.

Zhang, Y., Zhang, L., Abraham, S., Apparaju, S., Wu, T.C., Strong, J.M., Xiao, S., Atkinson, A.J., Jr., Thummel, K.E., Leeder, J.S., et al. (2009). Assessment of the impact of renal impairment on systemic exposure of new molecular entities: evaluation of recent new drug applications. *Clin Pharmacol Ther* *85*, 305–311.

PART II

APPLICATIONS TO DRUG DISCOVERY

Applications of Systems Biology Approaches to Target Identification and Validation in Drug Discovery

BART S. HENDRIKS

Merrimack Pharmaceuticals, Cambridge, Massachusetts

Summary

In the "systems biology era," pharmaceutical companies are seeking to develop a more holistic understanding of disease. New efforts are aimed at determining the drivers of disease in terms of cellular processes in multiple cell and tissue types, identifying and quantifying the signaling pathways involved, and then simultaneously choosing the optimal target within the pathways and the best modality for intervention. Work in academia and industry is beginning to accomplish this goal via integrated approaches that couple high-content and high-throughput data collection with a myriad of computational modeling approaches. These new methodologies are intended specifically to address attrition in phase II clinical trials, supplementing existing advances and expertise in drug discovery. Individual tools and their applications are discussed, including text mining, models of disease, biotherapeutics modeling, large multicontext data set collection, regression modeling, network modeling, and dynamic pathway modeling. Contributions from industry are highlighted to focus on real-world application.

5.1. INTRODUCTION

One can oversimplify the process of drug discovery into two steps: picking therapeutic targets and developing the corresponding therapeutic agents

Systems Biology in Drug Discovery and Development, First Edition.
Edited by Daniel L. Young, Seth Michelson.
© 2012 John Wiley & Sons, Inc. Published 2012 by John Wiley & Sons, Inc.

(e.g., small molecules, antibodies, peptides). As an industry, pharma is relatively good at developing therapeutic agents as a result of efforts in target- and structure-based drug design. The success in protein crystallography, understanding the druggability of various proteins with small molecules, and assessments of compound selectivity has shifted the industry's attention toward a better understanding of biology. If, for example, one knows the selectivity profile of two related kinase inhibitors, how does one decide which will have greater therapeutic benefit? Similarly, improved methods for generating antibody-based therapeutics has shifted the focus from generating the therapeutic itself to making even wiser choices regarding which targets to pursue. The process of selecting a therapeutic target and preclinically assessing its propensity to be safe and efficacious is known as *target identification and validation*.

With each successive stage of drug discovery and development comes a dramatic increase in cost. As an industry, only 10 to 20% of therapies that reach the first-in-human level ever get launched (Kola and Landis, 2004). If one can select targets with greater certainty and a higher probability of success, companies can put more resources behind them and move these projects along faster. With shorter time lines, there is generally a longer patent term remaining and a potential for greater returns on investments. The feasibility of this strategy is demonstrated by the speed at which companies are able to generate products in clinically precedented space (DiMasi and Paquette, 2004). Thus, improving our success rate at predicting valid targets can directly affect the bottom line, getting much-needed medicines or therapies to patients as quickly as possible.

Selecting targets with greater certainty and a higher probability of success amounts fundamentally to generating a deeper understanding of the roles of putative targets in both normal and disease physiology. It requires the integration of multiple competing processes and time scales as well as an understanding of contextual differences, from cell and tissue differences to genetic and environmentally driven patient variability. New systems-based perspectives aimed at integrating multiple technologies, diverse scientific disciplines, and experimental and computational approaches, termed collectively *systems biology*, have been offered as a possible means to improve target identification and validation (Butcher, 2005; Kumar et al., 2006; Michelson, 2006).

The past decade or more has seen the growth of numerous systems biology–related companies and targeted efforts within large pharma. In this chapter we stitch together the continuum of experimental and computational approaches that have been developed in both the academic and industrial sectors and highlight how they have been or might be applied to target identification and validation. Each section is intended as an introduction to basic concepts and provides a conceptual understanding of the types of scientific questions that they are well suited to answer. Particular attention is paid to highlighting examples from industry, although it should be recognized that there are many more examples that have not entered the public domain or have had only fleeting mention at conferences. Each topic itself is the subject of extensive further work, and in many cases numerous excellent reviews are cited that go into significant detail. In this chapter we focus exclusively on analysis at the protein level and omit some technologies that have fallen under the umbrella of systems biology, including genomics, metabolomics, metabolic flux analysis, bioinformatics, and "omics" profiling approaches (van der Greef and McBurney, 2005).

5.2. TYPICAL DRUG DISCOVERY PARADIGM

The primary goal of pharmaceutical drug discovery is to test such clinical hypotheses as "modulation of target X will affect clinical endpoint Y, where endpoint Y is, directly or indirectly, a marker for a disease." Although this is a simple concept, it is remarkably difficult to execute. One needs to have a means to modulate the desired target, typically a small molecule of some sort, and it must be of sufficient potency and selectivity that one may conclude that modulation of the intended target was responsible for the effect observed, rather than off-target effects. For this to be tested, the candidate drug must have adequate pharmacokinetic properties to cross various barriers (e.g., gut absorption, cell membrane permeability) and evade elimination or degradation for a sufficiently long time to reach the target of interest in the cell or tissue type of interest. In the clinic, one must have means to measure whether or not the target was modulated successfully as well as having a measurable clinical endpoint. Then, and only then, can one adequately test clinical hypotheses.

In general, clinically unprecedented targets (targets against which no drugs exist) enter the portfolio in one of the following ways:

1. *Literature.* Targets are initially identified from the literature elucidating fundamental aspects of biology that implicate a target in a cellular or disease process, usually via the use of a cell or animal model of disease or, more recently, via genetic associations in clinical populations. This is the point at which the clinical hypothesis is formally presented.

2. *Phenotypic screens.* Screening approaches can also be used to identify targets that modulate specific cellular behaviors. With these endpoint screening approaches, one can identify compounds or genes (via RNAi screens, for example) that alter cellular behavior without immediate knowledge of the target. The "hits" identified using this method require subsequent "deconvolution" to elucidate biological target(s), which can frequently prove very difficult, for a variety of technical reasons.

Once a target is identified and chosen, a cascade of events ensues that takes years and millions of dollars to complete for the sole purpose of making a potent, selective, and bioavailable compound. Biochemical assays are developed for screening compounds against the target protein of interest. Selection of the species and isoform of a target to screen against is of critical importance and has been the difference between failure and success. Additionally, significant protein production requirements may pose a challenge. Cell-based assays are developed to demonstrate that compounds are able to enter cells and hit the intended target. Selectivity is needed to ensure that effects are due to a known perturbation. Similarly, animal models are used to demonstrate that the compound may have adequate pharmacokinetic properties, yield clues for potential toxicity, and might also be able to shed light on possible efficacy. During this process there is virtually no opportunity to reassess the choice of target. Decisions regarding the mechanism of inhibition and drug modality all precede a deep understanding of the target, which typically evolves with the project for novel targets.

Experimental systems, including various *in vitro* and *in vivo* models, often fail to correlate with one another. Further, pharma's low success rate in phase II trials indicates that preclinical models are poorly predictive of clinical findings. This may be for a variety of reasons. For example, biochemical screens might be performed against a different conformation of an enzyme. In addition, experimental conditions may not accurately reflect *in vivo* conditions, often optimized for signal-to-noise ratios rather than optimally mimicking *in vivo* conditions. Moreover, dynamic effects, negative feedback, and interaction of multiple systems may make assays difficult to interpret. Further, assays measuring at a single time point following acute stimulation may yield misleading results due to complex interactions or the use of nonphysiologically relevant stimuli. Finally, interspecies differences, in every aspect from physical size to protein structures to metabolic enzymes, may also contribute to the lack of correlations. Ultimately, many target programs fail in the clinic, due either to unexpected safety concerns in phase I trials or lack of efficacy in phase II trials. Failure at these stages is expensive (hundreds of millions of dollars) (DiMasi et al., 2003) and failure without successful testing of the clinical hypothesis is especially wasteful. These are many of the reasons that are championing the rise of integrated systems biology approaches to identify and validate targets based on a deep understanding of health and disease.

It is worth noting that the path for biological therapies following target identification is substantially different (and can be faster), but is subject to many of the same challenges in terms of developing and applying experimental systems that are truly reflective of *in vivo* conditions. For the most part, the development of biologically based therapies has been pressed into the mold and workflow of small molecules, from target selection through pharmacokinetic modeling and decision making. Only recently are key differences between biotherapeutics and small molecules being fully appreciated and taken into account.

Despite all the challenges, it needs to be recognized that the target-based approach has delivered drugs to the patient successfully and is responsible for a variety of blockbuster drugs on the market today. However, as we tackle more challenging diseases and go after even more challenging targets, the inefficiency of what is fundamentally a trial-and-error approach cannot meet today's business needs or society's interest in novel medications to treat underserved patient populations. The goal moving forward is to make even better predictions of which targets are likely to succeed, by improving our ability to use preclinical models to predict clinical endpoints. Simultaneously, one must shorten the life cycle and resource burden from idea to marketed drug.

5.3. INTEGRATED DRUG DISCOVERY

In the systems biology era of drug discovery, the primary goal has not changed: One still seeks to test clinical hypotheses regarding the modulation of a specific target in a disease context. However, one seeks to make even better-informed decisions about target selection and to enable a more nimble decision-making environment where incremental biological knowledge and insight can inform portfolio decision making in real time. The systems biology approach to target identification and validation is different from the traditional approach in its explicit study of context, quantitative experimentation, and the application of cutting-edge computational technology and engineering approaches to the study of disease. In the target-based approach, one picks a target, develops compounds, and then takes them through a testing funnel of successively more complicated experimental systems that parallels the target-to-physiology continuum. In this approach, if the target fails, there often is no obvious backup plan in terms of what the next-best target would be. Also, decisions regarding the mechanism of inhibition and drug modality all generally precede a deep understanding of the target. Rather than pursue drug discovery from a target-based approach, systems biology utilizes what may be termed a "disease-centric" approach. One starts from the disease and successively digs deeper, building a quantitative understanding of the differences between health and disease states, building knowledge that leads simultaneously to the optimal target and mode of intervention (Figure 5.1). One takes advantage of top-down approaches to determine the major drivers of disease and bottom-up approaches to understand detailed target mechanisms. Knowledge is codified in the form of engineering diagrams and mathematical models to capture the essential behavior of healthy and disease physiology. Quantitative models are then analyzed to generate experimentally testable hypotheses.

There exists a spectrum of tools and computational techniques that can address specific questions. As these modeling techniques mature, the crux of the problem lies in integrating their individual contributions into multiscale efforts that are able to capture both the high-level essence of disease progression and the details of specific drug–target interactions. Below is one possible sequence by which leaps can be made across the various problem scales to identify, validate, and prioritize targets.

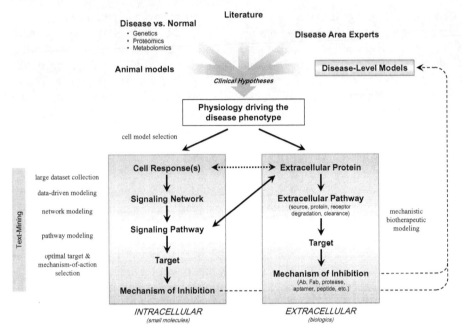

Figure 5.1 Conceptual workflow for integrating systems biology approaches across cell and disease scales.

5.4. DRIVERS OF THE DISEASE PHENOTYPE: CLINICAL ENDPOINTS AND HYPOTHESES

When approaching a disease indication, the first question that must be answered is: What is different between the healthy and disease states? In other words, what is the endpoint by which one measures success? For some diseases, this is readily apparent, such as hypertension or asthma, but for others it is not as clear, such as mental disorders. This is the point at which large "omics" experiments comparing disease versus normal states can bear fruit, yielding hypotheses regarding a causative gene or protein (van der Greef and McBurney, 2005). Additionally, *genome-wide association studies* are yielding hypotheses for targets and pathways in disease that are associated with clinical disease and distinct patient populations (McCarthy et al., 2008). Ultimately, one must formulate a clinical hypothesis as to what is the most sensitive and causative process leading to the disease phenotype. For example, lowering circulating TNF-α levels will stop disease progression in rheumatoid arthritis or antiapoptotic pathways that drive tumor progression in hepatocellular carcinoma. In their simplest form, these hypotheses arise from fundamental biology research and by stitching together pieces from the vast literature.

5.4.1. Literature Mining

The literature is the starting point for virtually all drug discovery efforts. At present, there are roughly 18 million abstracts in Medline, which continue to increase at an exponential rate. If one restricts his or her search to a particular disease, he or she can find thousands to millions of publications. Consequently, there is a great need for automated approaches to aid in identifying relevant literature and extracting information. These techniques, commonly referred to as *text mining*, encompass automated *literature retrieval, document classification*, and *natural language processing* (Cohen and Hersh, 2005; Cohen and Hunter, 2008; Erhardt et al., 2006; Roberts, 2006; Roberts and Hayes, 2005). These methods can supplement the vast array of public and private databases that are available as well. The following is focused explicitly on end-user application and highlights a narrow slice of the text-mining field. There are vast text-mining resources throughout the Internet, and many technical hurdles in identifying, extracting, structuring, and integrating information captured in biomedical texts are not covered here (Rzhetsky et al., 2008).

Most common search tools and databases index article abstracts and allow basic keyword searching to find articles of interest. On one level, this is a fine method to identify broad sets of articles of interest. However, as the literature increases in scale, this may become inefficient (e.g., searching "diabetes" on Medline pulls up about 300,000 items).

5.4.1.1. Literature Retrieval

As questions become more specific, the type of information and detail found in abstracts is not always sufficient to find targeted information. Consequently, it is often necessary to dive into full-text documents to find content of interest. Obtaining a literature corpus physically is the first step and can be time consuming if performed manually. To this end, there are literature retrieval software packages such as Quosa (Brighton, MA) specifically designed to obtain full-text documents in an automated fashion. These tools also enable keyword searching through full-text articles (Erhardt et al., 2006).

5.4.1.2. Document Classification

Enriching a collection of documents with the most relevant topics can greatly improve the performance of subsequent search methods. When a set of documents has been retrieved, efforts to group documents into smaller subgroups that are likely to contain specific or related information is known as *document classification* (Erhardt et al., 2006). This can be accomplished in either an unsupervised or a supervised manner. Unsupervised classification methods use various metrics to determine relatedness. For example, one might try to categorize documents about systems biology by looking for documents that have a high occurrence of words referring to computational approaches. Alternatively, supervised methods use sets of documents that have already been classified as training data to build statistical models to predict the classification of new documents. Once a collection of relevant documents has been assembled, one can begin to extract information.

5.4.1.3. Information Extraction

Keyword searching uses simple term co-occurrence within an abstract or entire document. For example, if you are searching for things that stimulate insulin production, you might use the search terms "stimulate" and "insulin production." With co-occurrence searching you may find some of what you are looking for but will also retrieve cases where the terms "insulin production" and "stimulate" occur in different sentences or completely different portions of the text. Similarly, a search for a kinetic rate constant, K_m, might return both the kinetic rate constant and authors with the initials "KM." A step beyond this is to utilize *natural language processing* (NLP) to enable the creation of increasingly complex and targeted queries against a literature corpus. These may come from a variety of sources, including Medline abstracts and collections of full-text articles. NLP addresses several of the querying issues by interpreting sentence structure. Sentences are broken into various parts: noun phrases, verb phrases, and prepositions. This enables a search for specific phrases and terms *within* a sentence. Furthermore, NLP tools such as Linguamatics I2E (Cambridge, UK) can make use of *ontologies* and thesauri to generate concise, powerful queries to extract information. Ontologies are simply term lists that provide some (biological) knowledge, often organized into a hierarchical tree (Schulze-Kremer, 2002). Each entry in an ontology consists of a preferred term and a list of synonyms as well as its relationship to other terms. For example, one could search for: [gene] that ("induces" or "causes") ("insulin resistance"), where [gene] would have a list of all gene names and synonyms. Similarly, one could generate ontologies of cellular or disease processes, or types of cancer. Gene ontology (Ashburner et al., 2000) is a particularly well-known effort to compile and organize information about genes and their function.

With literature retrieval, databases, and NLP tools, one can formulate specific queries to extract information of interest from literature and database sources. For example, what drugs already exist for my disease of interest? What are the phenotypic effects of those drugs? What are their targets? What are all the cellular processes associated with a disease? What are all the genes implicated in a cellular process? Which genes and/or proteins are altered in the diseased state? What is the knockout phenotype of a given gene?

Effective and comprehensive literature mining is critical to acquire the state of knowledge in a given disease area and determine quickly if opportunities exist. One can move from a disease to a list of cellular process or candidate target genes or proteins. In some cases the literature may lead immediately to promising target candidates; however, there is generally little literature that assembles a holistic view of physiological and disease processes that enable one to pinpoint the most sensitive points for novel intervention with great certainty. Further, one usually has to traverse several steps between target literature and whole animal physiology. Most papers do not make claims of a target altering a disease, but rather, altering a cellular process, with the cellular process being involved in an aspect of the disease. For example, heightened ERK activity causes increased cell motility → increased cell motility may confer an invasive phenotype → cell invasion is implicated in cancer metastasis → increased metastasis is correlated with poor prognosis in cancer. Thus, literature mining enables one to piece together all that is known regarding the intricate interplay between various cell types, physiological processes, signaling pathways, and putative targets to assemble disease-level understanding.

5.4.2. Computational Models of Disease

Computational models are quantitative representations that integrate our collective understanding of various molecular, cellular, and/or disease processes. Ideally, one would like to build a model of an entire human and understand how all of the various cells and tissues interact. While the *in silico* human is still beyond current capabilities, several groups have begun to assemble high-level models of specific diseases. High-level models encompass both simplified abstractions of disease processes and large-scale models with hundreds to thousands of entities.

5.4.2.1. Qualitative Models of Disease

Due to the challenge in quantifying aspects of biology, several groups and companies have adopted qualitative modeling approaches that utilize causal reasoning. Genstruct (Cambridge, MA) has developed systems-level models of molecular cause-and-effect relationships (Pollard et al., 2005). They have compiled disease-specific databases that contain cause-and-effect relationships between genes, proteins, and cellular processes and higher-level physiological responses, as well as their context (tissue, cell type, or subcellular compartment). For example, the data describe the fact that transcriptional activity of PPARGC1a positively influences the transcriptional activity of PPARG and NRF1 (Pollard et al., 2005). The magnitude of the interaction is not described, nor is how multiple influences should be integrated. Using genome-wide profiling and computer-aided causal reasoning, they are able to perform various analyses. Given a transcriptional profile, they can hypothesize a set of changes that could explain the data. Using this approach, they have hypothesized a collection of molecular causes for type 2 diabetes (Pollard et al., 2005), as well as a mechanism of androgen stimulation in prostate cancer (Pratt et al., 2006). This type of approach serves a role in hypothesis generation regarding which molecular players may be involved in a process, but is not able to provide quantitative insight.

5.4.2.2. Quantitative Models of Disease

These models aim to integrate multiple competing processes and dynamics. They tend to be top-down models that start with high-level endpoints and lumped rate parameters and successively dig deeper into the underlying physiological processes. Generally, the goal of these models is to capture the minimal essence of the disease so that one can identify the primary drivers of the disease phenotype and not get bogged down in molecular detail.

Entelos (Foster City, CA) has developed comprehensive models of several diseases, including rheumatoid arthritis, asthma, and diabetes. Entelos' large-scale differential algebraic equation model of type 1 diabetes represents cellular functions and biochemical interactions in the pancreatic lymph node, pancreatic islet, and blood compartments (Young et al., 2006). Their model includes the interaction of multiple cell types (CD4$^+$ T-cells, innate regulatory T-cells, CD8$^+$ T-cells, B-lymphocytes, endothelial cells, dendritic cells, macrophages, and pancreatic beta cells) and functions thought to be important for disease pathogenesis: cellular activation, proliferation, apoptosis, trafficking between compartments, mediator secretion, antigen presentation, beta cell killing, insulin secretion, and glucose regulation. Model parameters are estimated from quantitative data on cell populations, functions, and mediator activities. With this model, they are able to simulate the effects of anti-CD3 antibody treatment and to compare results for data obtained in a nonobese diabetic mouse. Further, they were able to determine requirements for sustained remission: rapid beta cell recovery and a more regulatory pancreatic infiltrate (Young et al., 2006).

Entelos has also developed a model of rheumatoid arthritis in a similar manner (Rullmann et al., 2005). Their model describes a prototypical rheumatoid joint in which a pannus of synovial-derived proliferative tissue grows over articular cartilage and osteoclast activity mediates bone erosion. The joint is modeled with multiple compartments, including synovial and articular spaces. The synovial tissue compartment contains multiple cell types, including macrophages, fibroblast-like synoviocytes, CD4$^+$ T-cells, and endothelial cells. Numerous soluble factors, including cytokines, proteases, and cell surface molecules, mediate intercellular communication that ultimately results in model outputs of synovial hyperplasia, cartilage degradation rate, bone erosion index, and levels of soluble factors. Together, these endpoints are combined to form an ACR score for direct comparison with clinical data. Using this model, Entelos and Organon (The Netherlands) evaluated prospective targets in rheumatoid arthritis, predicting that anti-IL-15 therapy will be effective in treating rheumatoid arthritis (Rullmann et al., 2005).

There is a vast literature of models describing insulin and glucose dynamics in the regulation of energy homeostasis in diabetes (Boutayeb and Chetouani, 2006; Cedersund and Stralfors, 2008; Pattaranit and van den Berg, 2008). These models are variations on a basic theme of positing simple relationships between glucose and insulin production and are often fit to clinical data to quantitatively characterize insulin resistance and glucose sensitivity. Such models have been in development for decades and the simplest models of glucose and insulin are gradually being expanded to include additional positive and negative regulators as well as multiple interacting organs.

Chow and Hall (2008) have developed elegant models of human body weight change. These models are based on macronutrient and energy flux balances and enable the partitioning of macronutrients in various lean and fat mass compartments. Using dynamic systems theory they were able to identify trajectories of weight change for different initial conditions. Their simulations allowed prediction of body weight change in response to changes in diet and/ or energy expenditure. Similarly, Hall and Baracos have used a model of human macronutrient metabolism to quantitatively understand involuntary weight loss in cancer-associated cachexia (Hall and Baracos, 2008). Simulations were able to show how known metabolic disturbances synergize with reduced energy intake. Importantly, one is able to use such a model to test, *in silico*, the effects of nutritional support and investigate effects of therapeutic intervention such as inhibition of lipolysis or proteolysis (Hall and Baracos, 2008).

In CancerSim (Abbott et al., 2006) an agent-based simulation implements the "hallmarks of cancer" from Hanahan and Weinberg's seminal paper (2000). The hallmarks include self-sufficiency in growth signals, sustained angiogenesis, insensitivity to growth-inhibitor signals, evasion of apoptosis, limitless replicative potential, and tissue invasion or metastasis. An agent-based model is a computational model that simulates the actions and interactions of autonomous individuals (cells or molecular species) in a network, with the aim of assessing their effects on the system as a whole (Materi and Wishart, 2007). CancerSim consists of cells and a circulatory system, both of which grow according to their own rules. Cell properties are expressed as phenotype traits and go through a primitive cell life cycle that balances several forces according to specific parameter values and stochastic variation. At each time step, the state changes by each cell are dictated by a set of complex rules and probabilities. This model is able to test the hypotheses put forth by Hanahan and Weinberg and, in particular, to test the likely sequences of precancerous mutations.

Spencer et al. (2004) also approached quantitative characterization of the balance of angiogenesis, cell death rates, genetic instability, and replication rates with an ordinary differential equation model. Their key findings predict that cancer develops fastest through a particular ordering of mutations, driven by early mutations in genes maintaining genomic integrity.

Wang et al. (2007) have simulated non-small cell lung cancer using a multiscale agent-based model. This model integrates mechanistic signaling pathway details with a two-dimensional virtual microenvironment containing epidermal growth factor, glucose, and oxygen tensions. A cell phenotype decision algorithm determines cell fate under various conditions, and a model of multicellular tumor expansion dynamics is responsible for calculating tumor size. With this model the authors were able to investigate the impact of cell phenotype decisions on cell numbers as well as to simulate the molecular effects of increased extrinsic epidermal growth factor concentration.

The purpose of these models is to build an integrated understanding of the system and enable hypothesis generation. The process of model building will help identify knowledge gaps in understanding and suggest areas of future research. Once a disease model has been built and validated with some degree of experimental or clinical data, one can begin to identify sensitive points of regulation and investigate possible means of intervention. In quantitative models, a *sensitivity analysis* can help determine which process is the most influential in altering the clinical endpoint. Sensitivity analysis is a technique that determines how much the output of a model changes following a small change in a parameter or initial condition while holding all other parameters and initial conditions fixed. For most moderately complex models, it is commonly found that many parameters will not have significant effects on the endpoint (i.e., not rate limiting), suggesting that not all components involved in disease regulation will be attractive targets for intervention. Sensitivity analysis may lead to nonintuitive hypotheses as a result of complex regulatory and feedback mechanisms. Explicit testing of the effects of perturbations will also enable the prioritization of hypothesis to guide experimental follow-up. Once a sensitive process has been identified, one must pursue experimental validation.

It is important to note that this approach will not identify completely novel targets (in the sense of new genes or proteins), as one can only put into the model what is known. However, such models may provide novel insights into regulatory processes and will identify gaps in current knowledge by determining the extent to which current dogma is consistent with the integrated view of all of the data. In some cases where model predictions are at odds with experimental data, it is possible to hypothesize additional components or processes required to obtain the behavior observed.

5.5. EXTRACELLULAR DISEASE DRIVERS: MECHANISTIC BIOTHERAPEUTIC MODELS

If the candidate target is an extracellular protein (such as a cytokine, secreted protein, or cell surface receptor), or the cellular process of interest is the production or inhibition of a secreted protein, biologically based therapies (i.e., recombinant proteins, antibodies, etc.) are possible. For these cases, the clinical goal tends to be clearly defined—for example, to lower the circulating level of TNF-α in rheumatoid arthritis—and one can build systemic models to describe the synthesis, distribution, and degradation of the protein of interest. These models are integrated with mechanism-based pharmacokinetic models (i.e., antibody dosing and clearance) of the biotherapeutics and can be used to answer specific drug discovery questions, such as:

- Is it better to pursue the protein itself or pathways regulating its synthesis or degradation?
- What is the optimal mechanism of intervention (i.e., Ab, Fab, recombinant protein, peptide, protease, aptamer, etc.)?

- What are the optimal properties? What is the optimal affinity or degree of intervention?
- To what extent does biology limit the maximum theoretical efficacy?

The answers to these questions can provide very direct actions for project teams and often generate proprietary insight into late-stage target selection decisions. Consequently, there are very few published examples of such models applied to real biotherapeutics.

In building such models, the biological details tend to be relatively well defined. The challenge often lies in informing models with values for rate parameters such as receptor ligand affinities and circulating protein half-lives. These are often available in the literature but can be difficult to find and may be calculated from other existing data. Text-mining approaches are a critical tool for finding parameter values, and specific approaches have been applied to classify papers that are likely to contain kinetic rate constants (Hakenberg et al., 2004).

For recombinant protein drugs, the models are in their simplest form, as the target and therapy are principally the same entity. To this end, Sarkar and Lauffenburger (2003) developed a cell-level pharmacokinetic model for granulocyte colony–stimulating factor (GCSF), a protein administered clinically to stimulate the production of white blood cells. In this work they modeled the dosing and clearance of GCSF as well as mechanistic interactions of GCSF with its receptor and its consequent intracellular trafficking. By incorporating receptor binding, endocytosis, and recycling rates, they were able to predict the effects of decreases in endosomal affinity. Further, they were able to compare the relative effects of receptor-mediated clearance versus nonspecific clearance mediated by protein modification such as conjugation with poly(ethylene glycol).

For cases where the desired goal is to lower the circulating protein level, one combines models of target regulation with antibody (or Fab fragment or aptamer) interaction and clearance. The complex clearance of antibodies and their high-affinity interaction with their targets pose unique challenges and opportunities with regard to pharmacokinetics. Due to their large size, antibody volumes of distribution tend to be relatively low, magnifying the importance of understanding antibody–target interactions (Lobo et al., 2004). IgG antibodies have low clearance rates that are driven by fluid-phase endocytosis in vascular endothelial cells. At the low pH of the endosome, IgG bind to the FcRn receptor and are protected from degradation by recycling with the unbound fraction sent for lysosomal degradation (Lobo et al., 2004). Garg and Balthasar (2007) have developed a physiologically based pharmacokinetic model to predict IgG tissue kinetics in wild-type and FcRn-knockout mice. Ferl et al. (2005) generated a model of antibody dynamics and regulation by the FcRn receptor and extended it to include antibody–target interactions within a tumor submodel. Their model correctly predicted antibody fragment biodistribution could be applied for optimizing dosing. Kamei et al. (2005)

have used molecular modeling approaches to predict the effect of mutations in the Fc region of antibodies on Fc–FcRn binding interactions. Further, mathematical models of Fc trafficking were developed to predict the effect of altered Fc–FcRn interactions on antibody half-lives. Experimental manipulation of antibody clearance via modulating Fc–FcRn interaction has further demonstrated this to be a feasible approach for anti-TNF-α antibodies, although with some species-specific effects (Datta-Mannan et al., 2007a,b). Thus, mechanism-based models of biotherapeutics enable one to study and predict the influence of various processes and parameters on antibody disposition and efficacy.

Lao et al. (2007) and Yadzi et al. (Yazdi and Murphy, 1994; Yazdi et al., 1995) have developed models for transferrin trafficking. Transferrin is frequently considered for conjugation to therapeutics in order to alter pharmacokinetics and/or aid in delivery. Lao's and Yadzi's models suggest that it may be possible to predict efficacy of certain anticancer therapies based on intracellular trafficking (Yazdi et al., 1995), and predict how iron release rates from transferrin will affect the cellular association of transferrin (Lao et al., 2007).

Interaction of an antibody with a target can fundamentally alter the clearance route of the target. Most small circulating proteins (<30 kDa) are cleared by glomerular filtration in the kidney (Venturoli and Rippe, 2005). Thus, small protein targets binding to an antibody will prevent renal clearance and can result in a large spike in circulating target–antibody complex levels by exclusion from glomerular filtration. Complex buildup has been observed multiple times in clinical trials for cytokine targets such as TNF-α, IL-6, and MCP-1 and could have been predicted readily using simple computational models (Dominguez et al., 2005; Haringman et al., 2006; Uchiyama et al., 2008). In some cases, accumulation of the antibody–target complex may lead to dangerous side effects or compromise efficacy and inadequately test the clinical hypothesis. Further, characterization of residual activity of the target–antibody complex can be used to address safety concerns as a result of complex buildup. Finally, simple models of biotherapeutics and target interactions can also be used to explore the effects of increased antibody affinity, altered dosing levels, and timing.

Combining cell-level properties with a mechanistic understanding of the unique clearance mechanisms into a mathematical framework can enable the improvement of protein therapeutics (Lao and Kamei, 2008; Rao et al., 2005). Implemented upfront, these methods can help determine design parameters a priori and help project teams decide when increasing antibody affinity has reached the point of diminishing returns. Dosing predictions can determine whether a proposed target is amenable to commercially feasible modulation. Detailed mechanistic information and rate parameters are not available for all targets and, consequently, incomplete literature knowledge can delay these projects. In these cases, the unfinished portions of the model will indicate which areas require further research, probably benefiting from integrated experimental and computational approaches to unravel complex biological regulation described below.

It is interesting to note that the predictions of which drugging modalities are likely to be less successful are extremely difficult to validate since pharma companies are generally not willing to expend resources to validate such predictions. However, there may be fortuitous external validation in the form of trials conducted by competitors.

5.6. RELEVANT CELL MODELS FOR CLINICAL ENDPOINTS

Depending on the cellular process identified from text mining or the disease-level models, one needs to identify appropriate experimental systems and should enlist the help of domain-expert biologists and disease-area specialists. In the traditional drug discovery paradigm, cell models are often chosen largely on the basis of signal-to-noise ratios for the purpose of assay development. In the integrated approach, it is preferable to examine multiple cell types under multiple experimental contexts to determine upfront which condition displays the most *in vivo*–like behavior and to better characterize assay limitations. Use of human primary cells is also preferred, as they are more likely to reflect *in vivo* conditions, but may provide limitations in terms of availability, ease of use, and amenability to genetic manipulation.

For extracellular targets described above that are pursued with biotherapeutics, animal models are typically needed to test model hypotheses due to the nature of the targets. Of course, depending on the target chosen and modality, there may be issues with the immunogenicity of antibody-based therapeutics, the sequence dissimilarity (of the target) between species, or simply the inability of animal disease models to recapture the true nature and etiology of human disease.

For intracellular targets, establishing relevant cell models is critical in ensuring that subsequent findings can be translated into confident clinical conclusions. If one pursues cell proliferation as a model for cancer, for example, one needs to weigh carefully the choice of cell type and cell culture conditions that are most reflective of *in vivo* conditions. The sheer nature of generating cell lines often selects for cells that generate their own growth factors. Consequently, one must be careful that the cell lines chosen for experimental studies accurately reflect the tumor microenvironment and that the *in vitro* drivers of proliferation are the same as those *in vivo*.

In cases where significant clinical literature is available, one can perform high-content screening and empirically determine cell endpoints that correlate best with clinical endpoints (Starkuviene and Pepperkok, 2007). For example, Xu et al. (2008) used high-content imaging to measure the response of cultured primary hepatocytes to various small molecule drugs to determine which measurements were most predictive of clinical hepatotoxicity. They used text-mining techniques to compile a list of over 300 known hepatotoxicants and safe compounds as well as corresponding clinical C_{max} values to set up the study design. Lipid context, glutathione content, reactive oxygen species, and mitochondrial membrane potential were measured using automated microscopy and quantitative measurements extracted with image analysis software. Finally, statistical models were constructed to identify the maximally informative measurements for predicting clinical hepatotoxicity.

In the case of rheumatoid arthritis, the clinical efficacy of anti-TNF biologics (Kievit et al., 2007) suggests that measurement of circulating TNF may be a good indicator of potential efficacy of small-molecule TNF inhibitors. Consequently, TNF production from peripheral blood mononuclear cells or macrophage cell lines is typically used. However, questions remain as to the most physiologically relevant stimuli to use in ex vivo experimental tests. More recent work from Espelin et al. (in preparation), Alexopoulos et al. (in preparation), and the Alliance for Cell Signaling (Gilman et al., 2002; http://www.signaling-gateway.org) have started to address some of these challenges in a more comprehensive manner, specifically comparing multiple stimuli alone and in combination with regard to cytokine production.

5.7. INTRACELLULAR DISEASE DRIVERS: SIGNALING PATHWAY QUANTIFICATION

For a given cellular endpoint, such as proliferation or cytokine production, one needs to determine and quantify the extent to which different signaling pathways regulate that endpoint. This analysis is often already seeded with hypotheses from the literature; however, it is rarely complete in terms of understanding differences in terms of both context and cell type. Large-scale experimental efforts are required to begin the process of unraveling complex and dynamic relationships between extracellular cues, intracellular signals, and cellular responses.

5.7.1. Large Data Set Collection

Initially, the advent of transcriptional profiling enabled researchers to gather some of the first large biological data sets. Although these data sets measure hundreds to thousands of endpoints, they tend to consist of few perturbations and time points, hampering their ability to provide functional insight into disease regulation. With the advent of medium- to high-throughput experimental methods for protein measurement, large experimental efforts are beginning to emerge in the literature (Albeck et al., 2006). Recent work at the protein level has begun to push the limits of scale of these data sets and emphasized multidimensional experimental design that involves measurements in response to multiple stimuli (and combinations), time points, compound treatment, cell types, and so on.

Perez and others have utilized polychromatic flow cytometry to measure multiple phosphoepitopes in single cells as determinants of kinase activity

(Perez and Nolan, 2002; Perez et al., 2004). They performed 11-color flow cytometry, monitoring thousands of cells, following cytokine stimulation with and without compound treatment, exploring five differentiation markers and following the activity of four kinases. This data collection provided the substrate for later Bayesian analysis aimed at reconstruction of intracellular signaling networks (Sachs et al., 2005).

Gaudet et al. (2005) combined kinase activity measurements, immunoblots, antibody arrays and flow cytometry to generate a self-consistent dataset of over 100,000 measurements in HT29 cells. They examined pro-apoptotic and pro-survival stimuli, monitoring 19 intracellular protein signals and four apoptotic response measurements over a 24-hour time course to lay the foundation for mining insight into cellular decision making. Using partial least-squares regression modeling (discussed further below), they were able to determine which measurements and time points were the most informative in describing cellular responses. Further, this work laid the foundation for subsequent analyses digging deeper in mechanisms of cellular decision making (Janes et al., 2005) and uncovering autocrine signaling cascades (Janes et al., 2004).

The Alliance for Cell Signaling has generated and made available an impressive data set in RAW 264.7 macrophages (Gilman et al., 2002; Natarajan et al., 2006). Their data set consists of a global profiling of intracellular signaling and cytokine responses following stimulation with 22 ligands alone or in pairwise combination. They measured 22 intracellular signals controlling the production of 7 cytokines. This work has supported numerous subsequent analyses, including the identification of signaling components required for prediction of cytokine release (Pradervand et al., 2006) and a global analysis of signaling crosstalk in cytokine production (Natarajan et al., 2006).

Work from Espelin et al. (2010) is an industry-based example of systematic, multivariate data collection, focusing on the quantitative comparison of small-molecule inhibitors of TNF production in U937 macrophages. They executed a complex experimental design with 15 stimulation conditions, with and without treatment with seven compounds, across a 24-hour period, measuring 23 phosphoprotein signals and 50 cytokine responses. In addition to attempting to link intracellular signals with individual cytokine responses, this work examined the global effects of kinase inhibitor treatment and highlighted context-dependent effects on efficacy.

It is worth noting that there are increasingly large data sets being generated via mass spectrometry approaches, offering far more individual measurements of phosphoproteins (White, 2008; Zhang et al., 2007). However, there are still limitations as to the number of experimental conditions that can be explored simultaneously in these data sets, limiting their utility for unraveling mechanism. Similarly, high-content imaging approaches are also gaining ground (Schultz et al., 2005) but still face limitations inherent to the specificity of affinity reagents or the need to generate custom constructs to image specific pathways (commercially available, for example, from Odyssey Thera (San Ramon, CA) (MacDonald and Westwick, 2007; Yu et al., 2003). Broad profiling services of signaling activities are commercially available from, for example, BioSeek (Berg et al., 2006), Kinexus (Vancouver, BC, Canada) (multiplexed immunoblotting), and Baypoint (Houston, TX) (reversed-phase protein arrays).

These works share a common theme of attempting to establish large, self-consistent data sets of protein-level measurements that span as much of the accessible signaling space as possible. This is accomplished by manipulating and perturbing the experimental system(s) in as many diverse ways as possible focusing on disease-relevant endpoints. Manipulations may track multiple dimensions, including generating dynamic time-course data, examining multiple combinations of multiple stimuli, co-treatment with pharmacological inhibitors at multiple concentrations, and multiple cell types. Due to the interconnected nature of intracellular signaling networks, measurement at key signaling nodes should yield insight into mechanisms of regulation for cellular responses, and intervention with compounds, even nonselective compounds, will help uncover true regulatory relationships from spurious collinearity. Time-course data are collected with the hope of identifying and teasing apart various regulatory relationships and feedback loops that may be present. In these works, the focus has been on protein measurements because they are more proximal to cellular response than genetic measurements. Proteins represent the site of action of drug molecules. The translation of the regulatory role of a protein in a cellular response to a drug is much more straightforward than for a gene. Thus, these approaches are meant to follow and complement early-stage genetic approaches for target identification and validation.

5.7.2. Statistical Data-Driven Approaches

Large self-consistent data sets enable data-mining and modeling efforts to uncover robust and context-specific information detailing how intracellular signals govern cellular responses. There are a wide variety of modeling techniques that have been adapted to specifically examine relationships between extracellular cues, intracellular signals, and cellular responses as a means to quantitatively characterize the contributions of signaling pathways to cellular endpoints (Janes and Yaffe, 2006).

5.7.2.1. Regression

One of the most basic ways to relate input and output data (or cell signals and responses) is to propose multilinear relationships of the form $y = \beta_1 x_1 + \beta_2 x_2 + \ldots + \beta_n x_n + \text{error}$, where y represents the output data, x_i the input data, and β_i the regression coefficients. When sufficient data have been collected, these relationships can be calculated via various regression techniques. There are numerous variations of regression techniques and related statistical approaches; the focus in this work is on approaches that have been applied directly to the interpretation of cell signaling data that may offer insights in target identification and validation. For most of these methods it is customary to perform some data scaling and/or normalization. Mean centering and variance scaling of data are typical (Geladi and Kowalski, 1986).

Multiple regression relates multiple input and output measurements. This method works well when all of the measurements are independent. In biological data, however, there is often strong covariation in the data (e.g., two measurements in the same pathway are very likely to covary). In these cases it is desirable to use data dimension reduction techniques such as principal components analysis (PCA) to eliminate data collinearity. PCA defines a new set of orthogonal axes, called *principal components*, such that the first axis explains the greatest variation in the data, the second axis explains the second most variation in the data, and so on (Janes and Yaffe, 2006). PCA is a good way to simplify data and calculate statistical distance between observations in the data set. Janes et al. (2004) demonstrate the utility of PCA in reducing the complexity of their HT29 signaling/apoptosis data set, discovering that four components were sufficient to capture 95% of the information contained in 20 measurements. Similarly, Espelin et al. (2010) use PCA to generate two-dimensional projections of their complex signaling–cytokine production data set. Although PCA enables easy visualization of complex data, it comes at the expense of easy interpretability—each component combines scores and loadings representing linear combinations of all measurements and stimulatory conditions.

The concept of PCA has been extended to principal components regression (PCR). In PCR, input and output data are decomposed in principal components, and then multiple regression is performed on the components rather than the raw data (Geladi and Kowalski, 1986). Pradervand et al. (2006) used PCR on the Alliance for Cell Signaling data set to define contributions signaling components to cytokine release. They identified the minimal measurements required for each PCR model and combined their results with an analysis of variance to correct for two-way interactions. The net result was a reconstruction of network topology governing cytokine release.

PCR has been improved upon by developing partial least-squares regression (PLSR), which ensures that the dimensionality reduction of the input and output data is done in a manner that maximizes the correlation between them (Geladi and Kowalski, 1986). Espelin et al. (2010) used PLSR to quantitatively describe the multivariate correlation between intracellular signals and cytokine release. Janes et al. (2004) used PLSR to quantitatively describe the contribution of signaling measurements for cell survival. They also applied PLSR models in a predictive fashion to simulate the effects of inhibitor treatment on TNF-induced apoptosis with experimental confirmation. They later extended these approaches to predict multiple apoptotic endpoints simultaneously (Janes et al., 2005). Examination of the model components yielded further insight into the role of stress and survival signals in dictating cell fate decisions and uncovered autocrine feedback mechanisms in the signaling network (Janes et al., 2006). Finally, they discovered that the PLSR models trained on HT-29 cell data were capable of predicting outcomes in other epithelial cell lines (i.e., HeLa and MCF-10a) in the context of adeno-viral- and TNF-stimulated apoptosis. These results indicated similar effector-processing machinery in these cell lines (Miller-Jensen et al., 2006). Their model also quantitatively predicted cell-specific responses to inhibition of the IKK–NF-κB pathway, suggesting that these approaches may have utility deconvoluting cell-specific responses to intervention.

There are few published industry examples of this type of work applied to understanding signal transduction and target identification and validation (Espelin et al., 2010). There are large hurdles in both the generation of large consistent data sets for analysis as well as the analysis or interpretation itself. Since most of these techniques are borrowed from chemometrics and standard statistics, most pharmaceutical companies are well equipped to perform and improve on these methods. At present, it appears that the blind application of standard statistical methodologies will yield only limited impact. Most likely, the augmentation of existing techniques based on current biological knowledge will be needed to translate these approaches into great scientific advances. As with all statistical techniques, the crux lies in posing the correct question and performing analyses that are appropriate to the data set and will yield mechanistic insight rather than mere correlative findings.

5.7.2.2. Decision Trees

Some efforts to unravel cellular response draw analogy with sequences of decision-making steps, known as *decision trees* (or *classification trees* or *regression trees*). With these models one attempts to describe a collection of response variables based on the hierarchical organization of input variables. Decision trees are statistical models that are constructed by going through the input (signaling) data systematically and asking which measurement is the best classifier for the output (response) data. This measurement is placed at the top of the tree and the process is repeated until all measurements have been used. Their strength lies in their graphical, easy-to-interpret output.

In work by Hua et al. (2006), decision tree analysis was used to describe the regulation of the Fas pathway in Jurkat cells. With such a model they were able to identify the minimal number of perturbations needed to change pathway behaviors and predict effectively how an alteration at the signaling level would affect caspase-3 activity under different cellular contexts.

Kharait et al. (2007) generated a decision tree model to describe how intra-cellular signaling measurements predicted EGF-induced fibroblast cell motility. Their model yielded the nonintuitive prediction that reducing myosin light chain kinase activity would increase motility on moderately adhesive surfaces. They confirmed their prediction experimentally and extended their findings more broadly in MDA-213 human breast carcinoma cells. Decision trees have been extended in the machine learning field to generate "forests" in which multiple trees are generated to improve the predictive power of such statistical models (Ho, 1995).

Together, large-scale data collection and data-driven modeling techniques provide an efficient means to assemble basic knowledge of signaling regulation of cellular response. Further, the works described above demonstrate that efforts to manipulate systems comprehensively form the foundations for subsequent follow-up work and lead invariably to serendipitous findings.

In target identification and validation, signaling measurements in these large data sets are best conceived as sentinels for specific pathways (or, more accurately, portions of the network) rather than as targets themselves. The ability to quantify the contribution of specific pathways to a given endpoint is a key step in target selection. At best, one is able to select pathways that play a dominant role in the cellular response of interest. At worst, one is able to set bounds on subsequent work. Knowledge of the secondary contributions of other pathways, or context dependence, may suggest alternative strategies including alternate targets or co-drugging opportunities or means by which to partition patient populations.

5.7.3. Network Approaches

Beyond looking for statistical association between measurements, it is desirable to be able to construct regulatory networks governing the cellular responses or phenotypes of interest. In some cases it may be necessary to build networks de novo, but in many cases there is prior knowledge regarding the relationships between signaling measurements. If possible, this knowledge should be incorporated and leveraged to derive further insight from experimental data.

5.7.3.1. Bayesian Networks

A *Bayesian network* is a graphical model that represents a set of variables and their probabilistic interdependencies. These approaches have had great utility in studying gene regulatory networks (Friedman, 2004; Friedman et al., 2000; Husmeier, 2003) and have recently found application in protein signal transduction. The term *Bayesian* (homage to Thomas Bayes) refers to the reliance to Bayes' conditioning to determine relationships and the subjective (or noisy) nature of the input data. Bayesian approaches are built from Bayes' theorem, which relates the conditional and marginal probabilities of two events, A and B: $P(A|B) = P(B|A) \cdot P(A)/P(B)$. Applied to model generation, one calculates the probability of a given model structure being correct given the data based on the probability of the data given the model and the prior probabilities of the data and the model (Pearl, 1988; Sachs et al., 2002). During the process of model building and evaluation, one specifies and calculates probabilities for possible two- and three-way (or higher-order) relationships between variables. Through the evaluation of three-way interactions, Bayesian networks are able to infer causality, enabling the reconstruction of signaling networks (Pearl, 2000). This technique is in contrast with correlative approaches that are able to determine the edges in a graph model, but not the directionality.

Consequently, the ability to explore and evaluate competing models quantitatively allows application for both model discovery and model selection (Sachs et al., 2002). It should be noted that Bayesian networks are constrained to be acyclic and, consequently, are not able to correctly infer negative feedback loops without extension into dynamic Bayesian networks (Lahdesmaki et al., 2006). In dynamic Bayesian models each measurement at each time point is considered a separate variable, effectively enabling feedback loops while maintaining acyclic structure. Finally, since a Bayesian network is a complete model for the variables and their relationships, it can be used to answer probabilistic queries about them. Once built, the networks can be used in a forward fashion to predict the state of a subset of variables (in a probabilistic fashion) when other variables are observed as well as to predict the effects of targeted intervention.

In the area of protein signal transduction, Bayesian networks have been used primarily for network reconstruction. Sachs et al. demonstrate the concepts of Bayesian network analysis on a small signaling data set from Asthagiri et al. (1999) evaluating the relationships between integrin binding, ERK, and FAK activation (Sachs et al., 2002). In later work, Sachs et al. (2005) analyzed multicolor flow cytometry data from thousands of human primary T cells to infer a causal protein signaling network using a Bayesian approach. They were able to infer most known interactions correctly, although missing two negative feedback loops, as expected from the static data. Their work provided support and experimental validation for two interactions that were not well known in the literature. Subsequently, Sachs et al. used their model to predict successfully the effects of siRNA of ERK on their other model variables. Woolf et al. (2005) have also applied Bayesian analysis to understanding signaling networks in the context of embryonic stem cell fate decisions. They were able to identify the role of LIF and STAT3 in maintaining undifferentiated mouse embryonic stem cell populations as well as to predict qualitative differences in stem cell differentiation following perturbation.

Using a Bayesian approach, GNS Biotech (Cambridge, MA) has built a network inference platform for the analysis of diverse types of data (Khalil and Hill, 2005; Pitluk and Khalil, 2007). Rather than generating a single best-fit model as others have done, GNS Biotech infers a distribution of models that are most likely given the data. Because of the challenge and expense of generating large data sets, GNS Biotech has focused on the ability to handle and integrate the diverse data, both discrete and continuous, already available from pharmaceutical companies. Through parallelization of their computations on supercomputing clusters, GNS Biotech is able to handle large data sets and generate ensembles of models rather than seek out the single best model. This approach appears to improve their ability to perform *forward simulation*, in which they are able to predict the effects of intervention and assign confidence metrics to their predictions. GNS Biotech has also recently expanded its ability to include dynamic Bayesian networks. While Bayesian networks are agnostic to the types of data being used, the ability to interpret model structure in a mechanistic fashion as Sachs et al. (2005) and Woolf et al. (2005) have done requires carefully constructed, self-consistent data sets. In the end, the ability to generate the proper data set for the question(s) at hand will dictate the ultimate success or failure of these approaches.

5.7.3.2. Boolean Networks

Boolean, or logical modeling, attempts to simplify signaling networks into simple on–off states and rules governing the dependence of one protein state on another [reviewed by Watterson et al. (2008)]. For example, a cascade of signaling events might be represented as follows: If protein A is "on," then protein B is "on"; if protein B is "on," then protein C is "off." Rules can be extended to represent more complex relationships, such as AND gates (if A is "on" and B is "on," then C is "on"), or OR gates, and so on. One must compose an underlying wiring diagram to describe the connectivity of the measurements and the rules governing them. To make experimental data amenable to logical modeling analyses, they must first be discretized, that is, converted to "on" or "off" states (this involves the loss of information) (Watterson et al., 2008). Following discretization, models and data can be compared directly.

Saez-Rodriguez et al. (2007) constructed a large-scale logical model of T-cell signaling, including 94 species, 123 interactions, and spanning two time scales. The global effect-of-interaction rules were then compared against experimental data to check for consistency. Once constructed, they were able to perform graph-based analyses on the network, identifying regulatory feedback loops. They were able to perform forward simulations, predicting the T-cell phenotype of a variety of previously described knockout mice. Finally, with the logical model they were able to explore missing interactions that are necessary to reconcile discrepancies between model predictions and experimental results.

Boolean network modeling facilitates predictions of the qualitative effect of interventions and, moreover, allows one to search for interventions that repress or provoke a certain logical response (Klamt et al., 2006). Furthermore, other important network properties, such as feedback loops, signaling paths, and network-wide interdependencies, can be evaluated that may provide hypotheses for sensitive points for intervention (Klamt et al., 2007). These models can be extended to offer more than simply on–off states in what are called *fuzzy logic models*, which offer additional complexity allowing for semi-quantitative dynamics [reviewed by Bosl (2007)].

5.8. TARGET SELECTION: DYNAMIC PATHWAY MODELING

With an understanding of the role of a pathway in the broader network (and higher-level) context, a detailed analysis of the pathway can be carried out. Although current dogma stresses that intracellular signals operate through networks, the pathway abstraction is a useful simplification when one has quantified the pathway contribution in the context of the network. One can think of a pathway as the minimal portion of the signaling network required to recapitulate the majority of the behavior observed experimentally.

For cases where a significant number of details of the molecular players have been described, detailed mechanistic models of signaling can identify optimal targets within that pathway and the optimal mode of intervention. From a target discovery perspective, these models are limited to known components of signaling pathways. Consequently, they cannot be used effectively to discover completely novel regulators of a given endpoint. Nonetheless, they can help unravel complex interactions and identify optimal points of intervention. The ultimate utility and impact of these models is based on being able reliably to tie the model output, such as ERK activity, to a clinical endpoint such as cancer progression.

Practically, pathways for which sufficient knowledge exists to build mechanistic pathway models often coincide with areas of intense drug discovery interest and contain multiple putative therapeutic targets: an ERK–MAPK pathway for oncology, an Akt pathway for diabetes and oncology, and p38 and NF-κB pathways for inflammatory disease.

5.8.1. Model Building/Validation

Mechanistic pathway models detail the interaction of pathway members with differential equations to describe the dynamics of signal transduction. Typically, pathway interactions are modeled using mass-action kinetics. For example, reversible receptor–ligand binding can be represented as: receptor + ligand ↔ complex, characterized by a forward rate constant with units of 1/concentration/time and a reverse rate constant with units of 1/time. Enzymatic events such as phosphorylation are represented as a two-step process: (1) kinase + substrate ↔ kinase–substrate complex, and (2) kinase–substrate complex → kinase + phosphorylated substrate. By connecting these simple constructs in various ways, one can build entire pathways and networks. Several good commercial software packages facilitate this type of modeling (e.g., Teranode Design Suite, MATLAB SimBiology, Jacobian OpenBio, Gepasi), [see also the article by Suresh Babu et al. (2006)].

There are several excellent reviews that describe both methodologies and tools for building these types of models (Aldridge et al., 2006; Kholodenko, 2006; Materi and Wishart, 2007). Pathway building tools are complemented by a myriad of public and private pathway databases (Bader et al., 2006; Cary et al., 2005), vendor Web sites, and most recently, wikis (Pico et al., 2008) that can provide excellent starting points for sketching out a pathway of interest.

A concise representation of combinatorial interactions is one of the emerging challenges in modeling signaling pathways. BioNetGen (Blinov et al., 2004) and Plectix Biosystems (Cambridge, MA) have built tools that make use of rule-based formalisms to enumerate possible interactions. There have also been attempts to represent these interactions visually with efficient circuit-style diagrams (Christopher et al., 2004); however, they have gained little momentum.

Once the model structure is codified, one needs to inform the model by specifying the parameter values. This is done by either finding reported values in the literature, by direct experimental measurement, or by parameter estimation (model fitting to experimental data). Models can be validated to various degrees by comparison with experimental data. In some cases, models seek to reproduce qualitative behavior seen in experimental findings; in others, quantitative reproduction of the data is sought. Ideally, models are further tested via prediction of unobserved behavior followed by experimental confirmation.

From the academic side, these models are generally built to test one's understanding of the biology: that is, to ask whether the experimental data observed are quantitatively consistent with the mechanistic understanding of the pathway. This is often married with a comparison of multiple structures to rule out specific mechanisms (Aksan Kurnaz, 2004; Cedersund et al., 2008; Hendriks et al., 2003, 2006a; Hua et al., 2005). By far, EGFR signaling and MAPK signaling cascades have been studied in the greatest detail using these approaches, although apoptosis, NF-κB signaling, and the cell cycle have also received considerable attention.

The EGFR system has been the prototype for application of computational modeling approaches (Wiley et al., 2003). It can be broken into four components: (1) receptor activation (ligand binding, dimerization, phosphorylation), (2) receptor trafficking (internalization, recycling, degradation), (3) adaptor protein interactions, and (4) downstream kinase signaling cascades. There are numerous trafficking models, ranging from the earliest model from Wiley and Cunningham (1981) to models incorporating the effects of EGFR family members on trafficking (Hendriks et al., 2003). The combinatorial interactions of receptor dimerization within the entire EGFR family were modeled explicitly in work from Hendriks et al. (2006a). Kholodenko et al. (1999) have pioneered modeling efforts aimed at short-term signaling and interaction of EGFR with adaptor proteins. MAPK signaling cascades have been the subject of countless models and mathematical analyses demonstrating properties of switchlike behavior and bistability (Asthagiri and Lauffenburger, 2001; Chapman and Asthagiri, 2004; Hornberg et al., 2005a,b; Huang and Ferrell, 1996; Mayawala et al., 2004; Qiao et al., 2007; Somsen et al., 2002). Finally, Schoeberl et al. (2002) were the first to assemble all the pathway pieces and demonstrate quantitative agreement with experimental signaling data. Additional models presented by Hatakeyama et al. (2003), Suresh Babu et al. (2006), and Birtwistle et al. (2007) have expanded the scope to include Akt activation as well.

There has been a similar progression in modeling efforts aimed at understanding signal transduction in apoptosis. Fussenegger et al. (2000) described FasL binding and the caspase activation cascade with a mechanistic model.

With their model they evaluated qualitative strategies for the prevention of caspase activation. Bentele et al. (2004) constructed a similar model quantitatively fit to experimental data. In their subsequent model analyses, they present a sensitivity analysis showing the importance of individual rate parameters and species concentrations on controlling the apoptotic response. Hua et al. (2005) evaluated competing hypotheses regarding the mechanism of Bcl-2 binding in an apoptosis model in Jurkat T cells. Subsequently, they predicted from a sensitivity analysis asymmetrical effects of Bcl-2 knockdown and overexpression that were validated experimentally with genetic manipulation. Most recently, Albeck et al. (2008) combined a model of apoptotic signaling with flow cytometry data to examine relationships between initiator and effector caspases. This work further identified parameters controlling the all-or-none apoptotic response.

There are several other pathways that have been modeled to various levels of detail and with varying degrees of validation: NF-κB [see the references in Cheong et al., (2008)], cell cycle (Haberichter et al., 2007), insulin signaling (Sedaghat et al., 2002; Wanant and Quon, 2000), TGF-β (Melke et al., 2006), PDGFR (Park et al., 2003), growth hormone (Haugh, 2004), and probably others as well, that may provide useful starting points for future efforts.

5.8.2. Model Exploitation

From a pharma industry perspective, dynamic pathway models are aimed not simply at understanding a given pathway in detail, but also at allowing quantitative assessment of optimal target selection within a pathway. A growing number of companies are involved in this space, including both small systems biology companies and large pharma.

GNS Biotech (Cambridge, MA) was an early pioneer in developing and applying mechanistic pathway models for aiding drug discovery (although their business model has since moved away from differential equation–based models). They created a model of an HCT 116 colon cancer cell line incorporating the major cellular interactions in determining the phenotypic fate of a cell, including apoptosis and cell cycle regulation (Christopher et al., 2004). They performed *in silico* knockdown experiments, changing protein expression levels for multiple prospective targets and evaluating predicted response in terms of the phase of cell cycle arrest or sensitivity to apoptotic stimuli.

Physiomics (Oxford, UK) has focused its models on an evaluation of specific compounds for oncology. They developed a model of cell cycle regulation including G1/S-phase transition control and timing of G1/S/G2/M transitions (Chassagnole et al., 2006). CDK inhibitors were represented implicitly by incorporation of inhibition terms (IC_{50} values) in the kinetic rates of the model. Importantly, they explicitly modeled compounds in a realistic fashion by allowing for imperfect selectivity. They evaluated multiple CDK inhibitors of varying selectivity against six CDKs in their model and were able to pinpoint the causes of cytotoxicity.

Merrimack Pharmaceuticals (Cambridge, MA) has leveraged their EGFR signaling network model for model-driven design of therapeutics. Using sensitivity analyses, they were able to evaluate various points in the pathway and support target identification efforts (Nielsen and Schoeberl, 2005). Further, they were able quantitatively to compare multiple therapeutic strategies in the EGFR pathway, including antiligand antibodies, antireceptor antibodies, and dimerization-blocking antibodies. Through varying model parameters, effects of varied receptor expression could also be evaluated and interpreted in the context of EGFR expression levels in cancer versus normal tissue. Most recently, Merrimack Pharmaceuticals identified ErbB3 as an attractive target using their network modeling approach and currently has a anti-ErbB3 antibody in clinical trials (http://www.merrimackpharma.com/newsEvents/2008/ MM-121_Phase_1_Initiation_11August08_FINAL.pdf).

AstraZeneca (Waltham, MA) applied mechanistic modeling in a retrospective fashion to aid in the interpretation of clinical findings of their EGFR kinase inhibitor, Iressa (Hendriks et al., 2006b). They constructed elaborate models of EGFR family interactions and signaling connecting existing models of EGFR family trafficking dynamics (Hendriks et al., 2006a) with ERK and Akt signaling models (Hatakeyama et al., 2003). Following reports of increased response rates in patients harboring a specific EGFR mutation, Hendriks et al. performed a sensitivity analysis on their EGFR model to predict possible changes that could explain altered intracellular signaling data. Their model correctly predicted impaired internalization rates in the EGFR mutants. This prediction was validated experimentally and led to a broader understanding of alternative mechanisms that could confer sensitivity to small-molecule EGFR inhibitors.

Pfizer's Research Technology Center (Cambridge, MA) developed a model of p38 signaling in the context of inflammatory disease (Hendriks et al., 2008). In this work, Hendriks et al. explicitly address large-scale parameter estimation challenges presenting novel concepts of finding collections of best-fit parameter sets and using them for subsequent analysis. They perform a multiparameter set sensitivity analysis to identify kinetic parameters controlling the model output and highlight specific challenges in its interpretation. For example, they found distinct differences in the relative ranking of targets, depending on whether one varied kinase expression levels versus kinase activities. Thus, the notion of the optimal target is inextricably connected to the intended mode of intervention. This work further demonstrated implicit methods for the representation of different mechanisms of action for kinase inhibition in model interpretation.

Mechanistic models of cell signaling pathways have also been used to simulate the effects of combination therapy (Araujo et al., 2004, 2007; Fitzgerald et al., 2006; Hendriks et al., 2008; Hopkins, 2008). With these pathway models, one can depart from traditional black-box models of synergy and predict points of synergy based on mechanistic simulation. The goal is to identify co-drugging opportunities that enable low dosing of multiple individual therapeutics so as to minimize off-target effects and potential safety concerns. For example, Fitzgerald et al. (2006) explored multiple variations of combination therapy: co-drugging a receptor with multiple modalities, co-drugging multiple receptors upstream of a common pathway, and co-drugging multiple points within a pathway. Additionally, one can also conceptualize co-drugging as the evaluation of (or prediction of optimal) "dirty" compounds that have activity against multiple targets, as done by Chassagnole et al. (2006). These efforts demonstrate important first steps in realizing aspirations of executing network pharmacology (Hopkins, 2008).

Thus far, most systems analysis for target identification and validation has focused on single endpoints for efficacy. Ultimately, one would like to be able to develop predictive assays for toxicology endpoints and understand their regulation in terms of molecular signaling events (Figure 5.2). One could then optimize for multiple endpoints simultaneously and analyze targets in terms of a therapeutic window and robustness against patient variability rather than solely an efficacy endpoint. The mechanistic understanding of key toxicological endpoints will need to be modeled for this approach to be realized completely (Mayne et al., 2006; Xu et al., 2008).

Finally, little work has been done to use these models to compare the differences between diseased versus normal states quantitatively or to examine cell type–specific differences. As one applies these models for target selection, the differences will be of increasing importance, especially in the area of oncology, where evaluation of therapies in the context of different genetic backgrounds is probably crucial to success.

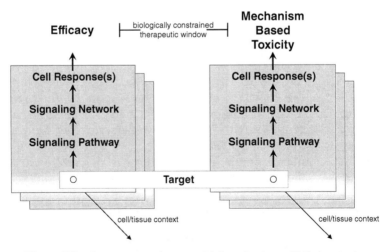

Figure 5.2 A target may have multiple roles in multiple contexts.

5.8.3. Model Limitations

Deterministic pathway models require that there be sufficient quantities (>1000 copies per cell as a rough guide) of each signaling component such that stochastic effects are not an issue. Stochastic models can be used for cases where species are in low quantity and require the incorporation of random fluctuations. Stochastic models have been especially useful to study gene regulatory networks and genetic noise. However, Resat et al. (2003) have also applied stochastic modeling to examine the ErbB receptor network and stochastic variation in receptor trafficking that could influence signal transduction.

Due to the inherent challenges of modeling transcriptional events, the majority of mechanistic pathway models are restricted to acute signaling and short time scales. Models of cell cycle dynamics, such as those by Physiomics (Chassagnole et al., 2006), and GNS Biotech (Christopher et al., 2004; Haberichter et al., 2007), are notable exceptions and appear to be adequately represented with deterministic modeling.

This modeling approach can also be used effectively to rule out proposed mechanisms of regulation (Aksan Kurnaz, 2004; Cedersund et al., 2008; Hendriks et al., 2003, 2006a; Hua et al., 2005). Unfortunately, it can never prove that a mechanism is correct; however, it can determine whether the current dogma is sufficient to describe the experimental data observed. If a model is inconsistent with the experimental data, it can form a starting point for proposing alternative models and inference of mechanisms required to obtain the behavior observed.

5.9. CONCLUSIONS

In this chapter we have outlined a sequence of approaches that span the spectrum from disease-level questions to using data-driven approaches to shed light on an area of biology, to network approaches to understanding regulation, and finally, to detailed pathway approaches to identify specific targets and subsequent modes of intervention (see Figure 5.1). At each stage there is a common thread of generating a quantitative understanding of biology and the use of models to codify the knowledge and generate hypotheses. Further, modeling efforts come in many forms, ranging from models that incorporate mechanistic knowledge to generate system-level understanding, to statistically based modeling approaches, and many more not presented.

By the very construction of the integrated systems approach, targets that emerge should carry a high degree of confidence in terms of their role in the disease phenotype. Nonetheless, targets will still require significant amounts of experimental testing in cell-based and animal models (if appropriate) to confirm findings. Depending on the assay system, target manipulation may be possible with RNAi approaches or may necessitate small-molecule compounds or antibodies to test concepts.

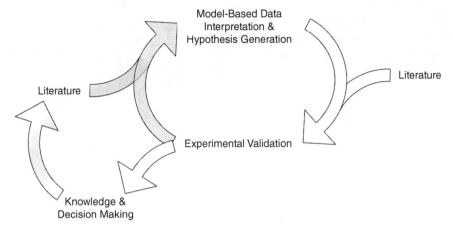

Figure 5.3 Experimental work and model-based interpretation are performed iteratively to enable decision making and knowledge generation.

The systems biology approach described here relies on putting the knowledge that we have in context to more deeply understand complex regulatory behavior of individual players. Thus, the hypothesis is that there still are many opportunities to further evaluate roles of known proteins in disease and to understand cell–tissue context and optimal selection of patients for trial design. The computational approaches described herein are not intended to replace experimental work, but rather to aid in focusing and prioritizing. In the end, experimental data in conjunction with model-based interpretation should drive decision making (Figure 5.3).

There are many small companies that are focusing on technology-specific aspects and methodologies of systems biology as it pertains to target identification and validation. These companies run the gamut from building large databases from literature extracted information to specializing in unique forms of data generation and experimental profiling to companies that specialize in modeling of disease, specific modeling approaches, or tool development. Covering the entire spectrum from disease to target requires significant financial resources, and currently, large pharma has served as a place to integrate many of these approaches. Systems biology groups within pharma have built many internal capabilities, but also served as important mediators with external collaborators from academia and industry. While systems biology may be the source of significant hype at present, there is no question that systems-level thinking and integrated experimental and computational approaches to unraveling biological complexity are here to stay by whatever name. The ultimate success of systems biology in target identification and validation relies on being able to identify the proper tools to answer the questions at hand and being able to span multiple problem scales:

physiology → organ → tissue → cell → pathway → target

This needs to be done in normal (health) and disease contexts for both efficacy and safety endpoints. The industry's ability over the next decade to reduce attrition in the clinic will be the final metric in gauging success.

Finally, target identification and validation is not the only part of a drug pipeline where systems biology efforts can make valuable contributions. Models of disease, particularly those incorporating aspects of pharmacokinetic modeling, can and have been employed in clinical trial design, aiding in the selection and optimization of dosing regimens as well as determining optimal time points for data collection. Companies such as Entelos and Optimata (Ramat Gan, Israel) have already demonstrated success in this area. Vertex Pharmaceuticals (Cambridge, MA) used a model of HCV viral dynamics for design and interpretation of their recent phase III trial (http://investors.vrtx.com/releasedetail.cfm?ReleaseID=190515). Early involvement and development of models as part of target identification is critical to ensuring that these tools are ready and validated for late-stage clinical application.

Acknowledgments

I would like to thank past and present colleagues of the systems biology group at Pfizer, and Jennifer Kispert, for careful review of the manuscript.

REFERENCES

Abbott, R.G., Forrest, S., and Pienta, K.J. (2006). Simulating the hallmarks of cancer. *Artif Life 12*, 617–634.

Aksan Kurnaz, I. (2004). Kinetic analysis of RSK2 and Elk-1 interaction on the serum response element and implications for cellular engineering. *Biotechnol Bioeng 88*, 890–900.

Albeck, J.G., MacBeath, G., White, F.M., Sorger, P.K., Lauffenburger, D.A., and Gaudet, S. (2006). Collecting and organizing systematic sets of protein data. *Nat Rev Mol Cell Biol 7*, 803–812.

Albeck, J.G., Burke, J.M., Aldridge, B.B., Zhang, M., Lauffenburger, D.A., and Sorger, P.K. (2008). Quantitative analysis of pathways controlling extrinsic apoptosis in single cells. *Mol Cell 30*, 11–25.

Aldridge, B.B., Burke, J.M., Lauffenburger, D.A., and Sorger, P.K. (2006). Physicochemical modelling of cell signalling pathways. *Nat Cell Biol 8*, 1195–1203.

Alexopoulos, L.G., Saez-Rodriguez, J., Cosgrove, B.D., Lauffenburger, D.A., and Sorger, P.K. (2010). Networks inferred from biochemical data reveal profound differences in toll-like receptor and inflammatory signaling between normal and transformed hepatocytes. *Mol Cell Proteomics 9*, 1849–1865.

Araujo, R.P., Doran, C., Liotta, L.A., and Petricoin, E.F. (2004). Network-targeted combination therapy: a new concept in cancer treatment. *Drug Discov Today Ther Strategies 1*, 425–433.

Araujo, R.P., Liotta, L.A., and Petricoin, E.F. (2007). Proteins, drug targets and the mechanisms they control: the simple truth about complex networks. *Nat Rev Drug Discov 6*, 871–880.

Ashburner, M., Ball, C.A., Blake, J.A., Botstein, D., Butler, H., Cherry, J.M., Davis, A.P., Dolinski, K., Dwight, S.S., Eppig, J.T., et al. (2000). Gene ontology: tool for the unification of biology. The Gene Ontology Consortium. *Nat Genet 25*, 25–29.

Asthagiri, A.R., and Lauffenburger, D.A. (2001). A computational study of feedback effects on signal dynamics in a mitogen-activated protein kinase (MAPK) pathway model. *Biotechnol Prog 17*, 227–239.

Asthagiri, A.R., Nelson, C.M., Horwitz, A.F., and Lauffenburger, D.A. (1999). Quantitative relationship among integrin-ligand binding, adhesion, and signaling via focal adhesion kinase and extracellular signal-regulated kinase 2. *J Biol Chem 274*, 27119–27127.

Bader, G.D., Cary, M.P., and Sander, C. (2006). Pathguide: a pathway resource list. *Nucleic Acids Res 34*, D504–D506.

Bentele, M., Lavrik, I., Ulrich, M., Stosser, S., Heermann, D.W., Kalthoff, H., Krammer, P.H., and Eils, R. (2004). Mathematical modeling reveals threshold mechanism in CD95-induced apoptosis. *J Cell Biol 166*, 839–851.

Berg, E.L., Kunkel, E.J., Hytopoulos, E., and Plavec, I. (2006). Characterization of compound mechanisms and secondary activities by BioMAP analysis. *J Pharmacol Toxicol Methods 53*, 67–74.

Birtwistle, M.R., Hatakeyama, M., Yumoto, N., Ogunnaike, B.A., Hoek, J.B., and Kholodenko, B.N. (2007). Ligand-dependent responses of the ErbB signaling network: experimental and modeling analyses. *Mol Syst Biol 3*, 144.

Blinov, M.L., Faeder, J.R., Goldstein, B., and Hlavacek, W.S. (2004). BioNetGen: software for rule-based modeling of signal transduction based on the interactions of molecular domains. *Bioinformatics 20*, 3289–3291.

Bosl, W.J. (2007). Systems biology by the rules: hybrid intelligent systems for pathway modeling and discovery. *BMC Syst Biol 1*, 13.

Boutayeb, A., and Chetouani, A. (2006). A critical review of mathematical models and data used in diabetology. *Biomed Eng online 5*, 43.

Butcher, E.C. (2005). Can cell systems biology rescue drug discovery? *Nat Rev Drug Discov 4*, 461–467.

Cary, M.P., Bader, G.D., and Sander, C. (2005). Pathway information for systems biology. *FEBS Lett 579*, 1815–1820.

Cedersund, G., and Stralfors, P. (2008). Putting the pieces together in diabetes research: Towards a hierarchical model of whole-body glucose homeostasis. *Eur J Pharm Sci 36*, 91–104.

Cedersund, G., Roll, J., Ulfhielm, E., Danielsson, A., Tidefelt, H., and Stralfors, P. (2008). Model-based hypothesis testing of key mechanisms in initial phase of insulin signaling. *PLoS Comput Biol 4*, e1000096.

Chapman, S., and Asthagiri, A.R. (2004). Resistance to signal activation governs design features of the MAP kinase signaling module. *Biotechnol Bioeng 85*, 311–322.

Chassagnole, C., Jackson, R.C., Hussain, N., Bashir, L., Derow, C., Savin, J., and Fell, D.A. (2006). Using a mammalian cell cycle simulation to interpret differential kinase inhibition in anti-tumour pharmaceutical development. *Biosystems 83*, 91–97.

Cheong, R., Hoffmann, A., and Levchenko, A. (2008). Understanding NF-kappaB signaling via mathematical modeling. *Mol Syst Biol 4*, 192.

Chow, C.C., and Hall, K.D. (2008). The dynamics of human body weight change. *PLoS Comput Biol 4*, e1000045.

Christopher, R., Dhiman, A., Fox, J., Gendelman, R., Haberitcher, T., Kagle, D., Spizz, G., Khalil, I.G., and Hill, C. (2004). Data-driven computer simulation of human cancer cell. *Ann NY Acad Sci 1020*, 132–153.

Cohen, A.M., and Hersh, W.R. (2005). A survey of current work in biomedical text mining. *Brief Bioinf 6*, 57–71.

Cohen, K.B., and Hunter, L. (2008). Getting started in text mining. *PLoS Comput Biol 4*, e20.

Datta-Mannan, A., Witcher, D.R., Tang, Y., Watkins, J., Jiang, W., and Wroblewski, V.J. (2007a). Humanized IgG1 variants with differential binding properties to the neonatal Fc receptor: relationship to pharmacokinetics in mice and primates. *Drug Metab Dispos: Biol Fate Chem 35*, 86–94.

Datta-Mannan, A., Witcher, D.R., Tang, Y., Watkins, J., and Wroblewski, V.J. (2007b). Monoclonal antibody clearance: impact of modulating the interaction of IgG with the neonatal Fc receptor. *J Biol Chem 282*, 1709–1717.

DiMasi, J.A., and Paquette, C. (2004). The economics of follow-on drug research and development: trends in entry rates and the timing of development. *PharmacoEconomics 22*, 1–14.

DiMasi, J.A., Hansen, R.W., and Grabowski, H.G. (2003). The price of innovation: new estimates of drug development costs. *J Health Econ 22*, 151–185.

Dominguez, H., Storgaard, H., Rask-Madsen, C., Steffen Hermann, T., Ihlemann, N., Baunbjerg Nielsen, D., Spohr, C., Kober, L., Vaag, A., and Torp-Pedersen, C. (2005). Metabolic and vascular effects of tumor necrosis factor-alpha blockade with etanercept in obese patients with type 2 diabetes. *J Vascular Res 42*, 517–525.

Erhardt, R.A., Schneider, R., and Blaschke, C. (2006). Status of text-mining techniques applied to biomedical text. *Drug Discov Today 11*, 315–325.

Espelin, C.W., Goldsipe, A., Sorger, P.K., Lauffenburger, D., de Graaf, D., and Hendriks, B.S. (2010). Elevated GM-CSF and IL-1beta levels compromise the ability of p38 MAPK inhibitors to modulate TNFalpha levels in the human monocytic/macrophage U937 cell line. *Mol Biolsyst 6*, 1956–1972.

Ferl, G.Z., Wu, A.M., and DiStefano, J.J., 3rd (2005). A predictive model of therapeutic monoclonal antibody dynamics and regulation by the neonatal Fc receptor (FcRn). *Ann Biomed Eng 33*, 1640–1652.

Fitzgerald, J.B., Schoeberl, B., Nielsen, U.B., and Sorger, P.K. (2006). Systems biology and combination therapy in the quest for clinical efficacy. *Nat Chem Biol 2*, 458–466.

Friedman, N. (2004). Inferring cellular networks using probabilistic graphical models. *Science 303*, 799–805.

Friedman, N., Linial, M., Nachman, I., and Pe'er, D. (2000). Using Bayesian networks to analyze expression data. *J Comput Biol 7*, 601–620.

Fussenegger, M., Bailey, J.E., and Varner, J. (2000). A mathematical model of caspase function in apoptosis. *Nat Biotechnol 18*, 768–774.

Garg, A., and Balthasar, J.P. (2007). Physiologically-based pharmacokinetic (PBPK) model to predict IgG tissue kinetics in wild-type and FcRn-knockout mice. *J Pharmacokinet Pharmacodyn 34*, 687–709.

Gaudet, S., Janes, K.A., Albeck, J.G., Pace, E.A., Lauffenburger, D.A., and Sorger, P.K. (2005). A compendium of signals and responses triggered by prodeath and prosurvival cytokines. *Mol Cell Proteom 4*, 1569–1590.

Geladi, P., and Kowalski, B.R. (1986). Partial least-squares regression: a tutuorial. *Anal Chim Acta 185*, 1–17.

Gilman, A.G., Simon, M.I., Bourne, H.R., Harris, B.A., Long, R., Ross, E.M., Stull, J.T., Taussig, R., Bourne, H.R., Arkin, A.P., et al. (2002). Overview of the Alliance for Cellular Signaling. *Nature 420*, 703–706.

Haberichter, T., Madge, B., Christopher, R.A., Yoshioka, N., Dhiman, A., Miller, R., Gendelman, R., Aksenov, S.V., Khalil, I.G., and Dowdy, S.F. (2007). A systems biology dynamical model of mammalian G1 cell cycle progression. *Mol Syst Biol 3*, 84.

Hakenberg, J., Schmeier, S., Kowald, A., Klipp, E., and Leser, U. (2004). Finding kinetic parameters using text mining. *Omics 8*, 131–152.

Hall, K.D., and Baracos, V.E. (2008). Computational modeling of cancer cachexia. *Curr Opin Clin Nutr Metab Care 11*, 214–221.

Hanahan, D., and Weinberg, R.A. (2000). The hallmarks of cancer. *Cell 100*, 57–70.

Haringman, J.J., Gerlag, D.M., Smeets, T.J., Baeten, D., van den Bosch, F., Bresnihan, B., Breedveld, F.C., Dinant, H.J., Legay, F., Gram, H., et al. (2006). A randomized controlled trial with an anti-CCL2 (anti-monocyte chemotactic protein 1) monoclonal antibody in patients with rheumatoid arthritis. *Arthritis Rheum 54*, 2387–2392.

Hatakeyama, M., Kimura, S., Naka, T., Kawasaki, T., Yumoto, N., Ichikawa, M., Kim, J.H., Saito, K., Saeki, M., Shirouzu, M., et al. (2003). A computational model on the modulation of mitogen-activated protein kinase (MAPK) and Akt pathways in heregulin-induced ErbB signalling. *Biochem J 373*, 451–463.

Haugh, J.M. (2004). Mathematical model of human growth hormone (hGH)-stimulated cell proliferation explains the efficacy of hGH variants as receptor agonists or antagonists. *Biotechnol Prog 20*, 1337–1344.

Hendriks, B.S., Opresko, L.K., Wiley, H.S., and Lauffenburger, D. (2003). Quantitative analysis of HER2-mediated effects on HER2 and epidermal growth factor receptor endocytosis: distribution of homo- and heterodimers depends on relative HER2 levels. *J Biol Chem 278*, 23343–23351.

Hendriks, B.S., Cook, J., Burke, J.M., Beusmans, J.M., Lauffenburger, D.A., and de Graaf, D. (2006a). Computational modelling of ErbB family phosphorylation dynamics in response to transforming growth factor alpha and heregulin indicates spatial compartmentation of phosphatase activity. *Syst Biol (Stevenage) 153*, 22–33.

Hendriks, B.S., Griffiths, G.J., Benson, R., Kenyon, D., Lazzara, M., Swinton, J., Beck, S., Hickinson, M., Beusmans, J.M., Lauffenburger, D., et al. (2006b). Decreased internalisation of erbB1 mutants in lung cancer is linked with a mechanism conferring sensitivity to gefitinib. *Syst Biol (Stevenage) 153*, 457–466.

Hendriks, B.S., Hua, F., and Chabot, J.R. (2008). Analysis of mechanistic pathway models in drug discovery: p38 pathway. *Biotechnol Prog 24*, 96–109.

Ho, T.K. (1995). Random decision forest. *Proceedings of the 3rd International Conference on Document Analysis and Recognition*, pp. 278–282.

Hopkins, A.L. (2008). Network pharmacology: the next paradigm in drug discovery. *Nat Chem Biol 4*, 682–690.

Hornberg, J.J., Binder, B., Bruggeman, F.J., Schoeberl, B., Heinrich, R., and Westerhoff, H.V. (2005a). Control of MAPK signalling: from complexity to what really matters. *Oncogene 24*, 5533–5542.

Hornberg, J.J., Bruggeman, F.J., Binder, B., Geest, C.R., de Vaate, A.J., Lankelma, J., Heinrich, R., and Westerhoff, H.V. (2005b). Principles behind the multifarious control of signal transduction. ERK phosphorylation and kinase/phosphatase control. *FEBS J 272*, 244–258.

Hua, F., Cornejo, M.G., Cardone, M.H., Stokes, C.L., and Lauffenburger, D.A. (2005). Effects of Bcl-2 levels on Fas signaling-induced caspase-3 activation: molecular genetic tests of computational model predictions. *J Immunol 175*, 985–995.

Hua, F., Hautaniemi, S., Yokoo, R., and Lauffenburger, D.A. (2006). Integrated mechanistic and data-driven modelling for multivariate analysis of signalling pathways. *J R Soc Interface 3*, 515–526.

Huang, C.Y., and Ferrell, J.E., Jr. (1996). Ultrasensitivity in the mitogen-activated protein kinase cascade. *Proc Natl Acad Sci USA 93*, 10078–10083.

Husmeier, D. (2003). Reverse engineering of genetic networks with Bayesian networks. *Biochem Soc Trans 31*, 1516–1518.

Janes, K.A., and Yaffe, M.B. (2006). Data-driven modelling of signal-transduction networks. *Nat Rev Mol Cell Biol 7*, 820–828.

Janes, K.A., Kelly, J.R., Gaudet, S., Albeck, J.G., Sorger, P.K., and Lauffenburger, D.A. (2004). Cue-signal-response analysis of TNF-induced apoptosis by partial least squares regression of dynamic multivariate data. *J Comput Biol 11*, 544–561.

Janes, K.A., Albeck, J.G., Gaudet, S., Sorger, P.K., Lauffenburger, D.A., and Yaffe, M.B. (2005). A systems model of signaling identifies a molecular basis set for cytokine-induced apoptosis. *Science 310*, 1646–1653.

Janes, K.A., Gaudet, S., Albeck, J.G., Nielsen, U.B., Lauffenburger, D.A., and Sorger, P.K. (2006). The response of human epithelial cells to TNF involves an inducible autocrine cascade. *Cell 124*, 1225–1239.

Kamei, D.T., Lao, B.J., Ricci, M.S., Deshpande, R., Xu, H., Tidor, B., and Lauffenburger, D.A. (2005). Quantitative methods for developing Fc mutants with extended half-lives. *Biotechnol Bioeng 92*, 748–760.

Khalil, I.G., and Hill, C. (2005). Systems biology for cancer. *Curr Opin Oncol 17*, 44–48.

Kharait, S., Hautaniemi, S., Wu, S., Iwabu, A., Lauffenburger, D.A., and Wells, A. (2007). Decision tree modeling predicts effects of inhibiting contractility signaling on cell motility. *BMC Syst Biol 1*, 9.

Kholodenko, B.N. (2006). Cell-signalling dynamics in time and space. *Nat Rev Mol Cell Biol 7*, 165–176.

Kholodenko, B.N., Demin, O.V., Moehren, G., and Hoek, J.B. (1999). Quantification of short term signaling by the epidermal growth factor receptor. *J Biol Chem 274*, 30169–30181.

Kievit, W., Fransen, J., Oerlemans, A.J., Kuper, H.H., van der Laar, M.A., de Rooij, D.J., De Gendt, C.M., Ronday, K.H., Jansen, T.L., van Oijen, P.C., et al. (2007). The efficacy of anti-TNF in rheumatoid arthritis, a comparison between randomised controlled trials and clinical practice. *Ann Rheum Dis 66*, 1473–1478.

Klamt, S., Saez-Rodriguez, J., Lindquist, J.A., Simeoni, L., and Gilles, E.D. (2006). A methodology for the structural and functional analysis of signaling and regulatory networks. *BMC Bioinf 7*, 56.

Klamt, S., Saez-Rodriguez, J., and Gilles, E.D. (2007). Structural and functional analysis of cellular networks with CellNetAnalyzer. *BMC Syst Biol 1*, 2.

Kola, I., and Landis, J. (2004). Can the pharmaceutical industry reduce attrition rates? *Nat Rev Drug Discov 3*, 711–715.

Kumar, N., Hendriks, B.S., Janes, K.A., de Graaf, D., and Lauffenburger, D.A. (2006). Applying computational modeling to drug discovery and development. *Drug Discov Today 11*, 806–811.

Lahdesmaki, H., Hautaniemi, S., Shmulevich, I., and Yli-Harja, O. (2006). Relationships between probabilistic Boolean networks and dynamic Bayesian networks as models of gene regulatory networks. *Signal Process 86*, 814–834.

Lao, B.J., and Kamei, D.T. (2008). Improving therapeutic properties of protein drugs through alteration of intracellular trafficking pathways. *Biotechnol Prog 24*, 2–7.

Lao, B.J., Tsai, W.L., Mashayekhi, F., Pham, E.A., Mason, A.B., and Kamei, D.T. (2007). Inhibition of transferrin iron release increases *in vitro* drug carrier efficacy. *J Control Release 117*, 403–412.

Lobo, E.D., Hansen, R.J., and Balthasar, J.P. (2004). Antibody pharmacokinetics and pharmacodynamics. *J Pharm Sci 93*, 2645–2668.

MacDonald, M.L., and Westwick, J.K. (2007). Exploiting network biology to improve drug discovery. *Methods Mol Biol 356*, 221–232.

Materi, W., and Wishart, D.S. (2007). Computational systems biology in drug discovery and development: methods and applications. *Drug Discov Today 12*, 295–303.

Mayawala, K., Gelmi, C.A., and Edwards, J.S. (2004). MAPK cascade possesses decoupled controllability of signal amplification and duration. *Biophys J 87*, L01–02.

Mayne, J.T., Ku, W.W., and Kennedy, S.P. (2006). Informed toxicity assessment in drug discovery: systems-based toxicology. *Curr Opin Drug Discov Dev 9*, 75–83.

McCarthy, M.I., Abecasis, G.R., Cardon, L.R., Goldstein, D.B., Little, J., Ioannidis, J.P., and Hirschhorn, J.N. (2008). Genome-wide association studies for complex traits: consensus, uncertainty and challenges. *Nat Rev Genet 9*, 356–369.

Melke, P., Jonsson, H., Pardali, E., ten Dijke, P., and Peterson, C. (2006). A rate equation approach to elucidate the kinetics and robustness of the TGF-beta pathway. *Biophys J 91*, 4368–4380.

Michelson, S. (2006). The impact of systems biology and biosimulation on drug discovery and development. *Mol Biosyst 2*, 288–291.

Miller-Jensen, K., Janes, K.A., Wong, Y.L., Griffith, L.G., and Lauffenburger, D.A. (2006). Adenoviral vector saturates Akt pro-survival signaling and blocks insulin-mediated rescue of tumor necrosis-factor-induced apoptosis. *J Cell Sci 119*, 3788–3798.

Natarajan, M., Lin, K.M., Hsueh, R.C., Sternweis, P.C., and Ranganathan, R. (2006). A global analysis of cross-talk in a mammalian cellular signalling network. *Nat Cell Biol 8*, 571–580.

Nielsen, U.B., and Schoeberl, B. (2005). Using computational modeling to drive the development of targeted therapeutics. *IDrugs 8*, 822–826.

Park, C.S., Schneider, I.C., and Haugh, J.M. (2003). Kinetic analysis of platelet-derived growth factor receptor/phosphoinositide 3-kinase/Akt signaling in fibroblasts. *J Biol Chem 278*, 37064–37072.

Pattaranit, R., and van den Berg, H.A. (2008). Mathematical models of energy homeostasis. *J R Soc Interface 5*, 1119–1135.

Pearl, J. (1988). *Probabilistic Reasoning in Intelligent Systems: Networks of Plausible Inference*. Morgan Kaufmann, San Francisco.

Pearl, J. (2000). *Causality: Models, Reasoning and Inference*. Cambridge University Press, Cambridge, MA.

Perez, O.D., and Nolan, G.P. (2002). Simultaneous measurement of multiple active kinase states using polychromatic flow cytometry. *Nat Biotechnol 20*, 155–162.

Perez, O.D., Krutzik, P.O., and Nolan, G.P. (2004). Flow cytometric analysis of kinase signaling cascades. *Methods Mol Biol 263*, 67–94.

Pico, A.R., Kelder, T., van Iersel, M.P., Hanspers, K., Conklin, B.R., and Evelo, C. (2008). WikiPathways: pathway editing for the people. *PLoS Biol 6*, e184.

Pitluk, Z., and Khalil, I. (2007). Achieving confidence in mechanism for drug discovery and development. *Drug Discov Today 12*, 924–930.

Pollard, J., Jr., Butte, A.J., Hoberman, S., Joshi, M., Levy, J., and Pappo, J. (2005). A computational model to define the molecular causes of type 2 diabetes mellitus. *Diabetes Technol Ther 7*, 323–336.

Pradervand, S., Maurya, M.R., and Subramaniam, S. (2006). Identification of signaling components required for the prediction of cytokine release in RAW 264.7 macrophages. *Genome Biol 7*, R11.

Pratt, D., Hahn, W., Matthews, A., Febbo, P., Berger, R., Duckworth, B., Levy, J., Segaran, T., Sun, J., Ladd, B., et al. (2006). Computational causal reasoning models of mechanisms of androgen stimulation in prostate cancer. *Conf Proc IEEE Eng Med Biol Soc 1*, 38.

Qiao, L., Nachbar, R.B., Kevrekidis, I.G., and Shvartsman, S.Y. (2007). Bistability and oscillations in the Huang–Ferrell model of MAPK signaling. *PLoS Comput Biol 3*, 1819–1826.

Rao, B.M., Lauffenburger, D.A., and Wittrup, K.D. (2005). Integrating cell-level kinetic modeling into the design of engineered protein therapeutics. *Nat Biotechnol 23*, 191–194.

Resat, H., Ewald, J.A., Dixon, D.A., and Wiley, H.S. (2003). An integrated model of epidermal growth factor receptor trafficking and signal transduction. *Biophys J 85*, 730–743.

Roberts, P.M. (2006). Mining literature for systems biology. *Brief Bioinf 7*, 399–406.

Roberts, P.M., and Hayes, W.S. (2005). Advances in text analytics for drug discovery. *Curr Opin Drug Discov Dev 8*, 323–328.

Rullmann, J.A., Struemper, H., Defranoux, N.A., Ramanujan, S., Meeuwisse, C.M., and van Elsas, A. (2005). Systems biology for battling rheumatoid arthritis: application of the Entelos PhysioLab platform. *Syst Biol (Stevenage) 152*, 256–262.

Rzhetsky, A., Seringhaus, M., and Gerstein, M. (2008). Seeking a new biology through text mining. *Cell 134*, 9–13.

Sachs, K., Gifford, D., Jaakkola, T., Sorger, P., and Lauffenburger, D.A. (2002). Bayesian network approach to cell signaling pathway modeling. *Sci STKE 148*, pe38.

Sachs, K., Perez, O., Pe'er, D., Lauffenburger, D.A., and Nolan, G.P. (2005). Causal protein-signaling networks derived from multiparameter single-cell data. *Science 308*, 523–529.

Saez-Rodriguez, J., Simeoni, L., Lindquist, J.A., Hemenway, R., Bommhardt, U., Arndt, B., Haus, U.U., Weismantel, R., Gilles, E.D., Klamt, S., et al. (2007). A logical model provides insights into T cell receptor signaling. *PLoS Comput Biol 3*, e163.

Sarkar, C.A., and Lauffenburger, D.A. (2003). Cell-level pharmacokinetic model of granulocyte colony–stimulating factor: implications for ligand lifetime and potency *in vivo. Mol Pharmacol 63*, 147–158.

Schoeberl, B., Eichler-Jonsson, C., Gilles, E.D., and Muller, G. (2002). Computational modeling of the dynamics of the MAP kinase cascade activated by surface and internalized EGF receptors. *Nat Biotechnol 20*, 370–375.

Schultz, C., Schleifenbaum, A., Goedhart, J., and Gadella, T.W., Jr. (2005). Multiparameter imaging for the analysis of intracellular signaling. *ChembioChem 6*, 1323–1330.

Schulze-Kremer, S. (2002). Ontologies for molecular biology and bioinformatics. *In Silico Biol 2*, 179–193.

Sedaghat, A.R., Sherman, A., and Quon, M.J. (2002). A mathematical model of metabolic insulin signaling pathways. *Am J Physiol Endocrinol Metab 283*, E1084–E1101.

Somsen, O.J., Siderius, M., Bauer, F.F., Snoep, J.L., and Westerhoff, H.V. (2002). Selectivity in overlapping MAP kinase cascades. *J Theor Biol 218*, 343–354.

Spencer, S.L., Berryman, M.J., Garcia, J.A., and Abbott, D. (2004). An ordinary differential equation model for the multistep transformation to cancer. *J Theor Biol 231*, 515–524.

Starkuviene, V., and Pepperkok, R. (2007). The potential of high-content high-throughput microscopy in drug discovery. *Br J Pharmacol 152*, 62–71.

Suresh Babu, C.V., Joo Song, E., and Yoo, Y.S. (2006). Modeling and simulation in signal transduction pathways: a systems biology approach. *Biochimie 88*, 277–283.

Uchiyama, Y., Yoshida, H., Koike, N., Hayakawa, N., Sugita, A., Nishimura, T., and Mihara, M. (2008). Anti-IL-6 receptor antibody increases blood IL-6 level via the blockade of IL-6 clearance, but not via the induction of IL-6 production. *Int Immunopharmacol 8*, 1595–1601.

van der Greef, J., and McBurney, R.N. (2005). Innovation: Rescuing drug discovery—*in vivo* systems pathology and systems pharmacology. *Nat Rev Drug Discov 4*, 961–967.

Venturoli, D., and Rippe, B. (2005). Ficoll and dextran vs. globular proteins as probes for testing glomerular permselectivity: effects of molecular size, shape, charge, and deformability. *Am J Physiol Renal Physiol 288*, F605–F613.

Wanant, S., and Quon, M.J. (2000). Insulin receptor binding kinetics: modeling and simulation studies. *J Theor Biol 205*, 355–364.

Wang, Z., Zhang, L., Sagotsky, J., and Deisboeck, T.S. (2007). Simulating non-small cell lung cancer with a multiscale agent-based model. *Theor Biol Med Model 4*, 50.

Watterson, S., Marshall, S., and Ghazal, P. (2008). Logic models of pathway biology. *Drug Discov Today 13*, 447–456.

White, F.M. (2008). Quantitative phosphoproteomic analysis of signaling network dynamics. *Curr Opin Biotechnol 19*, 404–409.

Wiley, H.S., and Cunningham, D.D. (1981). A steady state model for analyzing the cellular binding, internalization and degradation of polypeptide ligands. *Cell 25*, 433–440.

Wiley, H.S., Shvartsman, S.Y., and Lauffenburger, D.A. (2003). Computational modeling of the EGF-receptor system: a paradigm for systems biology. *Trends Cell Biol 13*, 43–50.

Woolf, P.J., Prudhomme, W., Daheron, L., Daley, G.Q., and Lauffenburger, D.A. (2005). Bayesian analysis of signaling networks governing embryonic stem cell fate decisions. *Bioinformatics 21*, 741–753.

Xu, J.J., Hendriks, B.S., Zhao, J., and de Graaf, D. (2008). Multiple effects of acetaminophen and p38 inhibitors: towards pathway toxicology. *FEBS Lett 582*, 1276–1282.

Yazdi, P.T., and Murphy, R.M. (1994). Quantitative analysis of protein synthesis inhibition by transferrin–toxin conjugates. *Cancer Res 54*, 6387–6394.

Yazdi, P.T., Wenning, L.A., and Murphy, R.M. (1995). Influence of cellular trafficking on protein synthesis inhibition of immunotoxins directed against the transferrin receptor. *Cancer Res 55*, 3763–3771.

Young, D.L., Ramanujan, S., Kreuwel, H.T., Whiting, C.C., Gadkar, K.G., and Shoda, L.K. (2006). Mechanisms mediating anti-CD3 antibody efficacy: insights from a mathematical model of type 1 diabetes. *Ann NY Acad Sci 1079*, 369–373.

Yu, H., West, M., Keon, B.H., Bilter, G.K., Owens, S., Lamerdin, J., and Westwick, J.K. (2003). Measuring drug action in the cellular context using protein-fragment complementation assays. *Assay Drug Dev Technol 1*, 811–822.

Zhang, Y., Wolf-Yadlin, A., and White, F.M. (2007). Quantitative proteomic analysis of phosphotyrosine-mediated cellular signaling networks. *Methods Mol Biol 359*, 203–212.

CHAPTER 6

Lead Identification and Optimization

SETH MICHELSON

Genomic Health Inc., Redwood City, California

Summary

Successful drug discovery and development require identification of the most appropriate compound for the most appropriate target in the most appropriate subpopulation of patients. This seemingly simple objective is central to the challenge of lead identification and drug optimization. Here we discuss systems approaches to the rational building of a bridge between a compound's chemical and biological activities. Hypothesis formation, experimental design, and model-based investigation increase the power of experimental designs and increase the likelihood of successful identification of a lead compound. The effects of genetic and environmental variations on the underlying disease physiology also have a critical effect on the optimal medicinal characteristics required for candidate compounds. Lead identification and optimization are thus enhanced by the systematic quantification of the optimal pharmacokinetic and pharmacodynamic compound profiles needed for specific patient populations.

6.1. INTRODUCTION

As noted in Chapter 1, discovering a new medicine is a highly risky undertaking that spans a number of development steps. Despite growing industry investment in research and development, approximately only 1 in 10 new drug candidates entering human clinical trials is likely to be approved (PhRMA, 2006). In fact, with greater than 53% failures, it is more likely that a compound in phase II clinical studies will fail than succeed. Failures, especially those

Systems Biology in Drug Discovery and Development, First Edition.
Edited by Daniel L. Young, Seth Michelson.
© 2012 John Wiley & Sons, Inc. Published 2012 by John Wiley & Sons, Inc.

suffered in late-stage clinical development, result in amortized costs of between $800 million and $1.7 billion per approved drug (DiMasi et al., 2003; Gilbert et al., 2003; PhRMA, 2006). To ameliorate this problem as efficiently as possible, one must clearly identify the most appropriate compound for the most appropriate target in the most appropriate subpopulation of patients, and then dose those patients as optimally as possible. This objective is the crux of lead identification and drug optimization and forms the philosophical cornerstone of the "learn and confirm" model of drug development suggested by Sheiner in 1997.

Building a successful medicine requires that one identify a cause–effect pathway (or pathways) inherent in the disease etiology and its subsequent pathophysiology. One must then associate that pathway or pathways with cellular and molecular entities (e.g., receptors, cytokines) that can be manipulated by an exogenous entity called a *drug*. These molecular entities are typically termed *targets*. Once a candidate drug target has been identified and validated, either *in vitro* or *in vivo* in an animal model of the disease, the focus of the drug discovery effort shifts to building a compound that will modulate that target to maximum therapeutic advantage. The relationship between chemical character and biological activity is termed the *structure–activity relationship* (SAR), and it is the job of the medicinal chemist to develop and exploit that relationship in the identification and optimization of lead compounds. How well researchers understand the biological impact of a compound on the most relevant pathways of a disease determines how successful (and efficient) the optimization process will be.

There are two basic strategies involved in building this bridge between chemical and biological activities. One may use a computer-based pattern recognition algorithm to identify those compounds that "look alike." The underlying assumption in this approach is that much compounds will behave similarly in a biological milieu. This process, in essence, segments the chemical character space and is depicted schematically in Figure 6.1. To perform this extrapolation, one must capture the shape and character of a molecule in a computer-readable format [e.g., Simplified Molecular Input Line Entry System (SMILES), Canonical SMILES] and then, using any number of multivariate techniques and pattern recognition algorithms (e.g., principal components analysis, hierarchical clustering, partial least-squares regression, support vector machines), identify that set of molecules that look alike. The collection, representation, and organization of these types of chemical data generate chemical information to which theories and models can be applied to create chemical knowledge. *En toto*, this set of tools makes up a discipline called *chemometrics* which complements systems biology, but whose details are beyond the scope of this chapter.

In particular, this process requires the development and application of computational methods for predicting "drug likeness." Typically, these methods are applied to *virtual* compounds or libraries, allowing the research chemist to eliminate poor candidates and optimize potential leads *in silico* rapidly (Clark

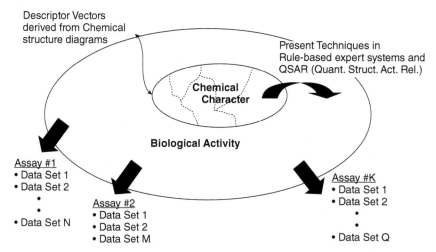

Descriptor Vectors
derived from Chemical
structure diagrams

Present Techniques in
Rule-based expert systems and
QSAR (Quant. Struct. Act. Rel.)

Chemical
Character

Biological Activity

Assay #1
• Data Set 1
• Data Set 2
•
•
• Data Set N

Assay #2
• Data Set 1
• Data Set 2
• Data Set M

Assay #K
• Data Set 1
• Data Set 2
•
•
• Data Set Q

Figure 6.1 Characterization of chemical character–based similarity measures and pattern recognition in the descriptor vector space is mapped to the biological activity space using SAR/QSAR models based on assumptive sampling of the biological activity space.

and Pickett, 2000). In particular, the computational scientist develops a series of filters to remove compounds deemed to be too chemically unsuitable for screening purposes. Such filters will typically incorporate substructure searches for toxic and/or reactive groups and can include other criteria, such as limits on molecular weight and the number of rotatable bonds. These types of filters are very useful for initial screening of the data, but by their very nature, they do not answer the question of what a drug looks like. Rather, they state that "a drug does not look like this." A more sophisticated approach to predicting drug likeness has been proposed in which two sets of compounds, one containing known positives (known drugs) and the other comprising negatives (compounds suspected of being non-drug-like) are compared and contrasted. The hypothesis is that those chemical properties or characteristics observed in the former successful set that best differentiate them from the latter negative set are those that best define druglike positive criteria.

Filtering facilities for ADMET (adsorption, distribution, excretion, metabolism, toxicity) screening have also been developed (Miteva et al., 2006). These models were tested by Miteva et al. for the calculation of log P values in an experimentally verified test set. Although no explicit r^2 was provided for this reported test, visual inspection of the plot of predicted versus that observed for over 100 test compounds suggests a significant correlation between the two [see Figure 1 of Miteva et al. (2006)].

Another area of particular interest in the optimization of a compound or lead is the calculation and prediction of polar surface area (PSA), which corresponds well with a molecule's ability to transport passively through lipid

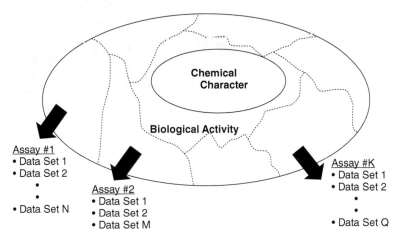

Figure 6.2 Appropriate sampling of the biological activity space and a reverse mapping back to the chemical character domain allows compounds that do not look alike but behave similarly to be clustered together in an activity descriptor space. The choice of assays now requires foreknowledge of the system to ensure that the sampling strategy is optimally informative.

membranes (Ertl et al., 2000). This facility of drug distribution and a compound's capacity to get to its site of action is fundamental to both identifying a valid lead and optimizing it for druglike characteristics.

An alternative strategy for lead optimization segments the biological activity space into regions of biologically relevant activity and provides an activity vector for each compound the medicinal chemist is interested in characterizing. In this strategy, compounds that "behave" the same are grouped together whether or not they "look alike". This strategy requires that the research team both understand and optimally sample the biological activity space. This process is depicted in Figure 6.2. The more completely that one understands a disease and its dynamic pathophysiology, the more likely it is that the most relevant bioassays will be developed. And the more effectively that one samples the biological activity space, the greater the probability will be of finding an optimally effective compound.

Equally important, the lead development team must understand and interpret these sample data within the context of the variations that one would expect to see in a clinical population. To achieve these objectives, one can use a systematic approach to both develop a set of hypotheses regarding the most pertinent aspects of an ideal activity [pharmacodynamic (PD)] and exposure [pharmacokinetic (PK)] profile for each compound, and based on these hypotheses, simulate that set of hypothetical dynamics that best represents the intended target population. These types of systems biology approaches help to establish a hypothetical concentration–response curve and, from that, a minimum level for PD and PK profiles for the "average" patient. Then, based on optimal sampling of the patient's actual activity profiles, the development team can refine the model assumptions and hypothetical constraints on the compound's optimality criteria. This highly directed and focused process of hypothesis formation, experimental design, and model-based feedback increases the power of the sampling scheme and increases the likelihood of identifying a lead compound successfully.

6.2. THE SYSTEMS BIOLOGY TOOL KIT

6.2.1. Pharmacokinetic Modeling

To predict clinical efficacy, one must be able to predict, and then optimize, the pharmacokinetics of a compound. A compound's pharmacokinetics is typically described by the parameters for well-defined exposure curves, each representing the time course of a compound in any number of body compartments. These compartments typically include those that are easily monitored with minimally invasive procedures such as the collection of serum, urine, and feces. Estimates of a compound's PK are achieved by fitting actual data to a theoretical model of a compound's concentration dynamics. The basis for developing these models is based on the compound's absorption, distribution, metabolism, and excretion (ADME) characteristics. Typically, a standard compartment model is developed and fit to the data observed (either in animal studies or during a phase I clinical trial). And although there are a multitude of such models from which to choose (Boobis et al., 2002), prior knowledge of a drug's dynamics are typically used to guide the fitting process (Hu et al., 2004). Once fit, a rigorous goodness-of-fit statistic is generated and the best model is chosen. For example, Norris et al. (2000) developed a physiology-based PK model to predict the oral bioavailability of ganciclovir, a well-known antiviral. On the basis of their *in silico* results, they determined that the poor bioavailability observed in the clinic resulted from compound solubility issues rather than from low permeability in the gut as hypothesized originally. In another study, Sarkar and Lauffenberger (2003) modeled the PK of granulocyte colony–stimulating factor (GCSF). As the PK of GCSF depends explicitly on its therapeutic effects, their model represents both normal clearance (renal and hepatic) and localized endocytosis (i.e., compound degradation by target cells). Simulation studies in this system suggested that a modified GCSF analog that eliminates renal clearance would best increase the therapy's potential efficacy by markedly improving peripheral neutrophil counts.

6.2.2. Characterizing the Relevant Patient Subpopulations

To optimize the chemical characteristics of a compound, one must first answer the question: "Optimal in which patients?" To be a medicine, a drug must be safe, effective, and biologically accessible; that is, it must remain at the target site in sufficient concentration for a sufficient period of time to exert its therapeutic effects. Patient-to-patient variability affects these aspects of medicinal character and must be accounted for when selecting and optimizing a candidate compound and its dosing regimen.

In 1997, Louis Sheiner proposed a strategy in which drug development is segmented into an inductive learning phase, followed by a complementary, deductive confirmatory phase. In the early stages of clinical development, phases I and IIa, one learns what doses are best tolerated in normal patients, and then confirms that this dose will probably be efficacious in a fairly circumscribed group of patients. If there is a sufficiently positive indication of efficacy (and lack of toxicity) to justify investing in the future development of the drug, one undertakes a larger series of learn-and-confirm studies. In phase IIb, the goal is to learn how best to dose the drug in a population of representative patients. Once an acceptable benefit/risk ratio is identified in a large enough segment of the patient population, one undertakes a confirmatory study in phase III or IV. The goal of these confirmatory studies is to demonstrate in a large and representative patient population that acceptable benefit/risk is achieved.

Sheiner depicts this process schematically as a response surface in three dimensions. The two independent axes (the support space) represent patient variability and drug dosing regimens. The dependent axis represents benefit or effect. The theoretical foundation for the learn-and-confirm strategy is to recognize that during the learn phase, one wants to sample the support space as widely and optimally as possible, and then, based on this sampling scheme, characterize the relationship between the patient variability axis and the dosing regimen. In principle, one can use the tools of systems biology to characterize both the patient variability axis and the hypothetical relationship to a set of criteria defining how an optimal compound should perform.

Based on this philosophy, the goal of every clinical development program is to prove that the effects which researchers observe in the laboratory can, in fact, be generalized to a reasonably large segment of the human clinical population. To do this, most compounds are typically developed in the context of *in vivo* models of the human disease. However, laboratory animals are typically derived from inbred strains, and thus the effects of genetic variation are relatively well controlled in the laboratory. By controlling this aspect of experimental variance, one improves the signal-to-noise ratio of the experiment, but pays for it by hampering one's ability to generalize these results to humans and their inherent variability (e.g., variable ADME characteristics). Additionally, the influence of environmental variability on test animals is further suppressed by housing them in controlled animal care facilities. Not so for humans. The fact that the human population is not composed of genetically controlled, environmentally sequestered subjects is a constant source of difficulty for the clinical researcher.

How, then, can pharmaceutical researchers account for patient variability during the drug discovery process, when the bulk of research and development is performed with cellular systems and test animals instead of human subjects? Three *in silico* methods for identifying and characterizing a compound's effects in potential responder populations are currently in use. They include the characterization of the most relevant covariates that drive population PD, pharmacogenomic pattern recognition, and development of virtual patient profiles in a biosimulation milieu.

6.2.2.1. Population Pharmacodynamics

An *in silico* technology that addresses patient variability across diverse subpopulations is termed *population pharmacodynamics* [see Chien et al. (2005), Ebling and Levy (1996), and Roy and Ette (2005) for excellent reviews of this subject]. This strategy employs a suite of statistical algorithms that define and estimate population-wide dose–response curves while accounting appropriately for statistical noise. Typically, these algorithms use mixed-effects models to fit observed data to a well-defined dose–response model. If the model is nonlinear (e.g., the Hill model of dose–response), it is fit with an algorithm termed NONMEM (nonlinear mixed-effect models). Based on a priori knowledge of the patient populations at hand, one can propose the existence of relevant blocking factors or covariates (e.g., age, weight, gender, race) to account explicitly for this variation during the model-fitting process. A general review of these modeling and simulation technologies in drug discovery and development has been presented by Chien et al. (2005).

6.2.2.2. Pharmacogenomics and Pharmacogenetics

One of the key characteristics in determining clinical efficacy in a particular subpopulation is how those patients metabolize and clear a compound (Ekins et al., 2005; Evans and McLeod, 2003; Weinshilboum, 2003). In the late 1950s and early 1960s, a series of familial studies were conducted to determine if a genetic component could account for the differences observed in the metabolism of several compounds (e.g., succinylcholine, isoniazid, hydralzine). These linkage analyses identified two classes of patients: fast acetylators and slow acetylators. Studies of this type have been termed *pharmacogenetic analyses*. With the advent of microarray technologies and high-throughput screening techniques, genome-wide scans of drug responses and metabolism have been generated. Analysis of these data is termed *pharmacogenomics*. This approach requires sophisticated multivariate analyses and pattern recognition technologies. Whether aimed at characterizing toxic potential (toxicogenomics) (see, e.g., Fielden et al., 2002), patient-specific ADME characteristics (see Ekins et al., 2005), or other aspects of subpopulation membership, the data are so massive and complex that the only way to exploit them in a predictive setting is to use a family of *in silico* algorithms for their analysis. These algorithms fall into two main categories: unsupervised and supervised.

Unsupervised pharmacogenomic tools typically include techniques developed from classical multivariate statistics (e.g., hierarchical clustering, discriminant function analysis) (Kari et al., 2003; Makretsov et al., 2004; Zhao and Karypis, 2005). Supervised pharmacogenomic tools require that guidance be provided to the algorithm before the first analysis (e.g., a training set of data [see Ludwig and Weinstein (2005) for details]. These techniques include support vector machines (Furey et al., 2000), self-organizing maps (Tamayo et al., 1999; Wang et al., 2002), recursive partitioning and decision trees (Zhang et al., 2003), and K-means clusters [see Wigle et al. (2004) for a detailed review]. Over the past 10 years, these tools have been used to characterize several disease-specific patient subpopulations. Chief among these are the staging, treatment, and prognosis of cancer patients (see, e.g., Wigle et al. (2004) in lung cancer, Furey et al. (2000) in leukemias and colon cancers, and Kari et al. (2003) in lymphomas].

6.2.2.3. Virtual Patients and Biosimulation

By explicitly linking a hypothesis of disease pathophysiology to an explicit set of biological mechanisms and equations, an image of a patient can be constructed in the context of a particular *in silico* model. These constructs are termed *virtual patients*. Michelson described how a multivariate response surface and support space (similar in principle to Sheiner's response surface) can be developed *in silico* to characterize patient responder types (Michelson, 2006). On the basis of that construct, biomarkers defining patient subpopulations can be identified and characterized.

To fully comprehend the impact of patient variability on the medicinal characteristics of candidate compounds, researchers must capture, in explicit, quantifiable form, the effects of genetic and environmental variations on the underlying disease physiology. In the context of the mathematical model and its biosimulation, the impact of each of these variable influences can be represented as a specific hypothesis and then translated mathematically into model-specific expressions. Michelson et al. (2006) detailed how one can use this strategy to explicitly represent patient variability in a predictive biosimulation to explore the impact of that variability on clinical trial design and execution.

Predictive biosimulation is one of the technologies used to characterize *in silico* the heterogeneity of the patient axis in Sheiner's response surface model. By explicitly representing the hypothetical variance of a compound's PK and PD profiles as a potential variation in an individual virtual patient, Kansal and Trimmer (2005) used a model of human metabolism to simulate a variety of clinical trial designs in different disease phenotypes to guide the design of actual experiments. Lead identification and optimization were thus enhanced by quantification of the optimal PK and PD profiles needed for each of the various patient subgroups.

6.3. CONCLUSIONS

Lead identification and lead optimization assume that one *knows* to some level of certitude:

- The clinical behavior one wants to effect and how best to effect it
- The dynamic character of the biology underlying that behavior
- How best to manipulate that biology to therapeutic advantage
- Whether the candidate compound achieves these objectives

These beliefs assume that:

- One understands enough about the biological activity space to sample it optimally
- The data derived are predictive of the desired effect one seeks to optimize against

Finally, these assume that one can:

- Characterize and quantify the processes underlying the disease and its dynamic pathophysiology
- Account for the complex dynamics controlling those processes
- Interpret one's data so as best to guide the medicinal chemistry efforts

When optimizing a lead, the primary challenge facing the pharmaceutical development team is how most efficiently to interpret the biological activity data in the context of a dynamic process we call human disease, while taking into account the heterogeneity of the patient–subject population at hand. For example, how much does a particular physiological pathway contribute to the overall physiology of the disease? Is there a feedback mechanism in place that amplifies or dampens this signal? Are there redundant or backup pathways that will mitigate attempts to inhibit the pathway? By systematically categorizing what one knows, and more important, what one does *not* know, and building testable hypotheses to explain each gap, one can use the tool kit of systems biology to optimally sample those data and systematically test the impact of each hypothesis on the decision at hand.

REFERENCES

Boobis, A., Gundert-Remy, U., Kremers, P., Macheras, P., and Pelkonen, O. (2002). *In silico* prediction of ADME and pharmacokinetics: report of an expert meeting organised by COST B15. *Eur J Pharm Sci 17*, 183–193.

Chien, J.Y., Friedrich, S., Heathman, M.A., de Alwis, D.P., and Sinha, V. (2005). Pharmacokinetics/pharmacodynamics and the stages of drug development: role of modeling and simulation. *AAPS J 7*, E544–E559.

Clark, D.E., and Pickett, S.D. (2000). Computational methods for the prediction of "drug-likeness." *Drug Discov Today 5*, 49–58.

DiMasi, J.A., Hansen, R.W., and Grabowski, H.G. (2003). The price of innovation: new estimates of drug development costs. *J Health Econ 22*, 151–185.

Ebling, W.F., and Levy, G. (1996). Population pharmacodynamics: strategies for concentration- and effect-controlled clinical trials. *Ann Pharmacother 30*, 12–19.

Ekins, S., Nikolsky, Y., and Nikolskaya, T. (2005). Techniques: application of systems biology to absorption, distribution, metabolism, excretion and toxicity. *Trends Pharmacol Sci 26*, 202–209.

Ertl, P., Rohde, B., and Selzer, P. (2000). Fast calculation of molecular polar surface area as a sum of fragment-based contributions and its application to the prediction of drug transport properties. *J Med Chem 43*, 3714–3717.

Evans, W.E., and McLeod, H.L. (2003). Pharmacogenomics: drug disposition, drug targets, and side effects. *N Engl J Med 348*, 538–549.

Fielden, M.R., Matthews, J.B., Fertuck, K.C., Halgren, R.G., and Zacharewski, T.R. (2002). *In silico* approaches to mechanistic and predictive toxicology: an introduction to bioinformatics for toxicologists. *Crit Rev Toxicol 32*, 67–112.

Furey, T.S., Cristianini, N., Duffy, N., Bednarski, D.W., Schummer, M., and Haussler, D. (2000). Support vector machine classification and validation of cancer tissue samples using microarray expression data. *Bioinformatics 16*, 906–914.

Gilbert, J., Henske, P., and Singh, A. (2003). Rebuilding big pharma's business model. *In Vivo 21*, 1–10.

Hu, Y., Akland, G.G., Pellizzari, E.D., Berry, M.R., and Melnyk, L.J. (2004). Use of pharmacokinetic modeling to design studies for pathway-specific exposure model evaluation. *Environ Health Perspect 112*, 1697–1703.

Kansal, A.R., and Trimmer, J. (2005). Application of predictive biosimulation within pharmaceutical clinical development: examples of significance for translational medicine and clinical trial design. *Syst Biol (Stevenage) 152*, 214–220.

Kari, L., Loboda, A., Nebozhyn, M., Rook, A.H., Vonderheid, E.C., Nichols, C., Virok, D., Chang, C., Horng, W.H., Johnston, J., et al. (2003). Classification and prediction of survival in patients with the leukemic phase of cutaneous T cell lymphoma. *J Exp Med 197*, 1477–1488.

Ludwig, J.A., and Weinstein, J.N. (2005). Biomarkers in cancer staging, prognosis and treatment selection. *Nat Rev Cancer 5*, 845–856.

Makretsov, N.A., Huntsman, D.G., Nielsen, T.O., Yorida, E., Peacock, M., Cheang, M.C., Dunn, S.E., Hayes, M., van de Rijn, M., Bajdik, C., et al. (2004). Hierarchical clustering analysis of tissue microarray immunostaining data identifies prognostically significant groups of breast carcinoma. *Clin Cancer Res 10*, 6143–6151.

Michelson, S. (2006). The impact of systems biology and biosimulation on drug discovery and development. *Mol Biosyst 2*, 288–291.

Michelson, S., Sehgal, A., and Friedrich, C. (2006). *In silico* prediction of clinical efficacy. *Curr Opin Biotechnol 17*, 666–670.

Miteva, M.A., Violas, S., Montes, M., Gomez, D., Tuffery, P., and Villoutreix, B.O. (2006). FAF-drugs: free ADME/tox filtering of compound collections. *Nucleic Acids Res 34*, W738–W744.

Norris, D.A., Leesman, G.D., Sinko, P.J., and Grass, G.M. (2000). Development of predictive pharmacokinetic simulation models for drug discovery. *J Control Release 65*, 55–62.

PhRMA (2006). *Pharmaceutical Industry Profile 2006*. Pharmaceutical Research and Manufacturers of America, Washington, DC.

Roy, A., and Ette, E.I. (2005). A pragmatic approach to the design of population pharmacokinetic studies. *AAPS J 7*, E408–E420.

Sarkar, C.A., and Lauffenburger, D.A. (2003). Cell-level pharmacokinetic model of granulocyte colony–stimulating factor: implications for ligand lifetime and potency *in vivo*. *Mol Pharmacol 63*, 147–158.

Sheiner, L.B. (1997). Learning versus confirming in clinical drug development. *Clin Pharmacol Ther 61*, 275–291.

Tamayo, P., Slonim, D., Mesirov, J., Zhu, Q., Kitareewan, S., Dmitrovsky, E., Lander, E.S., and Golub, T.R. (1999). Interpreting patterns of gene expression with self-organizing maps: methods and application to hematopoietic differentiation. *Proc Natl Acad Sci USA 96*, 2907–2912.

Wang, D., Ressom, H., Musavi, M., and Domnisoru, C. (2002). Double self-organizing maps to cluster gene expression data. Presented at the European Symposium on Artificial Neural Networks, Bruges, Belgium.

Weinshilboum, R. (2003). Inheritance and drug response. *N Engl J Med 348*, 529–537.

Wigle, D.A., Tsao, M., and Jurisica, I. (2004). Making sense of lung-cancer gene-expression profiles. *Genome Biol 5*, 309.

Zhang, H., Yu, C.Y., and Singer, B. (2003). Cell and tumor classification using gene expression data: construction of forests. *Proc Natl Acad Sci USA 100*, 4168–4172.

Zhao, Y., and Karypis, G. (2005). Data clustering in life sciences. *Mol Biotechnol 31*, 55–80.

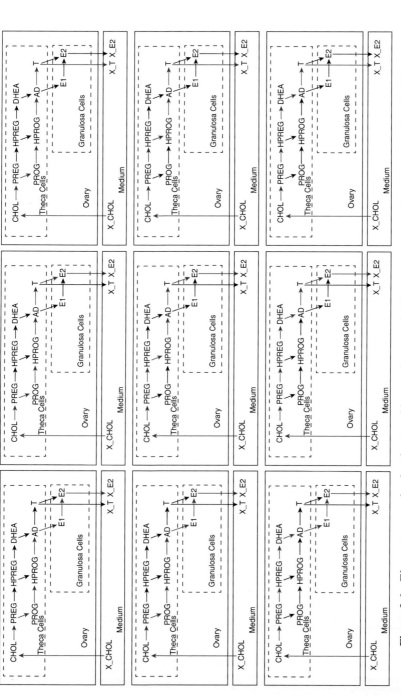

Figure 2.6 Elementary modes for the steroidogenesis network. Six elementary modes are responsible for E2 production, while three elementary modes are associated with T production. Red arrows indicate the active pathways, and black arrows indicate the inactive pathways in the network.

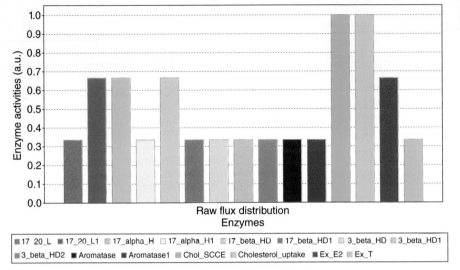

Figure 2.7 Enzyme activity diagram of the steroidogenesis process that can help guide drug development. Enzymes: cholesterol side-chain cleavage (Chol_SCCE); 17α-hydroxylase (17_alpha_H, 17_alpha_H1); 17, 20-lyase (17_20_L, 17_20_L1); 3β-hydroxysteroid dehydrogenase (3_beta_HD, 3_beta_HD1, 3_beta_HD2); 17β-hydroxysteroid dehydrogenase (17_beta_HD, 17_beta_HD1); and aromatase (Aromatase). Transport reactions: cholesterol uptake into inner mitochondrial membrane (Cholesterol_uptake); external E2 (Ex_E2); and external T (Ex_T).

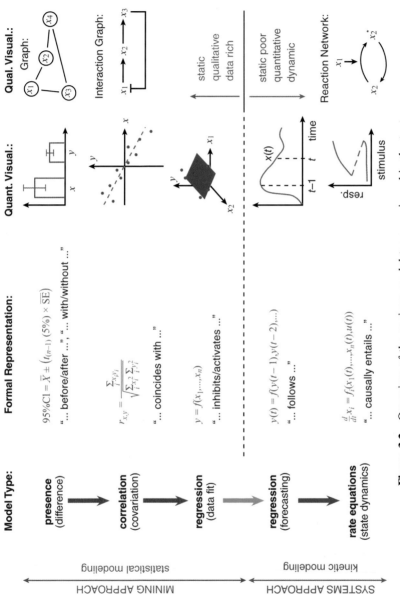

Figure 3.2 Overview of the various model types reviewed in the text.

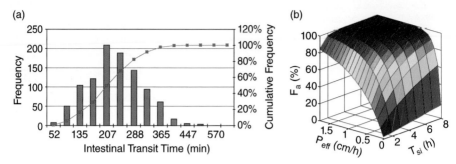

Figure 4.3 Small intestinal residence time: interindividual variability (A) and its impact on F_a (B). P_{eff} refers to effective intestinal permeability and T_{si} refers to the intestinal transit time shown in (A). [Adapted from Jamei et al. (2009b).]

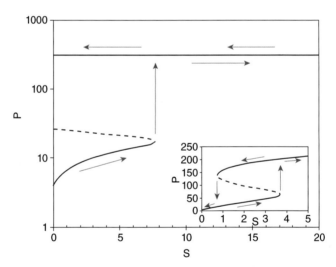

Figure 7.3 P–S bifurcation diagram showing the stable (solid curve) and unstable (dashed curve) steady states of the gene autoregulation model. Rightward- and leftward-pointing arrows indicate the dose–response curve, corresponding to increasing and decreasing dose, respectively, illustrating that the behavior of the system is an irreversible switch. The vertical arrow indicates the threshold value of the input signal S (= 7.64) at which the system switches from the low-protein expression ("off") state to the high-protein expression ("on") state. The inset shows the bifurcation diagram generated from the model with a different parameter set, where the system acts as a reversible switch.

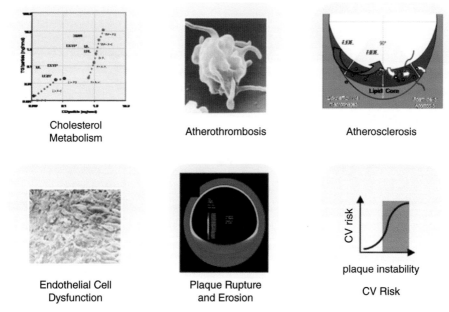

Figure 10.3 Overview of the main biological components of the Entelos human cardiovascular (CV) PhysioLab platform, a large-scale dynamic mechanistic model of cardiovascular disease. The platform enables prediction of the effects of dietary, lifestyle, and therapeutic interventions that modulate circulating lipids, serum inflammatory markers, and local vessel inflammation on relevant CV endpoints, including atherosclerotic plaque burden, stability, and the likelihood of a CV event.

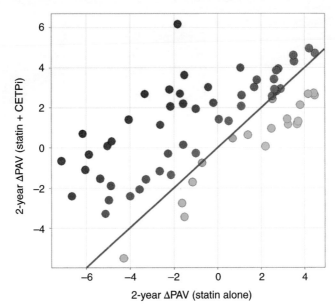

Figure 10.5 Predictions of changes in percent atheroma volume (ΔPAV) for individual VPs following two years of simulated therapy with statin alone (*x*-axis) or statin + CETPi. Each solid circle represents a single virtual patient. VPs below the blue line represent the "responder patients" who show an improved response to the combination therapy compared to atorvastatin alone, while those above the line are "adverse-responder patients," who exhibit exacerbation of atherosclerosis following addition of a CETPi. In this virtual cohort, there are a large number of adverse-responder VPs.

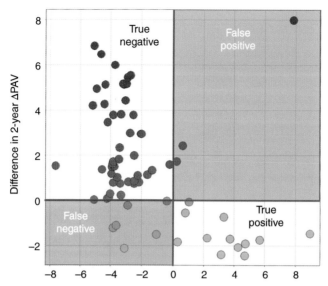

Figure 10.6 Predictions of the optimal multianalyte biomarker of patient response to addition of CETPi to a background statin, including pre-therapy analyte measurements only in the pool of possible analytes. The y-axis indicates the difference in ΔPAV between the combination therapy and the statin monotherapy arm following two years of simulation. The virtual patients with y-axis values greater than zero are the adverse responders; those with values less than zero are the responders. The x-axis indicates the output of the DFA algorithm applied to this analysis: values greater than zero indicate that the virtual patient is predicted to be a responder; values less than zero indicate that the virtual patient is predicted to be a nonresponder. In this case, the candidate biomarker effectively screens out adverse responders, as indicated by a few false positives (upper right quadrant), but is not as effective at identifying responders, as indicated by several false negatives (lower left quadrant).

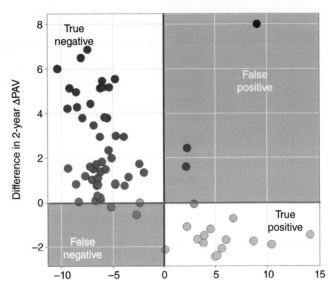

Figure 10.7 Predictions of the optimal multianalyte biomarker of patient response to addition of CETPi to a background statin, including both pre- and post-therapy analyte measurements in the pool of possible analytes. This figure should be interpreted in a manner similar to Figure 10.6. In this case, the candidate biomarker is highly predictive of both responders and adverse responders, as indicated by the presence of both few false negatives (lower left quadrant) and false positives (upper right quadrant).

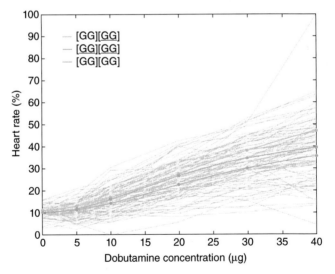

Figure 13.3 Profiles of heart rate in response to different dosages of dobutamine (indicated by dots) for three composite genotypes (thick curves) identified at two SNPs within the $_2AR$ gene. The profiles of 107 subjects studied from which the three composite genotypes were detected are also shown (thin curves).

CHAPTER 7

Role of Core Biological Motifs in Dose–Response Modeling: An Example with Switchlike Circuits

SUDIN BHATTACHARYA, QIANG ZHANG, and MELVIN E. ANDERSEN

Division of Computational Biology, The Hamner Institutes for Health Sciences, Research Triangle Park, North Carolina

Summary

By combining laboratory experiments and computational modeling, systems biology endeavors to examine quantitatively how components of biological systems are assembled to give rise to biological function. These components can be thought of as biological circuits whose perturbation by drugs and other chemicals can lead to either adverse responses (toxicity) or restoration of normal function in the compromised tissue (efficacy). By integrating a series of continuous and switchlike nonlinear dose–response behaviors in individual cells to describe the response at the tissue and organism level, systems biology can help provide a mechanistic basis for incidence-dose modeling. Specifically, this approach can be used to (1) predict the shape of dose–response curves in low-dose regions, and (2) enhance chemical risk assessment for compounds with varying modes of toxicity. In this chapter we examine biological circuit elements and response behaviors that are critical to dose–response modeling, with a particular focus on switchlike circuits.

7.1. INTRODUCTION: SYSTEMS PERSPECTIVES IN DRUG DISCOVERY

The advent of the "omics" era and the flood of data it generated at the molecular level raised hopes for a revolution in the field of drug discovery. In

Systems Biology in Drug Discovery and Development, First Edition.
Edited by Daniel L. Young, Seth Michelson.
© 2012 John Wiley & Sons, Inc. Published 2012 by John Wiley & Sons, Inc.

particular, the detailed characterization of protein interaction networks accompanied by a comparison of networks in normal and diseased patients was expected to accelerate the identification of critical nodal points (proteins) in the networks that could serve as novel drug targets (Hood and Perlmutter, 2004). But as noted by reports of a 30-year decline in productivity in pharmaceutical research and development, the rate of approval of new drugs, especially those that act against novel targets, has not kept pace with ever-increasing investments in drug discovery research (Booth and Zemmel, 2004; Butcher, 2005; Couzin, 2002; DiMasi et al., 2003; Drews, 2003).

A systems biology approach, which aims to understand physiology and disease by integrating information from molecular pathways, regulatory networks, cells, tissues, and organs, all the way to the whole-organism level, may help move beyond this bottleneck in the drug discovery process. Such an approach would have to be interdisciplinary, comprising (1) integration of "omic" data sets, (2) direct experimental investigation of the biological effects of drugs with cell-based assays, and (3) computational modeling based on information about responses at the cell and organ levels (Butcher et al., 2004). While the large data sets generated from "omics" technologies can provide a scaffold for identifying signaling, regulatory, and metabolic pathways (Ideker and Lauffenburger, 2003), the data sets may not themselves provide insight into the cellular mechanisms that control initiation of cellular responses and coordinate activation of therapeutically important pathways.

For such insights, systems biologists have focused on the signaling modules or "motifs" (Alon, 2007; Bhalla and Iyengar, 1999; Tyson et al., 2003) that make up the control circuitry of cells. These circuits give rise to nonlinear responses and may serve as prioritized points of intervention in regulatory networks. Understanding the organization and function of these circuits would predict the cellular outcome of perturbations (both the desired pharmaceutical activity and side effects) introduced by specific drug molecules. Although specific aberrations in signaling may be specific to particular disease states or individual patients, the underlying functional modules that govern the behavior of protein pathways—for example, negative feedback mechanisms that give rise to homeostasis, and positive feedback loops responsible for switching between distinct cellular states—are universal properties of cell signaling networks (Araujo et al., 2007).

7.2. SYSTEMS BIOLOGY AND TOXICOLOGY

A similar challenge is faced in the field of toxicology and risk assessment. The overarching goal of toxicity testing is to assess, with minimum uncertainty, the risks posed to human populations by exposure to specified concentrations of potentially toxic compounds. Toxicology studies serve the public health objective by (1) providing measures to determine if individual compounds (or their reactive metabolites, e.g., acetaminophen and NAPQI) are themselves likely to lead to harm in a specific population; and (2) providing a means to compare one chemical with another (i.e., to assess relative risks), thereby aiding in selecting particular chemicals for a specific societal use. These risk assessment activities are only as reliable as the data that are available for the decision-making process, and require contributions from a variety of biological disciplines, including toxicology and molecular biology.

Risk assessment for chemical hazards in the workplace and in the general environment has become increasingly formalized over the past several decades, with an emphasis on introduction of "best available" science into the risk assessment process (Lehman and Fitzhugh, 1954; NAS/NRC, 1983, 1994; USEPA, 1996). Modern toxicology has incorporated research and testing strategies from the clinical and biological sciences, with increasing use of *in vitro* cell systems for assessing chemical interactions in living cells and application of molecular techniques emerging from the field of molecular biology in the 1980s and 1990s.

Although the molecular approaches to assessing modes of action and targets have kept pace with advances in cell biology, genomics, and other areas, the continued reliance on organism-level responses (e.g., hepatotoxicity, cancer, reproductive–developmental toxicity, neurotoxicity) in high-dose studies with homogeneous groups of laboratory animals has increasingly come into question. The use of these high-dose animal toxicity test results as a basis for predicting risks posed to humans at much lower environmental exposures requires extrapolations to (1) predict the shape of the dose–response curve at low levels of response, and (2) adjust for species differences in response. The central question in interpreting most toxicological data is: *Is the response expected to be low-dose linear, or is it expected to have a threshold or other more complex shape?* Noncancer endpoint risk assessments have been based on the belief that there is a level of exposure, a *threshold*, below which the risks should be negligible. The difficulty in practice is defining objectively how these thresholds should be established (Daston, 1993). Estimation of nonlinear dose–response behavior in the low-dose region requires the use of uncertainty factors, usually employed in a highly subjective manner without sufficient biological basis. These and other concerns have led many practicing toxicologists over the decades to consider chemical risk assessment as a process determined primarily by policy rather than as a process representing a rigorous science well grounded in biological and toxicological principles. *There is an urgent need to integrate molecular toxicology and "omics"-based information to strengthen the scientific basis of the current risk assessment process.*

A recent National Academy of Sciences committee evaluated alternative approaches to toxicity testing (NAS/NRC, 2007). This report listed the key criteria for a modern toxicity testing strategy. The toxicity testing approach should be (1) capable of testing the large number of existing and new compounds; (2) broad-based, to assess responses for multiple endpoints, life stages, and various mixtures of compounds; (3) timely and cost-effective in providing results for regulatory decision making; and (4) focused on human biology and modes of action of chemicals in human cells and tissues at relevant exposures. In addition, the tests should use as few animals as possible.

Based on these criteria, a new approach was recommended in which virtually all routine toxicity testing would be conducted in human cells or cell lines *in vitro* by evaluating cellular responses in a suite of *toxicity pathway* assays using high-throughput tests, implemented with robotic assistance (NAS/NRC, 2007). Toxicity pathways are normal cellular signaling pathways that may be perturbed by test compounds. Risk assessment would shift toward the avoidance of significant perturbations of these pathways in exposed human populations. This redirection of toxicity testing would use smaller numbers of animals, improve knowledge of modes of action, enhance human relevance, and provide higher throughput than is possible with current toxicological testing strategies. Although such a wide-ranging change of toxicity testing in risk assessment remains a work in progress, we suggest that the transition would benefit by the expansion of molecular toxicity studies in human tissues and by computational modeling of the targeted pathways.

During the year 2000, a monthly series of articles celebrating the millennium was published by the journal *Science*. The review that appeared in March, "Genomics: Journey to the Center of Biology" (Lander and Weinberg, 2000), noted the overall goals of genomic studies, goals that apply equally well to toxicology and drug discovery:

> The long-term goal is to use this information to reconstruct the complex molecular circuitry that operates within the cell—to map out the network of interacting proteins that determines the underlying logic of various cellular biological functions including cell proliferation, responses to physiologic stresses, and acquisition and maintenance of tissue-specific differentiation functions. A longer term goal, whose feasibility remains unclear, is to create mathematical models of these biological circuits and thereby predict these various types of cell biological behavior.

Toxicologists study the manner in which excesses of various exogenous chemicals lead to physiological stress, alterations in gene batteries, and resulting degradation or alteration of function. This approach, pursued in a comparative manner, resembles studies in cancer in which the final aggressive transformed cell is compared with the initial normal cell to see the differences in characteristics between the two states. Such a strategy could help categorize compounds in relation to modes of action. However, these studies may still say little about the dose–response behaviors of the molecular alterations that move the cell from the initial to the final altered state.

Uncovering the circuitry involved in these transitions will tell us more about the network context of the molecular targets for the toxic responses. Coupled with novel computational systems biology methods, these approaches should produce improved dose–response assessment of the toxic actions of the compounds through biologically based dose–response (BBDR) modeling at the level of cellular responses. The actions of many circuit elements and motifs—

cell surface receptors, cytosolic transcriptional factors, kinase/phosphatase cascades—are now more completely understood than just a few years ago. Studies of the human health risks posed by chemicals should focus on normal function and how normal function becomes perturbed by exogenous compounds. This strategy, espoused in the NAS report (NAS/NRC, 2007), is a perturbation approach to molecular and cellular toxicology. A reorientation to focus on initial perturbations of normal biological pathways rather than an emphasis on final pathology or altered state should provide new avenues to evaluate dose–response relationships both in chemical risk assessment and drug discovery.

7.3. MECHANISTIC AND COMPUTATIONAL CONCEPTS IN A MOLECULAR OR CELLULAR CONTEXT

One of the most significant advancements that could arise from combining molecular toxicology and pharmaceutical sciences with analysis of cellular circuitry is the ability to understand the molecular basis of dose–response relationships for toxic compounds and drugs. In the case of toxicology, there is a particular need for biologically plausible methods for low-dose risk assessment. Current dose–response assessment tools have largely been empirical or driven by assumed defaults. The commentary in *Science* (Lander and Weinberg, 2000) addressed the long-term goal of creating mathematical models of biological circuits that describe responses to physiological (and/or chemical) stress and the acquisition and maintenance of tissue-specific differentiation function. Similarly, there is the desire to create biological circuit models of dose–response curves for toxicity based on alterations in cell and tissue function. The linkage of these biological parameters with a dose of an exogenous compound may be highly nonlinear and associated with alterations in suites of gene products in the cells. Whereas most dose–response assessment models tend to assume smooth continuous changes in response to dose, the molecular circuitry in the real world of cells demonstrates a more complex array of responses.

Chemical kinetics is generally described using deterministic equations because the number of entities involved in these reactions is typically large. At the cellular level, however, behaviors are more likely to be stochastic (Kaern et al., 2005). A cell either divides or it does not; it differentiates or remains in a precursor state. A challenge in formulating the mathematical models of cellular functions is to reproduce the manner in which continuous changes of chemical variables within the cellular machinery lead to dichotomous, discontinuous responses such as apoptosis, proliferation, differentiation, or activation of global cellular circuitry by exposure to chemicals. Stochastic, nonlinear models of cellular-level responses are likely to provide the basis for developing tools that will predict threshold behavior under exposure to toxic chemicals or drugs, as well as predict low-dose regions where the proportionate response to increasing dose varies considerably from the dose–response structure at high doses. Mechanistically, dose–response relationships are unlikely to be simple continuous functions and will depend on the molecular targets of test chemicals and the molecular circuitry in which the targets are embedded.

7.4. RESPONSE MOTIFS IN CELL SIGNALING AND THEIR ROLE IN DOSE RESPONSE

Response motifs are relatively simple building blocks that appear frequently in complex molecular networks and possess a specific input/output (I/O) signaling property (Alon, 2007; Bhalla and Iyengar, 1999; Tyson et al., 2003). It follows that different network motifs serve specific biological functions. In the remainder of this chapter we discuss one such motif used by organisms to enable ligand-mediated switching between different cellular states: gene autoregulation. We will also see how stochastic gene expression interacts with the I/O property of a network motif to create a particular dose–response profile.

To activate suites of genes coordinately, cells in all living organisms have evolved molecular modules to allow transitions, or *switching*, between distinct functional states over a small range of signal (dose of hormone or other ligand concentration), as well as mechanisms to stabilize the new state. In many cases, such coordinated control of sets of gene products leads to an extensive change in the properties of the cell: for example, irreversible differentiation, or a reversible phenotypic alteration that persists until the activation signal falls back to a very low concentration. Molecular control processes for switching are inherently nonlinear and often utilize autoregulatory feedback loops. Some of the biological processes that contribute to switching phenomena are receptor autoinduction, induction of enzymes for ligand synthesis, mRNA stabilization or activation, and receptor polymerization (Bhalla and Iyengar, 1999; Lisman and Fallon, 1999). Specifically, switching phenomena require a response motif containing an overall positive feedback loop architecture. Switching in this context does not refer simply to a process with "off" and "on" states but, rather, a dynamic process where small changes in the concentration of the active ligand lead to relatively large changes in cellular response. A typical example is the all-or-none regional induction of metabolizing enzymes in the liver by xenobiotics (Andersen et al., 1997a,b). The presence of switches for concerted transcriptional regulation of gene batteries and their nonlinear I/O properties have important consequences for the shape of dose–response curves.

7.4.1. The Gene Autoregulation Motif

In the gene autoregulation response motif (Figure 7.1a, Box 7.1) a protein activates its own gene, either directly as a transcription factor, or indirectly,

BOX 7.1: MATHEMATICAL MODEL OF GENE AUTOREGULATION

In this chapter we use a simplified mathematical representation of a transcriptional regulatory circuit with both constitutive activation and autoregulatory induction of a gene (Figure 7.1a). The equations that describe the model dynamics are

$$\frac{dM}{dt} = k_0 + \frac{k_1 S}{k_{d1} + S} + \frac{k_2 P^n}{k_{d2}^n + P^n} - k_3 M$$

$$\frac{dP}{dt} = k_4 M - k_5 P$$

In these equations, M and P are the variables representing amounts of the mRNA and protein, respectively, and S represents a saturable input signal (hormone/ligand) that activates the gene. The parameter k_0 is the basal (constitutive) transcription rate; k_1 and k_{d1} are the transcription rate constant and the effective affinity constant, respectively, for the input signal S acting on the gene, and k_2 and k_{d2} represent the transcription rate constant and the effective affinity constant, respectively, for the protein P acting as a transcription factor to induce activation of the gene. The parameter n is the Hill coefficient, which describes an ultrasensitive activation of gene transcription by P. P and S are assumed to act on two independent promoters, leading to an additive effect on the transcription rate. The parameter k_4 denotes the basal translation rate constant, and k_3 and k_5 represent the first-order degradation rate constants for mRNA and protein, respectively. For this simplified model we use dimensionless parameters with the following values: $k_0 = 4, k_1 = 15, k_{d1} = 5, k_2 = 300, k_{d2} = 50, k_3 = 1, k_4 = 1, k_5 = 1$, and $n = 4$. These values were optimized to ensure bistable switching behavior in the model. The value of S is varied to explore the dynamic behavior of the model. Initial values of the variables M and P (i.e., initial amounts of mRNA and protein) need to be specified for each "run" (simulation) of the model. The action of the protein P to activate its own gene forms a positive feedback loop that gives the module its switching properties (see the text). All deterministic simulations were run on the Berkeley Madonna program; bifurcation diagrams were generated with XPPAUT. To implement the stochastic version of the model, we used the BioNetS program [Biochemical Network Stochastic Simulator (Adalsteinsson et al., 2004)], which is based on the Gillespie stochastic simulation algorithm for coupled chemical reactions (Gillespie, 1977).

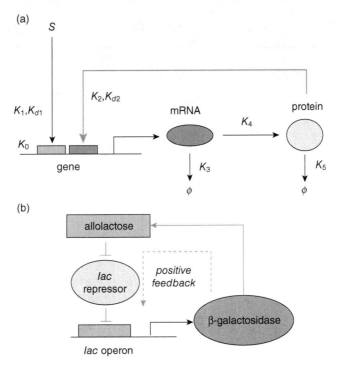

Figure 7.1 (a) Gene autoregulation module. The symbols S and ϕ denote activating input signal and mRNA/protein degradation, respectively. Other symbols are explained in Box 7.1. (b) *lac* operon module in the bacterium *E. coli*: see the text for a description. Arrows denote activation; T-shaped pointers denote repression.

thereby implementing a positive feedback loop. An example of this motif is the operon structure common in bacterial systems, where a set of genes is controlled simultaneously to regulate a particular physiological process. In the *lac* operon of the bacterium *Escherichia coli*, the transcription of the set of genes that produce proteins responsible for lactose metabolism is controlled by the *lac* repressor, which binds to the promoter in the absence of ligand and blocks transcription of the genes in the operon. One of the gene products of the operon, the enzyme β-galactosidase, converts lactose to allolactose, which binds the repressor, causing it to dissociate from the promoter and allow transcription of the genes in the operon (Figure 7.1b). Here the positive feedback is implemented indirectly by inhibition of a repressor. Another example can be found in the regulation of the *comK* gene in the soil bacterium *Bacillus subtilis*. The *comK* gene is the master regulator for the transition from a "vegetative" state to a "competent" state where the bacterium can take up DNA from the environment. The ComK protein itself acts as a transcription factor for the *comK* gene, thus forming a direct autoregulatory positive feedback

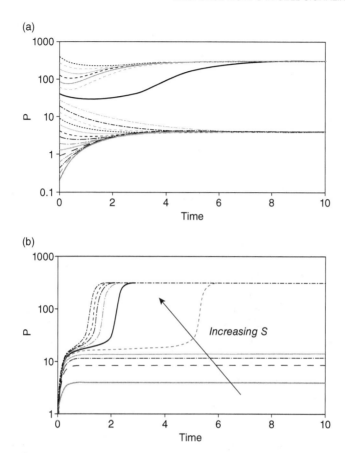

Figure 7.2 Simulations of the gene autoregulation model with protein amount P plotted against time, demonstrating bistable behavior as: (a) initial value of P is varied from 0 to 400, with initial value of $M = 1$, and input signal $S = 0$; (b) S is varied from 0 to 20, with the initial values of P and M fixed at 1.

loop (Hamoen et al., 1998; Vansinderen and Venema, 1994; Vansinderen et al., 1995).

The dynamic behavior of our generalized gene autoregulation model was first explored by running simulations with a range of initial conditions for protein amount P, with input signal S set to 0, and then plotting the time course of P (Figure 7.2a). The curves show that the system settles into one of two different stable steady states, depending on the initial condition, thus exhibiting "bistable" behavior even in the absence of the signal S. One of the steady states corresponds to low protein expression (an "off" state) and the other to high protein expression (an "on" state). This bistable dynamics can also be demonstrated by keeping the initial amount of protein fixed at a low level and varying the strength of the input signal S (Figure 7.2b). Again, the system

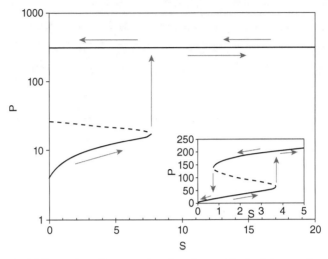

Figure 7.3 P–S bifurcation diagram showing the stable (solid curve) and unstable (dashed curve) steady states of the gene autoregulation model. Rightward- and leftward-pointing arrows indicate the dose–response curve, corresponding to increasing and decreasing dose, respectively, illustrating that the behavior of the system is an irreversible switch. The vertical arrow indicates the threshold value of the input signal S (= 7.64) at which the system switches from the low-protein expression ("off") state to the high-protein expression ("on") state. The inset shows the bifurcation diagram generated from the model with a different parameter set, where the system acts as a reversible switch. (See insert for color representation.)

settles into a low- or high-expression state, depending on the signal strength: there is a threshold value of S below which it settles into the "off" state and above which it settles into the "on" state, showing that the system acts as a threshold-dependent switch.

This switching behavior can be examined in greater detail by plotting a "bifurcation diagram" which shows the steady states of the system plotted against a parameter—here we plot steady states of P versus the input dose S (Figure 7.3). The bifurcation diagram thus represents the dose–response curve of the bistable system. The solid blue lines in the figure correspond to stable steady states of the system, and the dashed blue line corresponds to unstable steady states that are predicted theoretically (by solving the system equations) but can never be attained in practice. As the dose is increased from zero, the system switches from the "off" to the "on" state at a threshold dose of $S = 7.64$. The system also exhibits *hysteresis*, a characteristic feature of any bistable system, where different dose–response curves are obtained depending on whether the dose is increasing or decreasing, as indicated by the arrows in Figure 7.3 (Bagowski and Ferrell, 2001; Ferrell, 2002). Stated otherwise, over a certain dose range, a bistable system exhibiting hysteresis will reside in one of two alternative steady states for a given dose, depending on the history of the system. The bistable switching behavior arises from the nonlinearity (embodied by the Hill function in the current model) and positive feedback inherent in the system (Angeli et al., 2004; Ferrell, 2002; Ferrell and Xiong, 2001; Tyson et al., 2003), and has been demonstrated in a number of natural biological systems (Bagowski and Ferrell, 2001; Chang et al., 2006; Xiong and Ferrell, 2003) as well as in synthetic biological circuits (Becskei et al., 2001; Gardner et al., 2000; Ozbudak et al., 2004). Bistability is likely to be an important biological mechanism in the control of cellular differentiation processes (Chang et al., 2006; Chickarmane et al., 2006), where a cell needs to reside in one of two mutually exclusive phenotypic states.

The other notable feature of the switch portrayed in the bifurcation diagram (Figure 7.3) is that it is irreversible; that is, the system stays in the "on" state even after the triggering stimulus (S) is removed, as indicated by the leftward-pointing arrows in the figure. Irreversibility arises from the strength of the feedback loops involved in the regulatory circuit (Bagowski and Ferrell, 2001; Ferrell, 2002). In the context of the gene autoregulation module, the irreversibility in the switch implies that the system will remain in the high protein-expression state even after the input signal S (hormone or other ligand) is removed (an outcome consistent with cellular differentiation). It should be noted that biological switches need not be irreversible; weaker feedback in the model would allow the system to return to the "off" state as the stimulus is decreased. An example of a "reversible" switch that still exhibits hysteresis is illustrated in the inset in Figure 7.3.

7.4.1.1. Effect of Stochasticity
In the deterministic model described above, the occurrence and timing of the switching event are determined uniquely by the dose of the input signal S (see Figure 7.2b). However, for a population of cells, the presence of intrinsic and extrinsic fluctuations in mRNA and protein concentrations (Kaern et al., 2005; Raser and O'Shea, 2004, 2005) introduces a probabilistic element to both the occurrence and the timing of the switch; that is, a particular cell may or may not switch from the "off" state to the "on" state within a given time window at a given dose of S. We have modeled this scenario with a *stochastic* version of the gene autoregulation model, which allows for "noise": intracellular variation in the mRNA and protein content, and intercellular variation in the dose of input signal S. Stochasticity introduces distributional characteristics to the timing and probability of switching among a population of cells. As we shall see, this cell-to-cell variability is a key determinant of the sensitivity of individual cells to switching and dose–response at the population level.

Figure 7.4 compares the time courses of protein amount P obtained from the deterministic model and multiple simulations of the stochastic model with input dose $S = 1$. The thick red line shows the deterministic result; the thin lines represent time courses from five stochastic simulations—equivalent to tracking the protein level in five different cells. The distributional characteristic of the occurrence and timing of switching is evident. While in the

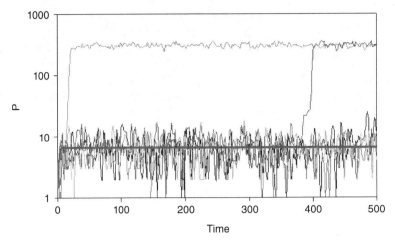

Figure 7.4 Comparison of time-course plots of protein amount P, obtained from deterministic and stochastic simulations. The thick dark line corresponds to the deterministic time course; the thin lines denote five stochastic time courses. Input signal $S = 1$ in each case.

deterministic version of the model a cell never switches from the "off" state to the "on" state at dose $S = 1$; in the stochastic version a cell may or may not switch in a given time window. In this case, two of the five cells switch to the "on" state at different time points within a time window $t = 0$ to 500, while the other three cells remain in the "off" state.

The distributional characteristics of switching in the stochastic model can also be examined by simulating a large number of cells and tracking the populations of cells that inhabit the "off" and "on" states, respectively, at different doses of the input signal S. We simulated a total population of 10,000 cells and recorded the protein level P in each cell at time $t = 1000$. In Figure 7.5, we have plotted the histograms of protein-level distribution at values of S ranging from 0 to 2.5, and then overlaid them on the P-axis in the P–S bifurcation diagram generated from the deterministic model.

At dose $S = 0$, the entire population of cells is in the "off" (low-protein-expression) state (Figure 7.5a). As the dose S is gradually increased (Figure 7.5b to f), we see a population of "on" cells (expressing high levels of protein) emerge, producing the *bimodal* population distribution characteristic of bistable systems (Becskei et al., 2001; Ferrell and Machleder, 1998; Gardner et al., 2000; Ozbudak et al., 2004), until at $S = 2.5$, all cells are in the "on" state (Figure 7.5f). Note that the histograms depicting the "off" and "on" populations are centered around the low- and high-P steady states, respectively, for a particular applied dose of S on the P–S bifurcation diagram. The unstable steady state (dashed line) at each value of S represents the threshold protein level above which a cell would be likely to switch from the "off" to the "on" state.

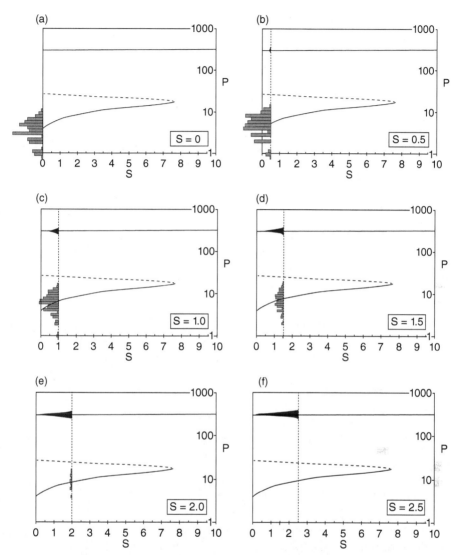

Figure 7.5 Histograms of protein-level distribution for different values of S, overlaid on the P–S bifurcation diagram: (a) $S = 0$; (b) $S = 0.5$; (c) $S = 1.0$; (d) $S = 1.5$; (e) $S = 2.0$; (f) $S = 2.5$. Vertical dashed lines indicate the S-value (also labeled on panels). For each panel, the total population of cells = 10,000 and the observation time $t = 1000$.

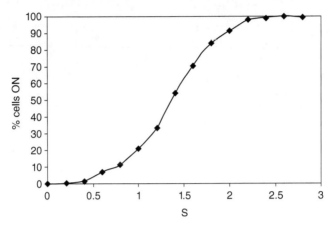

Figure 7.6   Dose–response curves generated by counting the proportion of cells that switch to the "on" state (using a cutoff value of 50 for P) as a function of input dose S (based on stochastic simulations with a total cell population of 1000 and in observation time $t = 1000$).

Based on these results, one can generate a dose–response curve by calculating the proportion of cells that end up in the "on" state as a function of input dose S (Figure 7.6). For these calculations, if the protein level in a cell was higher than the defined cutoff level $P = 50$, we considered the cell to be "on." The sigmoidal shape of the dose–response curve arises from a combination of the underlying deterministic switch and the stochastic fluctuations in amounts of protein and mRNA. A measure of the steepness of the dose–response curve is provided by the effective Hill coefficient n_H (Goldbeter and Koshland, 1981; Legewie et al., 2005), calculated as

$$n_H = \frac{\log(81)}{\log(S_{90}/S_{10})} \tag{7.1}$$

where S_{10} and S_{90} represent the doses required to get 10% and 90% of the maximal response, respectively. Equation (7.1) yields an effective Hill coefficient $n_H = 4.4$ for the dose–response curve in Figure 7.6.

The probabilistic nature of switching in the stochastic model implies that the percentage of cells switching "on" should increase as the signal S is applied for longer time. This raises a question: *How would the dose–response behavior vary if we increase or decrease the observation time?* We addressed this issue by calculating the dose–response at different observation times t and measuring the effective Hill coefficient in each case. The results are shown in Figure 7.7, where the dose (horizontal axis) is plotted on a logarithmic scale to facilitate visual comparison of the steepness of the dose–response curves. For each curve, the response is normalized with respect to the maximal response observed. The numbers next to the curves show the corresponding effective

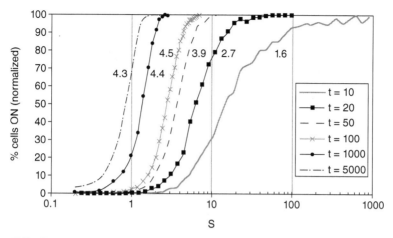

Figure 7.7 Dose–response curves corresponding to different observation times t. The numbers next to each curve denote the corresponding effective Hill coefficient (based on stochastic simulations with a total cell population of 1000).

Hill coefficient n_H, calculated from Eq. (7.1). A gradual increase in the Hill coefficient occurred as the observation time is increased from $n_H = 1.6$ at $t = 10$ to $n_H = 3.9$ at $t = 50$, until it stabilizes at $n_H \cong 4.4$ for values of $t \geq 100$. These results illustrate that observation time is an important experimental parameter when characterizing and comparing dose–response in a biological system subject to stochastic fluctuations.

7.4.1.2. Effect of Dose Distribution

So far we have assumed that all cells in our model are subject to the same input dose S. However, in a physiological scenario, there would be some cell-to-cell variation in the input signal. We model this scenario by drawing the dose that each cell "sees" from a lognormal distribution. We first examine the effect of this dose distribution on the deterministic version of our gene auto-regulation model, where there is no other source of fluctuation.

The noise η in a distribution can be characterized by its coefficient of variation, the ratio of the standard deviation to the mean (Kaern et al., 2005; Raser and O'Shea, 2005). We have generated dose–response curves from the deterministic model for various noise values (Figure 7.8a), where the response is measured by the proportion of cells that switch to the "on" state as a function of the mean dose of the distribution. For noise $\eta = 0$, which corresponds to solving the deterministic model with an identical dose for all cells, the response undergoes a discontinuous, 0-to-100% switching transition at the deterministic threshold dose $S = 7.64$ (thin line in Figure 7.8a). As the noise level in the dose distribution is increased, the steepness of the response gradually decreases, making the response less switchlike. We calculated the effective Hill coefficient

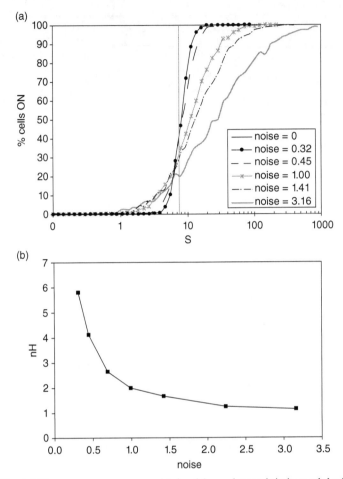

Figure 7.8   (a) Dose–response curves obtained from deterministic model with lognormal dose distributions corresponding to different noise levels for S; (b) effective Hill coefficient n_H of the dose–response curves in Figure 7.8a plotted as a function of noise in dose (S) distribution (based on simulations with a total cell population of 1000).

n_H of the dose–response curves from Eq. (7.1) as a function of the noise level. The Hill coefficient decreases with increasing noise level (Figure 7.8b), reflecting the decrease in the steepness of the response. The diminished steepness characterizes the aggregate response of a population of cells to a noisy input: The response of individual cells is still all-or-none.

The shape of the dose–response curves in Figure 7.8a can be explained by considering the shape of the dose distribution itself at a given noise level. In Figure 7.9 we have plotted the dose distribution histograms corresponding to a noise level $\eta = 0.32$ for three values of the mean dose: 0.5, 5, and 50. The

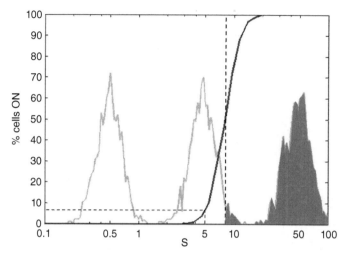

Figure 7.9 Relation between dose distribution and dose–response curves. Dose distribution histograms are plotted for three values of the mean dose: 0.5, 5, and 50, corresponding to a noise level $\eta = 0.32$. The vertical dashed line represents the deterministic threshold dose $S = 7.64$. The response at each mean dose is given by the proportion of the area (shaded) under the corresponding histogram that is to the right of the threshold dose; the horizontal dashed line denotes the response corresponding to a mean dose of 5. The solid dark line is the dose–response curve thus obtained (based on simulations with a total cell population of 1000).

response at each mean dose is given by the proportion of the area (shaded in the figure) under the corresponding histogram that is to the right of the threshold dose $S = 7.64$ (indicated by the vertical dashed line), since this area represents the cells that are exposed to doses higher than the switching threshold. With increasing mean dose, more of the area under the dose histogram would fall to the right of the threshold dose, leading to progressively higher levels of response until all cells switch. Thus in Figure 7.9, for a mean dose of 0.5, we get no response; for a mean dose of 5, we get a response of about 6% of cells switching; and for a mean dose of 50, all cells have switched, giving a 100% response.

This behavior also implies that the steepness of the response is determined by the breadth of the dose distribution: The broader the distribution (i.e., the higher the noise), the more graded (or less switchlike) is the response. This relationship is illustrated in Figure 7.10, where we have plotted the dose distributions for four different noise levels with mean dose set equal to the deterministic threshold dose $S = 7.64$, together with the corresponding dose–response curve.

Once we know the deterministic threshold dose, we should be able to derive the dose–response directly by calculating the proportion of the dose-distribution histogram to the right of the threshold dose as a function of the

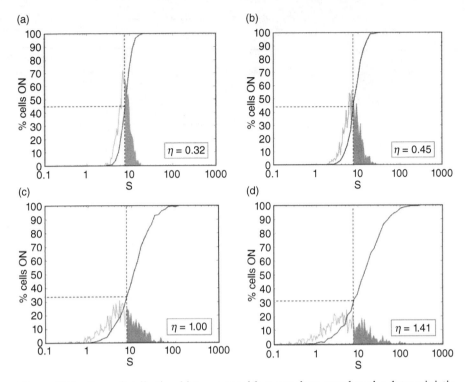

Figure 7.10 Dose-distribution histograms with mean dose equal to the deterministic threshold dose $S = 7.64$ for different levels of noise η: (A) $\eta = 0.32$; (B) $\eta = 0.45$; (C) $\eta = 1.00$; (D) $\eta = 1.41$. In each panel, the solid dark line represents the dose–response curve, while the vertical and horizontal dashed lines represent the (deterministic) threshold dose and the response corresponding to the threshold dose, respectively. The shaded area under the distribution contributes to the response.

mean dose, without having to solve the deterministic model for each dose. We have verified that this is indeed the case by comparing the dose–response obtained by this direct method and the response obtained by solving the model (Figure 7.11); the results from the two approaches are identical.

7.4.1.3. Effect of Stochasticity Coupled with Dose Distribution

Finally, we consider the effect of a dose distribution on the stochastic version of our gene autoregulation model. Here the sources of fluctuation in the system are both the cell-to-cell variation in dose and the probabilistic nature of the reaction steps involved in the switching of an individual cell. As in the preceding section, doses are drawn from a lognormal distribution when solving the stochastic model.

We have plotted the stochastic dose–response for various levels of noise in Figure 7.12a. The results are qualitatively similar to that obtained with the

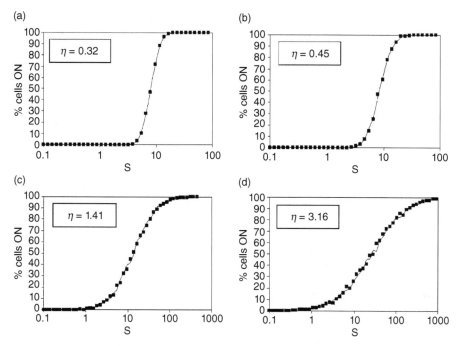

Figure 7.11 Comparison of dose–response obtained by solving deterministic model (squares) and directly from the dose-distribution (line) for different levels of noise η: (a) $\eta = 0.32$; (b) $\eta = 0.45$; (c) $\eta = 1.41$; (d) $\eta = 3.16$. For each panel, the total population of cells = 1000.

deterministic model: The higher the noise level in the dose distribution, the less steep the response. The effective Hill coefficient n_H of the aggregate response thus decreases with increasing noise level (Figure 7.12b), although the response of individual cells is still all or none.

7.5. DISCUSSION AND CONCLUSIONS

In this chapter we have looked at a common biological response motif, the gene autoregulation module, and examined its dose–response behavior in detail. We discussed the role of bistability and hysteresis in enabling switching phenomena and stabilization of induced states. We also demonstrated the importance of stochastic modeling in describing the probabilistic nature of cellular switching, and showed that observation time and the degree of cell-to-cell variation in the input dose can be critical determinants of the shape of the dose–response curve.

The gene autoregulation module is representative of a broader range of positive feedback control processes found in both bacteria and eukaryotes.

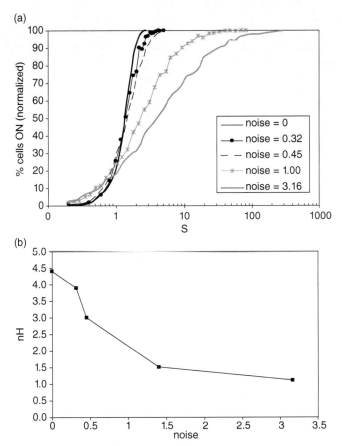

Figure 7.12 (a) Dose–response curves obtained from stochastic model with lognormal dose (S) distributions corresponding to different noise levels; (b) effective Hill coefficient n_H of the dose–response curves in (a) plotted as a function of noise in dose distribution (based on simulations with a total cell population of 1000 and observation time $t = 1000$).

Although the Hill coefficient n in our model formulation (Box 7.1) ostensibly describes cooperative binding of a transcription factor to its own promoter, it can also implicitly represent more common forms of nonlinear positive feedback, including receptor-mediated effects (Andersen and Barton, 1999) or signaling through ultrasensitive protein kinase cascades (Ferrell, 1996). The combination of ultrasensitivity and positive feedback in signal transduction is responsible for all-or-none switchlike cellular responses (Ferrell and Machleder, 1998). Such cellular switches are likely to be the basis of dose thresholds observed in biological responses to both environmental agents and pharmaceuticals. Biological switches abound in nature and some examples are discussed below.

1. *Xenopus laevis* oocytes undergo a switch from a state of G_2 arrest to metaphase arrest in response to the maturation-inducing hormone progesterone. The biochemical basis of this all-or-none response at the level of individual oocytes is signaling through a mitogen-activated protein kinase (MAPK) cascade (Ferrell, 1999a,b; Ferrell and Machleder, 1998). A combination of ultrasensitivity in MAPK signaling, which filters out small stimuli, and positive feedback in the cascade, which prevents the oocyte from getting stuck in intermediate states, is responsible for converting a continuously variable stimulus (progesterone) to a highly switchlike, quantal response, with effective Hill coefficients $\cong 42$ for individual oocytes (Ferrell and Machleder, 1998).

2. The induction of cytochrome P450 (CYP450) enzymes in the liver by the environmental contaminant 2,3,7,8-tetrachlorodibenzo-*p*-dioxin (TCDD) involves binding of TCDD to the aryl hydrocarbon receptor (AhR), followed by migration of the AhR–TCDD complex to the nucleus, where it forms a heterodimer with the aryl hydrocarbon receptor nuclear translocator (ARNT) protein. The heterodimer binds to specific DNA sites to initiate transcription of several genes, including members of the CYP450 family of xenobiotic-metabolizing enzymes. Induction of one member of the family, CYP450 1A1, in liver cells by TCDD *in vitro*, is switchlike, with some cells fully induced and others not induced at all (Bars et al., 1989). Patterns of induction *in vivo* also appear to be switchlike (Bars and Elcombe, 1991; Tritscher et al., 1992). Pharmacokinetic models of CYP1A1 induction in the liver showed that ultrasensitivity, in the form of a Hill coefficient higher than 4.0, was required to explain this all-or-none response (Andersen et al., 1997a), implying the existence of a dose threshold. Use of the Hill term in these models to generate ultrasensitivity is a mere convenience, accounting for other intrinsically ultrasensitive biochemical processes that probably include MAP-kinase cascades and multiple transcription factor activation. Receptor-mediated feedback mechanisms are also likely to be involved in this induction process, as Ah receptor levels in the liver increase following treatment by TCDD (Sloop and Lucier, 1987).

3. A biological switch appears to underlie temperature-dependent gender determination in many species of egg-laying reptiles, where the incubation temperature of the egg determines the gender of the offspring. Here the continuously varying external signal of temperature must be transduced into an all-or-none genetic response that determines gonadal sex (Crews et al., 1994, 1995; Pieau, 1996). Temperature acts on genes encoding hormone receptors and steroid-synthesizing enzymes, activating either the ovary-determining cascade or the testis-determining cascade. In one hypothesis, estradiol- or dihydrotestosterone-forming enzymes compete for testosterone, a precursor common to both sex steroids (Crews et al., 1994). Either estradiol or dihydrotestosterone can take part in a positive feedback loop, increasing the amount of the enzyme (aromatase or reductase, respectively) responsible for its own synthesis. Depending on the temperature, one or the other feedback

loop is activated first. Once a loop is initiated, because of the common precursor (testosterone), the formation of the other sex steroid is inhibited, locking the direction of gonadal development toward either an ovary or a testis.

4. A computational model of the transcriptional circuitry that regulates the fate of embryonic stem cells showed that a network of three transcription factors, OCT4, SOX2, and NANOG, connected by multiple positive feedback loops can generate a bistable switch, alternating between two phenotypic states of the system: self-renewal and differentiation (Chickarmane et al., 2006). Curiously, these positive feedback loops, like many others in developmental processes, appear to comprise double-negative feedback processes to provide the positive feedback required.

5. Similar theoretical models (Huang et al., 2007; Roeder and Glauche, 2006) have been used to show that mutual inhibition of the two transcription factors GATA-1 and PU1 coupled with positive autocatalytic regulation can help explain lineage choice (myeloid vs. erythroid differentiation) in hematopoietic stem cells. This system switches from a "primed" state representing the stem cell fate with low-level coexpression of the two transcription factors, to a differentiated state where one factor dominates at the expense of the other.

Most of these switches are yet to be analyzed with a sufficient level of mechanistic detail, particularly with regard to their dose–response behavior. Our study of the gene autoregulation module suggests that a proper understanding of the dose–response of these and other biological switches will probably require stochastic modeling, with particular attention to the observation time and the extent of cell-to-cell variation in dose.

A positive-feedback loop motif, which underlies most cellular switches, can be implemented in double-positive form with two mutually activating components, as in the gene autoregulation model. This network architecture is useful in situations where a cell needs to execute an on–off switch. However, positive feedback can also be implemented in the form of a double-negative loop with two mutually inhibiting components, which acts as a "toggle switch," helping a cell choose between two alternative states (Becskei et al., 2001; Ferrell, 2002; Gardner et al., 2000) (as in example 4). Both architectures are common in biological systems.

Besides the positive-feedback loop motif, investigation of the transcriptional regulatory networks in the bacterium *Escherichia coli* (Shen-Orr et al., 2002) and the budding yeast *Saccharomyces cerevisiae* (Lee et al., 2002) have revealed a core set of recurring regulatory motifs, each with a characteristic structure and the capacity to perform specific information-processing functions (Alon, 2007). These motifs include negative autoregulation, which enables homeostasis and a speedup of response time in gene circuits (Rosenfeld et al., 2002). Other common motifs include the coherent feedforward loop, which can introduce a time delay in activation as well as detect persistence in the activation signal; and the incoherent feedforward loop, which can function as a pulse generator and response accelerator (Mangan and Alon, 2003; Mangan et al., 2003, 2006). These motifs can also act in combination to generate more complex regulatory patterns in transcriptional networks (Alon, 2007). Similar motifs have been identified in the cells of higher organisms: for example, in the circuits that control gene expression in the pancreas and liver (Odom et al., 2004) and in the regulatory circuits of human embryonic stem cells (Boyer et al., 2005) and hematopoietic stem cells (Rothenberg, 2007; Swiers et al., 2006).

In recent years, new technologies such as genome-wide functional screening and other bioinformatic tools have complemented traditional experimental techniques in mapping out the molecular circuitry underlying cellular behavior. As our understanding of the architecture of network motifs is enhanced, computational modeling of these circuits should help us better understand their inherent functions, as well as the alterations in their behavior under perturbation by drugs and xenobiotics. With environmental agents, these models are likely to provide new insights into the basis of dose–response curves and transform low-dose extrapolations. For drug safety assessment, these models can unravel the underlying components in circuit function, which may lead to variability among patients in response to drugs, either limiting efficacy or initiating low-incidence adverse responses in the total patient population.

REFERENCES

Adalsteinsson, D., McMillen, D., and Elston, T.C. (2004). Biochemical Network Stochastic Simulator (BioNetS): software for stochastic modeling of biochemical networks. *BMC Bioinf 5*, 24.

Alon, U. (2007). Network motifs: theory and experimental approaches. *Nat Rev Genet 8*, 450–461.

Andersen, M.E., and Barton, H.A. (1999). Biological regulation of receptor–hormone complex concentrations in relation to dose–response assessments for endocrine-active compounds. *Toxicol Sci 48*, 38–50.

Andersen, M.E., Birnbaum, L.S., Barton, H.A., and Eklund, C.R. (1997a). Regional hepatic CYP1A1 and CYP1A2 induction with 2,3,7,8-tetrachlorodibenzo-*p*-dioxin evaluated with a multicompartment geometric model of hepatic zonation. *Toxicol Appl Pharmacol 144*, 145–155.

Andersen, M.E., Eklund, C.R., Mills, J.J., Barton, H.A., and Birnbaum, L.S. (1997b). A multicompartment geometric model of the liver in relation to regional induction of cytochrome P450s. *Toxicol Appl Pharmacol 144*, 135–144.

Angeli, D., Ferrell, J.E., and Sontag, E.D. (2004). Detection of multistability, bifurcations, and hysteresis in a large class of biological positive-feed back systems. *Proc Natl Acad Sci USA 101*, 1822–1827.

Araujo, R.P., Liotta, L.A., and Petricoin, E.F. (2007). Proteins, drug targets and the mechanisms they control: the simple truth about complex networks. *Nat Rev Drug Discov 6*, 871–880.

Bagowski, C.P., and Ferrell, J.E. (2001). Bistabillity in the JNK cascade. *Curr Biol 11*, 1176–1182.

Bars, R.G., and Elcombe, C.R. (1991). Dose-dependent acinar induction of cytochromes-P450 in rat-liver: evidence for a differential mechanism of induction of P4501A1 by beta-naphthoflavone and dioxin. *Biochem J 277*, 577–580.

Bars, R.G., Mitchell, A.M., Wolf, C.R., and Elcombe, C.R. (1989). Induction of cytochrome-P-450 in cultured rat hepatocytes: the heterogeneous localization of specific isoenzymes using immunocytochemistry. *Biochem J 262*, 151–158.

Becskei, A., Seraphin, B., and Serrano, L. (2001). Positive feedback in eukaryotic gene networks: cell differentiation by graded to binary response conversion. *EMBO J 20*, 2528–2535.

Bhalla, U.S., and Iyengar, R. (1999). Emergent properties of networks of biological signaling pathways. *Science 283*, 381–387.

Booth, B., and Zemmel, R. (2004). Prospects for productivity. *Nat Rev Drug Discov 3*, 451–457.

Boycr, L.A., Lcc, T.I., Cole, M.F., Johnstone, S.E., Levine, S.S., Zucker, J.R., Guenther, M.G., Kumar, R.M., Murray, H.L., Jenner, R.G., et al. (2005). Core transcriptional regulatory circuitry in human embryonic stem cells. *Cell 122*, 947–956.

Butcher, E.C. (2005). Can cell systems biology rescue drug discovery? *Nat Rev Drug Discov 4*, 461–467.

Butcher, E.C., Berg, E.L., and Kunkel, E.J. (2004). Systems biology in drug discovery. *Nat Biotechnol 22*, 1253–1259.

Chang, H.H., Oh, P.Y., Ingber, D.E., and Huang, S. (2006). Multistable and multistep dynamics in neutrophil differentiation. *BMC Cell Biol 7*.

Chickarmane, V., Troein, C., Nuber, U.A., Sauro, H.M., and Peterson, C. (2006). Transcriptional dynamics of the embryonic stem cell switch. *PLoS Comput Biol 2*, 1080–1092.

Couzin, J. (2002). Cancer drugs: smart weapons prove tough to design. *Science 298*, 522–525.

Crews, D., Bergeron, J.M., Bull, J.J., Flores, D., Tousignant, A., Skipper, J.K., and Wibbels, T. (1994). Temperature-dependent sex determination in reptiles: proximate mechanisms, ultimate outcomes, and practical applications. *Dev Genet 15*, 297–312.

Crews, D., Bergeron, J.M., and Mclachlan, J.A. (1995). The role of estrogen in turtle sex determination and the effect of PCBs. *Environ Health Perspect 103*, 73–77.

Daston, G.P. (1993). Do thresholds exist for developmental toxicants? A review of the theoretical and experimental evidence. In: *Issues and Reviews in Teratology*, Vol. 6 (Kalter, H., ed.). Plenum Press, New York.

DiMasi, J.A., Hansen, R.W., and Grabowski, H.G. (2003). The price of innovation: new estimates of drug development costs. *J Health Econ 22*, 151–185.

Drews, J. (2003). Strategic trends in the drug industry. *Drug Discov Today 8*, 411–420.

Ferrell, J.E., Jr. (1996). Tripping the switch fantastic: how a protein kinase cascade can convert graded inputs into switch-like outputs. *Trends Biochem Sci 21*, 460–466.

Ferrell, J.E. (1999a). Building a cellular switch: more lessons from a good egg. *Bioessays 21*, 866–870.

Ferrell, J.E. (1999b). *Xenopus* oocyte maturation: new lessons from a good egg. *Bioessays 21*, 833–842.

Ferrell, J.E. (2002). Self-perpetuating states in signal transduction: positive feedback, double-negative feedback and bistability. *Curr Opin Cell Biol 14*, 140–148.

Ferrell, J.E., and Machleder, E.M. (1998). The biochemical basis of an all-or-none cell fate switch in *Xenopus* oocytes. *Science 280*, 895–898.

Ferrell, J.E., and Xiong, W. (2001). Bistability in cell signaling: how to make continuous processes discontinuous, and reversible processes irreversible. *Chaos 11*, 227–236.

Gardner, T.S., Cantor, C.R., and Collins, J.J. (2000). Construction of a genetic toggle switch in *Escherichia coli. Nature 403*, 339–342.

Gillespie, D.T. (1977). Exact stochastic simulation of coupled chemical-reactions. *J Phys Chem 81*, 2340–2361.

Goldbeter, A., and Koshland, D.E. (1981). An amplified sensitivity arising from covalent modification in biological-systems. *Proc Natl Acad Sci Biol 78*, 6840–6844.

Hamoen, L.W., Van Werkhoven, A.F., Bijlsma, J.J.E., Dubnau, D., and Venema, G. (1998). The competence transcription factor of *Bacillus subtilis* recognizes short A/T-rich sequences arranged in a unique, flexible pattern along the DNA helix. *Genes Dev 12*, 1539–1550.

Hood, L., and Perlmutter, R.M. (2004). The impact of systems approaches on biological problems in drug discovery. *Nat Biotechnol 22*, 1215–1217.

Huang, S., Guo, Y.P., May, G., and Enver, T. (2007). Bifurcation dynamics in lineage: commitment in bipotent progenitor cells. *Dev Biol 305*, 695–713.

Ideker, T., and Lauffenburger, D. (2003). Building with a scaffold: emerging strategies for high- to low-level cellular modeling. *Trends Biotechnol 21*, 255–262.

Kaern, M., Elston, T.C., Blake, W.J., and Collins, J.J. (2005). Stochasticity in gene expression: from theories to phenotypes. *Nat Rev Genet 6*, 451–464.

Lander, E.S., and Weinberg, R.A. (2000). Genomics: journey to the center of biology. *Science 287*, 1777–1782.

Lee, T.I., Rinaldi, N.J., Robert, F., Odom, D.T., Bar-Joseph, Z., Gerber, G.K., Hannett, N.M., Harbison, C.T., Thompson, C.M., Simon, I., et al. (2002). Transcriptional regulatory networks in *Saccharomyces cerevisiae. Science 298*, 799–804.

Legewie, S., Bluthgen, N., and Herzel, H. (2005). Quantitative analysis of ultrasensitive responses. *FEBS J 272*, 4071–4079.

Lehman, A.J., and Fitzhugh, O.G. (1954). 100-Fold margin of safety. *Assoc Food Drug Off US Q Bull 18*, 33–35.

Lisman, J.E., and Fallon, J.R. (1999). Neuroscience: What maintains memories? *Science 283*, 339–340.

Mangan, S., and Alon, U. (2003). Structure and function of the feed-forward loop network motif. *Proc Natl Acad Sci USA 100*, 11980–11985.

Mangan, S., Zaslaver, A., and Alon, U. (2003). The coherent feedforward loop serves as a sign-sensitive delay element in transcription networks. *J Mol Biol 334*, 197–204.

Mangan, S., Itzkovitz, S., Zaslaver, A., and Alon, U. (2006). The incoherent feed-forward loop accelerates the response-time of the gal system of *Escherichia coli. J Mol Biol 356*, 1073–1081.

NAS/NRC (1983). *Risk Assessment in the Federal Government: Managing the Process.* National Academy of Sciences Press, Washington, DC.

NAS/NRC (1994). *Science and Judgment in Risk Assessment.* National Academy of Sciences Press, Washington, DC.

NAS/NRC (2007). *Toxicity Testing in the 21st Century: A Vision and a Strategy.* National Academy of Sciences Press, Washington, DC.

Odom, D.T., Zizlsperger, N., Gordon, D.B., Bell, G.W., Rinaldi, N.J., Murray, H.L., Volkert, T.L., Schreiber, J., Rolfe, P.A., Gifford, D.K., et al. (2004). Control of pancreas and liver gene expression by HNF transcription factors. *Science 303,* 1378–1381.

Ozbudak, E.M., Thattai, M., Lim, H.N., Shraiman, B.I., and van Oudenaarden, A. (2004). Multistability in the lactose utilization network of *Escherichia coli. Nature 427,* 737–740.

Pieau, C. (1996). Temperature variation and sex determination in reptiles. *Bioessays 18,* 19–26.

Raser, J.M., and O'Shea, E.K. (2004). Control of stochasticity in eukaryotic gene expression. *Science 304,* 1811–1814.

Raser, J.M., and O'Shea, E.K. (2005). Noise in gene expression: origins, consequences, and control. *Science 309,* 2010–2013.

Roeder, I., and Glauche, I. (2006). Towards an understanding of lineage specification in hematopoietic stem cells: a mathematical model for the interaction of transcription factors GATA-1 and PU.1. *J Theor Biol 241,* 852–865.

Rosenfeld, N., Elowitz, M.B., and Alon, U. (2002). Negative autoregulation speeds the response times of transcription networks. *J Mol Biol 323,* 785–793.

Rothenberg, E.V. (2007). Cell lineage regulators in B and T cell development. *Nat Immunol 8,* 441–444.

Shen-Orr, S.S., Milo, R., Mangan, S., and Alon, U. (2002). Network motifs in the transcriptional regulation network of *Escherichia coli. Nat Genet 31,* 64–68.

Sloop, T.C., and Lucier, G.W. (1987). Dose-dependent elevation of Ah-receptor binding by Tcdd in rat-liver. *Toxicol Appl Pharmacol 88,* 329–337.

Swiers, G., Patient, R., and Loose, M. (2006). Genetic regulatory networks programming hematopoietic stem cells and erythroid lineage specification. *Dev Biol 294,* 525–540.

Tritscher, A.M., Goldstein, J.A., Portier, C.J., McCoy, Z., Clark, G.C., and Lucier, G.W. (1992). Dose–response relationships for chronic exposure to 2,3,7,8-tetrachlorodibenzo-*p*-dioxin in a rat-tumor promotion model: quantification and immunolocalization of Cyp1A1 and Cyp1A2 in the liver. *Cancer Res 52,* 3436–3442.

Tyson, J.J., Chen, K.C., and Novak, B. (2003). Sniffers, buzzers, toggles and blinkers: dynamics of regulatory and signaling pathways in the cell. *Curr Opin Cell Biol 15,* 221–231.

USEPA (1996). *Proposed Guidelines for Carcinogen Risk Assessment.* Office of Research and Development, U.S. Environmental Protection Agency, Washington, DC.

Vansinderen, D., and Venema, G. (1994). Comk acts as an autoregulatory control switch in the signal-transduction route to competence in *Bacillus-subtilis. J Bacteriol 176,* 5762–5770.

Vansinderen, D., Luttinger, A., Kong, L.Y., Dubnau, D., Venema, G., and Hamoen, L. (1995). Comk encodes the competence transcription factor, the key regulatory protein for competence development in *Bacillus-subtilis*. *Mol Microbiol 15*, 455–462.

Xiong, W., and Ferrell, J.E. (2003). A positive-feedback-based bistable "memory module" that governs a cell fate decision. *Nature 426*, 460–465.

CHAPTER 8

Mechanism-Based Pharmacokinetic–Pharmacodynamic Modeling During Discovery and Early Development

HANS PETER GRIMM

F. Hoffmann–La Roche Ltd., Basel, Switzerland

YING OU and MICAELA REDDY

Roche Palo Alto LLC, Palo Alto, California

PASCALE DAVID-PIERSON and THIERRY LAVÉ

F. Hoffmann–La Roche Ltd., Basel, Switzerland

Summary

Assuming drug metabolism, pharmacokinetics, and physicochemical properties to be part of the drug discovery and development process has substantially improved the quality of drug candidates. The main reason for attrition in development is now related to safety and efficacy, and the current challenge is to establish a relationship between pharmacokinetic and pharmacological/safety endpoints starting from early discovery stages. Historically, empirical models were applied to address these questions. However, we suggest that more mechanistic-based models are needed to support preclinical drug discovery and early development.

8.1. INTRODUCTION

Assuming drug metabolism and pharmacokinetics (DMPK) and physicochemical properties to be part of the drug discovery and development process has substantially improved the quality of drug candidates with respect to

Systems Biology in Drug Discovery and Development, First Edition.
Edited by Daniel L. Young, Seth Michelson.
© 2012 John Wiley & Sons, Inc. Published 2012 by John Wiley & Sons, Inc.

pharmacokinetic properties. The main reason for attrition in development is now related to safety and efficacy and the current challenge is to establish a relationship between pharmacokinetic and pharmacological safety endpoints starting from the early discovery stages. Mechanism-based pharmacokinetic–pharmacodynamic (PK–PD) modeling is being employed successfully throughout all discovery and drug development stages for data interpretation, study design, and enhanced decision making. Mechanism-based PK–PD modeling is motivated by the mechanistic understanding of biology and disease processes. A mechanism-based PK–PD model can cover a simple PK–PD model, a physiologically based pharmacokinetic–pharmacodynamic (PBPK–PD) model, as well as more complicated systems biology. Because the models are developed to resemble the biological pathways and disease processes, they have several salient features. For example, they provide the opportunity to separate system-specific parameters from compound specific parameters (Danhof et al., 2007, 2008). They also enable extrapolation from *in vitro* to *in vivo* settings, from animals to humans, from healthy volunteers to a disease population, and from one compound to similar compounds. In addition, unlike empirical models, the model parameters in mechanism-based PK–PD model can be measured experimentally and in some cases estimated *in silico*.

The specific set of questions to be addressed using PK–PD modeling depends on the stage of drug development. For late-stage preclinical and clinical development, PK–PD modeling is used to affect the selection of dose regimens and more generally to support optimal study design. For the discovery and early development stages, an understanding of the PK–PD relationship helps to better define the target profile, support the selection of lead compounds to advance into clinical studies, predict safe starting doses for first-in-human studies, and provide a basis for optimal design of proof-of-concept studies (usually, phase IIa) in relevant patient populations.

In this chapter we focus on the application of mechanism-based PK–PD modeling during discovery and early drug development supported by specific case studies as well as examples from the literature.

8.2. CHALLENGES IN DRUG DISCOVERY AND DEVELOPMENT

8.2.1. Challenge 1: Data Integration

Drug discovery is increasingly "data rich," with high-throughput chemistry generating numerous compounds which are rapidly screened for pharmacological and pharmacokinetic properties. This vast amount of data is used to drive decision making for compounds to be moved into development. Successful integration of discovery data is a key to selecting good compounds for development.

The most common method for selecting compounds is by eliminating the compounds that fail to meet criteria for DMPK, safety, and pharmacological screens, then picking the best candidate from the remaining compounds based on efficacy and other concerns. For example, consider a choice between the following compounds: compound A has excellent efficacy in a rat pharmacology bioassay and good permeability but low solubility, and has much higher protein binding in humans than in rats. In contrast, compound B has good efficacy and good permeability and solubility, but has protein binding in humans similar to that in rats. Which compound should be chosen to move forward in development?

We suggest integrating all available preclinical data into a single interpretable context by using PBPK modeling, and, whenever feasible, further integrating pharmacology data into the model so as to develop the PK–PD relationship and to come up with the most accurate and quantitative interpretation of the data set. Biological mechanism-based PK–PD models are especially relevant at this early stage because these PK–PD models allow separation of biological system-specific and compound-specific components and are thus, by design, capable of integrating information about various processes. This PBPK–PD approach can deal with a diverse set of physicochemical, pharmacokinetic, and pharmacodynamic data and the high throughput with which drug candidates are produced; it is scientifically driven by relying on validated mechanistic models, thereby eliminating a large portion of the usual bias in data interpretation. Ultimately, by comparing projections at the human level for multiple drug candidates, it provides a rational basis for improved compound selection (Lavé et al., 2007).

8.2.2. Challenge 2: Relevance of *In Silico, In Vitro*, and *In Vivo* Preclinical Data to the Situation in Human

Biological mechanism–based models built on the basis of human physiologically relevant parameters provide the opportunity to translate *in silico, in vitro*, and *in vivo* preclinical data into knowledge that is relevant to the situation in humans. This approach provides the possibility of optimizing compounds based on the profile *expected* in the relevant species (i.e., human) rather than on direct observations in mice or rats, which might prove to be misleading for human patients.

As a simple example, take a measured value for the solubility of a compound. Alone, this data item tells us little about the absorption of the compound in humans. Only when combined with permeability, pK_a, and other physicochemical properties can one start to make predictions (i.e., the first necessary step is data integration). Yet, without any model (be it physiology based or statistics based), the data make little sense (i.e., the second step must be the construction of a suitable model). With appropriate data and a trustworthy model, predictions can be attempted. However, to gain additional confidence, comparison of model predictions and *in vivo* outcomes in animal species should be attempted. After this third step, predictions can be made with reasonable confidence.

As another example, consider an *in vivo* test fundamental for the evaluation of central nervous system compounds: namely, the induction of locomotor activity (LMA) or variants thereof. Per se, a dose–response of LMA in mice is of little value when it comes to predictions of efficacy against a psychiatric condition in humans. On the one hand, LMA needs to be linked to receptor occupancy *in vitro* and to measured target affinity; this allows one to account for species differences (e.g., in protein binding and affinity). On the other hand, LMA needs to be connected to some functional experiment in animals, which in turn has been linked to the psychiatric disorder under investigation, possibly based on other compounds (e.g., competitor information in the public domain). Ultimately, this knowledge has to be combined with pharmacokinetics. Modeling is indispensable as the "glue" between these pieces. Furthermore, mechanistic- or physiological-based models have the capability to capture the strongly inherent nonlinear processes, which are often problematic in purely statistics-driven approaches.

8.2.3. Challenge 3: Uncertainty in Models and Data

Another challenge is related to the uncertainty in the data and the unknown in the processes driving the pharmacokinetic and efficacy profiles of drug candidates. The dimensions of uncertainty can be (1) from *in vitro* to *in vivo* extrapolation, (2) from cross-species extrapolation, (3) from preclinical model to clinical efficacy prediction, and (4) from healthy volunteers to disease population.

Mathematical (PBPK, PK–PD) modeling enforces the explicit formulation of hypotheses; based on a given set of hypotheses, predictions can be made and later—hopefully—tested. Several hypotheses can coexist, and the resulting predictions delimit the range of probable outcomes. In this way, models offer the possibility of explicitly incorporating uncertainty into the decision-making process and translating that uncertainty into a measure of confidence in the simulation and/or prediction. Unlike other empirical models, the assumption and uncertainty in a mechanistic PK–PD model may be reduced by further experimental data collection. Quantifying key uncertainties and providing a range of possible outcomes based on current knowledge of the PK properties of the compound will allow for more informed decision making. In addition, biologically based mechanistic models offer a nice platform for incorporating the known variability among patient populations (Rostami-Hodjegan and Tucker, 2007).

8.2.4. Challenge 4: The Need to Systematically Translate Findings from Clinical Studies Back to Preclinical Discovery and Development

One of the most powerful applications of mechanism-based modeling and simulation is the ability to integrate the information from different studies, especially findings from clinical studies, to advance the best compounds at preclinical development. Mechanism-based PK–PD models allow separation of system parameters from compound-specific parameters; thus, the same "system" parameter from studies of other compounds in humans on the same pharmacology or disease process can be used to model similar compounds in the same system. This is particularly useful considering the challenge of translating research from the animal model to human efficacy and safety.

In preclinical discovery and development, the key activity is to use certain "predictive" or "evaluative" tools to help screen out those candidates most likely to have serious undesired side effects, and to identify those most likely to become safe and effective treatments. Because of the predictive nature of the type of modeling needed in preclinical development, such models ideally would be mechanistic as opposed to empirical. That is, the mechanistic model can provide better capacity for credible extrapolations. For example, *in silico* models based on a large clinical safety database such as adverse drug reactions are now used in preclinical development (Krejsa et al., 2003). The learning and confirming phases of drug development as defined by Sheiner and Steimer (2000) also apply to learning from clinical data and clinical experience back into drug discovery to better design predictive models at the preclinical stage. There are vast amounts of clinical data from compounds with similar structures or from a similar class that can help in the selection of lead compounds or backup molecules at an early development stage. Model-directed drug development processes should be bidirectional. Successful prediction and application of a preclinical model for phase I and early proof-of-concept clinical studies should not be seen as an end unto itself. As compounds move through subsequent development stages, new learning from the clinical study of compounds should be incorporated into the model, and an updated model should be a better "predictive" model for the backup program or a similar class of targets. In summary, the mechanistic PK–PD model provides a quantitative framework for translation and systematic integration of data and learning from clinical studies to preclinical development.

8.3. METHODOLOGICAL ASPECTS AND CONCEPTS

8.3.1. Cascading Drug Effects

The principle of cascading models to relate processes on the causal path between drug administration and response has been described recently (Danhof et al., 2007, 2008). With this approach the effect of drugs from one process to the next in the chain of events can be described. With such an approach, pharmacokinetics can be used to estimate target exposure, which can then be related to pharmacodynamics. Target effect considerations represent the initial steps in PK–PD model building, which can then be extended to include downstream effects such as molecular target activation, physiological measures, pathophysiological measures, and clinical ratings (Danhof et al.,

2007, 2008; Mager et al., 2003) as drug candidates move through the discovery and development process. The relationships between the various processes are solely dependent on the functioning of the biological system and are therefore independent of the drug.

Mechanism-based PK–PD modeling constructed on the basis of cascading models therefore constitutes the scientific basis for prediction of the ultimate clinical effects of novel drugs based on the response obtained at the various stages of the chain of biological events.

8.3.2. Linking Exposure and Effect

In many cases, PK predictions can be made with reasonable confidence for small molecules using, for example, physiologically based models (Jones et al., 2006). Physiologically based models are useful to simulate exposure in plasma and in individual tissues, including target tissues. The target exposure can be linked to efficacy parameters measured *in vitro* in order to estimate receptor occupancy, which provides the link between the exposure and effect. Lack of solid understanding of target exposure can invalidate prior PK–PD modeling. Target exposure can be challenging to estimate when active transport processes are involved in, for example, tissue uptake. Recently, improved estimation of the transporter Michaelis–Menten parameters in the *in vitro* assay for quantitative predictions of transporter dynamics *in vivo* has opened the door for the possibility of incorporating transporter kinetics in a PBPK model for improved prediction of target tissue concentration (Poirier et al., 2008).

Many biological responses can show a delay relative to drug concentrations in plasma, often referred to as *hysteresis*. When distribution to the site of action becomes rate limiting and determination of drug concentration at the target site is difficult, the *effect compartment model* (or *link model*), for example, provides a useful way of estimating concentration at the effect site (Sheiner et al., 1979). The model assumes that drug in the effect compartment does not contribute to the pharmacokinetics of drug in plasma. Effect compartment modeling is useful when response delays are due to drug distribution from plasma to the effect site. Use of the effect compartment allows collapse of the hysteresis loop and estimation of effect concentration at the target site, and subsequently leads to an improved estimation of *in vivo* potency of compounds.

8.3.3. Receptor Occupancy and Enzyme Inhibition

The potency (i.e., the EC_{50}) and the intrinsic activity (i.e., the maximal effect, E_{max}) of a drug are functions of compound-specific (i.e., receptor affinity and intrinsic efficacy) and system-specific properties (i.e., the receptor density and the function relating receptor occupancy to pharmacological effect). Classical receptor theory explicitly separates drug- and system-specific properties as determinants of the drug concentration–effect relationship and therefore constitutes a theoretical basis for the prediction of this relationship. Not surprisingly, receptor theory is used increasingly in mechanism-based PK–PD modeling to explain and predict (variability in) *in vivo* drug concentration–effect relationships (Danhof et al., 2007, 2008).

8.3.4. Transduction of *In Vivo* Response

Transduction refers to the processes of the translation of the receptor activation into the ultimate pharmacological response. Specifically, the binding of a drug to a biological target initiates a cascade of biochemical and/or electrophysiological events, resulting in an observable biological response (Danhof et al., 2007, 2008). When transduction is fast (i.e., operating with rate constants in the range of milliseconds to seconds) relative to the rate constants governing the disposition processes (typically, minutes to hours), the transduction process does not influence the time course of the drug effect relative to the plasma concentration. *In vivo* transduction can also be slow, operating with rate constants on the order of hours to days, in which case transduction becomes an important determinant of the time course of drug action (Danhof et al., 2007, 2008).

8.3.4.1. Indirect Response Models
A widely used mechanism-based modeling approach for describing delayed biological response is the *indirect response model* (IDR). IDR is based on the concept of homeostasis; that is, physiological entities (e.g., proteins, body temperature) are kept in dynamic equilibrium by balancing their buildup and their loss. Pharmacological activity can either stimulate or inhibit either of these processes, as well reviewed by Mager and Jusko (2001) and Mager et al. (2003).

8.3.4.2. Transit Compartment Models
Models have been proposed in which transduction is modeled mechanistically on the basis of intermediary processes between pharmacokinetics and response. The *transit compartment model* (TCM) has been proposed for this purpose. This model relies on a series of differential equations to describe the cascade of events between receptor activation and final response (Lobo and Balthasar, 2002; Mager and Jusko, 2001; Sun and Jusko, 1998). As with the IDR, traditional TCMs are motivated physiologically but are often phenomenological descriptions of pharmacodynamic response.

An interesting application of a transduction model in drug development is the model for describing the time course of myelosuppression (Friberg et al., 2002). The model consists of a proliferating, drug-sensitive compartment, a series of transit compartments representing maturation, and a compartment of circulating blood cells. A key feature of this model is the separation of fixed system-specific parameters (such as proliferation and transit time) and a small number of drug-related parameters that have to be estimated. The model, "calibrated" with known compounds (Friberg et al., 2002), can be used to translate the myelosuppression of new compounds from animals to humans. Clearly, the model is semiphenomenological in the sense that it does not aim at profound understanding of the complex processes in blood cell maturation. Rather, it is tuned with a minimum of parameters required to capture the most important aspects of interindividual differences, as well as drug action.

8.3.4.3. System Biology Mechanistic Models

When dealing with complex systems, combining knowledge and data from various sources generated in different experiments is indispensable. As mentioned earlier, these models should clearly separate drug-related parameters and physiology-related parameters. In the past this approach was often hampered by a scarcity of detailed data. With the explosion of systems biology, the development of dynamic mechanistic models for selected biological response and transduction processes has become easier. One recent example is the development of a model describing the effect of corticosteroid (dexamethasone) on multiple proinflammatory cytokine levels, as well as physiological endpoints (bone density, paw edema) in the context of collagen-induced arthritis in rats (Earp et al., 2008a,b). Quantitative analysis of corticosteroid effects on proinflammatory cytokine mRNA was performed and used to explain differences in concentrations necessary for treatment effects on paw edema versus bone mineral density, potentially providing insight for optimizing the use of corticosteroid in the clinical setting. Although mechanistic models are a key to improved understanding of pharmacology, there are still many limitations in their application in drug development. This limitation often lies with the availability of data: Can all relevant entities be assayed? Are all dynamic parameters known? Can species differences be bridged? Such modeling efforts need to be initiated very early in drug discovery and developed in parallel with the project, in order to deliver timely input and to support important decisions.

8.3.5. Disease Modeling

One of the key challenges in early drug discovery and development, especially for novel first-in-class compounds, is that we often do not know whether a highly potent compound that inhibits a specific receptor function or alters a specific pathway bears any relevance to efficacy in the disease population (e.g., modulation of disease progression or symptomatic relief). Without a doubt, efforts in the development of new compounds are directed toward drugs that can halt or alter disease progression. Therefore, it is important that PK–PD modeling be extended to include the effects on disease progression. Understanding disease progression is critical, as the optimal pharmacodynamic response needs to be defined in the context of the effects of a compound on the process of disease progression. In early drug discovery and development, compounds that target a specific pathway are often assumed to have an impact on the ultimate disease process. For a complex disease, this target could be difficult to validate until a proof-of-concept study is performed in a disease population.

Disease progression modeling was listed in the Critical Path Initiative developed by the U.S. Food and Drug Administration (Woodcock and Woosley, 2008). Development of new biomarkers for disease processes was identified as the highest priority for scientific effort and quantitative modeling of the disease process, and incorporating what is known about biomarkers would be an obvious next step. Disease progression modeling has been used in modeling clinical studies into Alzheimer's disease, Parkinson's disease, and viral dynamics in HIV- or HCV-infected patients (Bonhoeffer et al., 1997; Chan et al., 2007).

Disease modeling is defined here as mathematical modeling describing the dynamic changes or progression of clinically relevant disease endpoints. In the case of diabetes, a disease model would include time-course changes in β-cell function and insulin sensitivity. A PK–PD disease model will be able to link the changes in glucose and insulin regulation to the overall disease progression and its associated clinically relevant endpoints. De Winter et al. (2006) developed a mechanism-based disease progression model for type 2 diabetes. The model includes the interaction of glucose, insulin, and HbA1c and the effects of drugs with different mechanisms of action (pioglitazone, metformin, and gliclazide) on the disease process. Once this model is validated using available clinical data from compounds with diverse mechanisms, this disease model should also be very useful for preclinical lead selection and study design of new compounds.

In the context of antiviral drugs, PK–PD models have been developed to describe the effect of compounds on viral replication using empirical E_{max} models (Rosario et al., 2005) as well as PK–PD disease models to link the viral and cell dynamics in patients as a function of time. Useful disease models for viral dynamic changes in patients have recently been reported for compounds targeting HIV and HCV (Bonhoeffer et al., 1997; Dixit et al., 2004; Neumann et al., 1998). The development of an HCV viral dynamic model to describe viral load changes in patients has helped us to understand the mechanism of the antiviral efficacy of interferon-α and ribaviron (Bonhoeffer et al., 1997; Dixit et al., 2004; Neumann et al., 1998). Subsequently, these initial models were extended to account for the presence of both wild-type virus and a low level of telaprevir-resistant variants in estimating the treatment duration required to eradicate the virus (Khunvichai et al., 2007).

In the following section we describe and illustrate by examples the application of PK–PD modeling within the discovery and development process.

8.4. USE OF PK–PD MODELS IN LEAD OPTIMIZATION

During lead optimization, high-throughput chemistry generates numerous compounds, and the physicochemical, pharmacokinetic, and pharmacological properties targeted within a particular project need to be defined. Since PK–PD models integrate all properties in a single framework, they can be extremely useful in defining the range of properties needed to achieve a desired clinical outcome in terms of extent and duration of effect.

8.4.1. Example: Ex Vivo Binding and PK Simulation to Predict Efficacy in an Obesity Model During Lead Optimization

In a recent Roche antiobesity project, PBPK–PD simulations, including target effects, were performed to get a better understanding of the efficacy, or lack thereof of compounds tested in a subchronic food intake model. A PK–PD model was able to simulate brain receptor occupancy for all compounds tested in a three-day *in vivo* food intake model in the rat. These simulations were performed based on *in vitro* parameters for DMPK and efficacy (*in vitro* K_i, *in vitro* microsomal clearance, buffer solubility, log$D$, pK_a, and unbound fraction in plasma), using a PBPK model to predict *in vivo* concentration–time profiles in the rat. The simulations of receptor occupancy were performed under the assumption that the unbound concentration in the plasma is close to the unbound concentration in the brain. Interestingly, these PK–PD simulations indicated that *in vivo* active compounds exhibited high (>60%) and sustained (>8 hours) receptor occupancy, while lower or less sustained receptor occupancies were predicted for inactive compounds (Figure 8.1). A cross-validation of predicted receptor occupancy with observed ex vivo receptor occupancy was also carried out, proving the validity of the simulations and of the assumptions used.

Such extension of PBPK simulations for the prediction of target effects is very powerful for generating insights into the efficacy or lack of *in vivo* efficacy

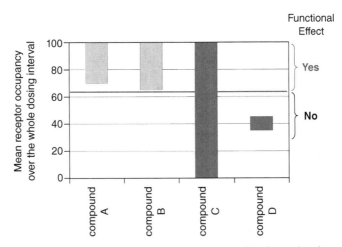

Figure 8.1 Simulations of receptor occupancy for active (gray bars) and inactive compounds (black bars) between two consecutive doses.

in relation to receptor occupancy. Consequently, such PBPK–PD simulations can be used as a filter between high-throughput screening and *in vivo* efficacy in order to prioritize compounds expected to be active *in vivo*.

8.4.2. Example: Viral Disease Model to Support Definition of Target Product Profile

PK–PD modeling has been especially useful for the development of compounds for viral disease due to the lack of robust animal models for efficacy. Before lead optimization, the target product profile (TPP) needs to be carefully defined, as it has considerable influence on subsequent screening, optimization strategy, and development time. In this antiviral project, the goal was to define a target concentration at the end of the dosing interval (C_{min}) in relation to the IC_{90} measured *in vitro* and protein binding. Review of clinical data of antiviral compounds revealed a wide range for the ratio C_{min}/IC_{90} with approximately 2 to 3 order-of-magnitude differences, depending on the compound. A PK–PD–viral disease model incorporating mechanistic understanding of each class of compound was developed based on available clinical data to guide the team in setting a competitive target. This model was developed to include relevant preclinical data inputs, such as predicted C_{min} levels in humans by PBPK modeling and IC_{50} from the *in vitro* assay. This combined PBPK–PD model was able to predict successfully the viral kinetics in the two-week treatment period for at least two classes of antiviral compounds in disease populations (Figure 8.2). This validated model was then used to help define the TPP for the project and to address the questions posed above.

The benefits of applying a PBPK–PD and disease progression model in early drug lead optimization are multiple. First, the learning from developing a model based on available clinical data (including competitor compounds) can be effectively and quantitatively translated into lead optimization efforts. Second, the potency in an *in vitro* assay and pharmacokinetic properties for a compound can be stated in the context of the clinical efficacy predicted in a relevant disease population. Third, the PBPK–PD–disease mechanism model allows identification of sensitive parameters for further optimization efforts. Thus, the model allows one to understand the relative impact of potency versus PK on the expected outcomes.

8.4.3. Example: PK–PD Modeling for Identifying the Therapeutic Window Between an Efficacy and a Safety Response

This example demonstrates the use of PK–PD modeling in a lead optimization stage project to determine the relationship between plasma concentrations and both an efficacy and safety PD effect, to determine which candidate compound has a large enough margin of safety for clinical success. Investigators have shown that selective agonists of the α_{1a} receptor can cause increased pressure in the urinary tract (Blue et al., 2004), which could lead to decreased

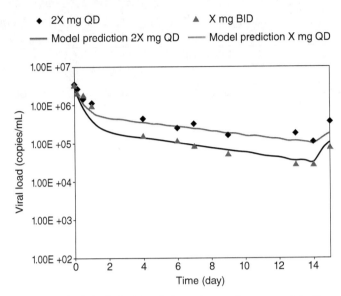

Figure 8.2 Observed clinical viral load data observed compared to those predicted from a PBPK–PD–disease model. Model predictions showed that the twice-daily dose regimen was more efficacious than the once-daily dose regimen having the same total daily dose. Drug treatment started at day 0 and lasted for 14 days.

symptoms from stress urinary incontinence (SUI). However, agonism of the α_{1a} receptor can also cause increased blood pressure (e.g., the α_{1a} agonist midodrine treats orthostatic hypotension but can cause dangerously increased supine blood pressure if taken too soon before bedtime). Blood pressure is a carefully regulated physiological phenomenon, and, at low doses of an α_{1a} agonist, as the blood pressure increases, the heart rate decreases rapidly to compensate, resulting in no net change in blood pressure. But with increasingly high doses of an α_{1a} agonist, the ability of the heart rate to compensate is swamped and the blood pressure will start to increase. The project described here was aimed at developing an α_{1a} partial agonist that could increase pressure in the urinary tract while avoiding any increase in blood pressure effects, which would make it a promising medicine for SUI (Musselman et al., 2004).

The first compound evaluated, referred to as compound 1, had been used in a clinical trial to demonstrate that this class of compounds has the potential to improve the symptoms of SUI (Musselman et al., 2004). Data pertinent to cardiac safety for compound 1 in humans (i.e., heart rate and supine systolic blood pressure) were available (Musselman et al., 2004). A preclinical model, the conscious minipig, showed increased urethral tone at low doses with candidate partial agonists as determined using a catheter that determined pressure throughout the length of the urethral tract. With increasing doses of compound 1 in humans, the conscious minipig showed first a decreased heart rate and, eventually, increased blood pressure (Blue et al., 2004). To assess the predictivity of the preclinical animal model, PK–PD modeling was used to compare the cardiac safety of the compound in clinical development, compound 1, in both the minipig model and in humans. Once the predictivity of the model was verified, the model was used to assess the margin of safety in lead optimization candidates to determine which compounds to move forward into clinical development.

The PK–PD analysis was begun by plotting PD response as a function of plasma concentrations for individual minipigs. No hysteresis was observed for intraurethral pressure (IUP), blood pressure (BP), or heart rate (HR), indicating that the time course of the effect could be related to the time course of plasma concentrations. The data for multiple animals and dosage levels were pooled to establish the PK–PD relationship. Sigmoidal E_{max} models were used to fit the data observed for PD effects (i.e., ΔIUP, ΔHR, and ΔBP, where the Δ symbol indicates change from baseline) as functions of plasma drug concentration (C_p):

$$\Delta \text{IUP} = E_{\text{max}_{\text{IUP}}} \frac{C_p^\gamma}{\text{EC}_{50\text{IUP}}^\gamma + C_p^\gamma} \tag{8.1}$$

$$\Delta \text{BP} = E_{\text{max}_{\text{BP}}} \frac{C_p^\gamma}{\text{EC}_{50\text{BP}}^\gamma + C_p^\gamma} \tag{8.2}$$

$$\Delta \text{HR} = E_{\text{max}_{\text{HR}}} - \left(E_{\text{max}_{\text{HR}}} - E_{0\text{HR}} \right) \frac{C_p^\gamma}{\text{EC}_{50\text{HR}}^\gamma + C_p^\gamma} \tag{8.3}$$

The resulting models were used to determine the plasma concentrations that would result in an efficacious response (i.e., a high enough value of ΔIUP to result in efficacy) or that would result in a 5-bpm drop in HR or a 5-mmHg increase in BP, which would be considered an unacceptable change in heart rate or blood pressure.

This PK–PD assessment was useful for the project for several reasons. First, the modeling allowed a clear assessment of compound efficacy and of the safety window between the plasma concentrations required for efficacy and those that would result in cardiac safety issues. For compound 1, the safety margin was about ninefold; that is, the C_p value resulting in a 5-mmHg ΔBP was about nine times higher than the C_p required for efficacy. For candidate compound 2, the safety margin was lower (5.9) than for compound 1, but for all other candidates the safety margin was higher. Second, the PK–PD modeling could be combined with a human PK extrapolation to provide a clear prediction as to whether efficacy could be achieved in the clinic while avoiding the cardiac safety effect. For example, compound 3 had rapid clearance, and initially there were doubts that it would be a good clinical candidate. But using the PK–PD models coupled with a prediction of human PK for the compound, it was determined that the margin of safety was high enough that even with a large peak-to-trough ratio, compound 3 would not only be efficacious in the clinic, but would also have a large margin of safety. These parameters have been used to select compounds for preclinical development. Finally, PK–PD modeling was used to provide guidance for the design of some clinical studies. For this guidance, a PK model was combined with the PK–PD models to simulate certain dosage regimens and dose levels to determine an optimal clinical trial design.

8.5. USE OF PK–PD MODELS IN CLINICAL CANDIDATE SELECTION

PK–PD has a great potential to assist clinical candidate selection when numerous factors must be considered and data related to the PK and PD of a compound need to be combined and compared in a rational way. This potential is illustrated below by a number of examples. Examples are also available in the literature: for example, Parrott et al. (2005) demonstrated the use of combined PBPK and PK–PD modeling to select the best clinical lead from among five candidates. The preclinical data for the five candidates were integrated and the efficacious human doses and associated exposures were estimated. The PBPK models were linked to a PD model so that the dose resulting in a 90% effect could be identified. This example showed that the PBPK approach facilitates a sound decision on the selection of the optimal molecule to be progressed by integrating the available information and focusing attention on the properties expected in humans. Importantly, the method can include estimates of variability and uncertainty in the predictions to allow decisions to be based on significant differences between the compounds.

In another example, a mechanism-based PK–PD model incorporating target-mediated binding and clearance of an antibody was developed for the candidate selection stage of backup molecules for omalizumab (Agoram et al., 2007). The challenge addressed by the modeling was to understand the relationship between dose, *in vitro* affinity, and *in vivo* efficacy in humans for the follow-on compounds. The PK–PD model was developed based on clinical data of omalizumab, and *in vivo* efficacy was based on a surrogate marker of maximum reduction in the free IgE level. Unlike other empirical models, the construction of such a mechanism-based model makes it easy to separate the system–disease parameter from the drug parameter. As such, the model was flexible enough to account for different properties from another antibody, including different interactions of the antibody in the system, on–off rates from the antigen, and capacity-limited distribution and elimination of antibody. A critical finding based on the sensitivity analysis of the model was that similar maximum reduction of free IgE could be achieved by half the dose if the antibody affinity for IgE was 5- to 10-fold higher than omalizumab. Further increase in affinity would not increase *in vivo* efficacy. This insight from the modeling could avoid expensive affinity maturation steps. The resulting model was able to help clinical lead selection of backup mAb. In addition, the model could easily be adapted for other follow-up compounds and used to model different disease populations (e.g., different beseline IgE levels).

8.6. ENTRY-INTO-HUMAN PREPARATION AND TRANSLATIONAL PK–PD MODELING

Translational PK–PD is a continuous process starting with human projections during preclinical development and stretching as far as into phase II. Whereas compound selection is the focus at discovery stages, in the entry-into-human (EIH) phase, attention shifts more to questions of safety and study design. In particular, concerned studies are GLP toxicology (phase 0), single ascending dose/multiple ascending dose (phase I), and proof of concept (phase II).

The EMEA (European Medicines Agency) "Guideline on the Clinical Investigation of the Pharmacokinetics of Therapeutic Proteins" (http://www.emea.europa.eu/pdfs/human/ewp/8924904enfin.pdf) recommends evaluating the relationship between drug concentration and pharmacodynamic response (PK–PD) and considers it to be an important tool for drug development:

> Early pre-clinical and clinical data can be evaluated using appropriate models for a mechanistic understanding of the disease and the PK–PD relationship. PK–PD models may be developed accounting for the time-delay between plasma concentrations and measured effect. The model might also need to take into account the pharmacokinetics of the therapeutic target. PK–PD models may allow extrapolation from volunteers to target population given that suitable assumptions have been made, e.g., regarding pathological factors. These models may provide guidance for dose selection and are helpful when interpreting changes in the pharmacokinetics in important subpopulations or when evaluating comparability. Effort to explore relevant biomarkers and their link (surrogacy) to safety and efficacy endpoints is encouraged.

The extrapolation from healthy volunteers to the target population as noted here is similar to the extrapolation from single-dose PK in animals to toxicology study design and for the extrapolation from animals to humans for dose estimation.

8.7. USE OF PK–PD MODELS IN TOXICOLOGY STUDY DESIGN AND EVALUATION

Among the various observations made in toxicology studies, often only a few are amenable for PK–PD modeling, and even fewer can be predicted beforehand to improve the toxicology study design. Therapeutic proteins and monoclonal antibodies in particular are an important exception to that rule, since toxicity is often driven by exaggerated pharmacology.

8.7.1. Example: Target-Related Toxicity

For compound A, target-related toxicity was anticipated based on observations from different compounds sharing the same or a similar mechanism of action. However, the signs of toxicity seen in the study appeared later and were much less pronounced than expected. Retrospective comparison to two similar compounds showed that (1) for compound B, which has about a 10-fold higher affinity than A, the time to appearance of toxicity seemed to decrease with dose (with a lag of about two months at the lowest dose); and (2) for compound C, which has a more than 100-fold higher affinity than A, the time of appearance of toxicity did not depend on dose and was similar to that reported for the highest dose of compound B (one to two weeks), suggesting that the appearance of this type of toxicity depends on the ratio of exposure and the dissociation constant at the target (i.e., on target occupancy).

8.7.2. Example: Impact of Dynamic Physiological Processes on Toxicity Readouts

Compound M, a monoclonal antibody, depletes its target from the blood. The original toxicology study was planned based on a 13-week period with weekly dosing at 100 mg/kg and a 13-week washout and recovery phase. With the data available from a single-dose PK study in which the target was monitored and compared to existing models for similar compounds, it was possible to construct a turnover model for the target with a stimulated depletion by the compound. With this model it was shown that clinical observation had to extend until at least week 40 of the study to see partial recovery of the target, which was later confirmed. This also showed that the slow recovery of the target was not due to any unexpected toxicity but was probably the normal result of pharmacological activity. This knowledge is somewhat counterintuitive and would have been difficult to predict without quantitative modeling.

8.7.3. Example: Modeling Downstream Compound and Metabolite Effects

Rich PK–PD data are usually available in telemetry studies monitoring cardiac safety. Accurate interpretation of such studies is complicated by interindividual variability of PK, interindividual variability of PD baseline values and PD susceptibility, circadian baseline variations, and the time lag of the PD response with respect to PK. A PK–PD modeling approach was used in two recent projects with the benefit of objectively quantifying the exposure–response relationship. In this example, the compound was efficacious in an animal model of depression and pain. The compound was found to be a moderate inhibitor based on an *in vitro* hERG assay and was estimated to have a sufficient safety margin. However, the compound showed a tendency to prolong the QTc interval in a dog telemetry study. The challenge was to understand the mechanism of QT liability and to devise a strategy/screening assay for the backup compounds. There appeared to be some dissociation between the concentration profile of the parent compound (T_{max}: 1 to 2 hours) and the onset of the QT effect (7 to 8 hours post-dose). A major metabolite was identified (with exposure of 30 to 40% of parent exposure in dogs), where the QT effect coincided more closely with the metabolite exposure profile.

The impacts of PK–PD modeling on the investigation into key mechanistic effects in this example can be seen from several aspects. Perhaps most significantly, the compartment modeling collapsed the hysteresis loop (effect vs. concentration profile of parent compound), resulting in a profile more closely related to the concentration–time profile of the metabolite. Hence, this analysis strongly supported the key hypothesis that the metabolite was responsible for the QT effect observed *in vivo*.

8.8. JUSTIFICATION OF STARTING DOSE, CALCULATION OF SAFETY MARGINS, AND SUPPORT OF PHASE I DESIGN

Dose selection depends crucially on safety and efficacy projections. For example, the EMEA guideline regarding the first dose in humans states: "The estimation of the first dose in human is an important element to safeguard the safety of subjects participating in first-in-human studies. All available information has to be taken in consideration for the dose selection and this has to be made on a case-by-case basis." At the simplest level, this is done by projecting PK (using PBPK or other approaches) and relating C_{max} and the area under the course (AUC) for safety (typically, from the no observable adverse effect level, adjusted for species differences and with additional safety factors applied) or to C_{min} and AUC for efficacy (typically inferred from an animal model). Even though quantities such as C_{min} for efficacy might be derived from PK–PD in animal models, this approach does not deserve the label of PK–PD since it falls short of many important aspects of drug action. PK–PD modeling using safety endpoints has been used successfully to analyze ECG alterations during telemetry studies in animals, as described in Section 8.7.

With respect to compounds for which *factors of risk* have been identified according to the EMEA "Guideline on Strategies to Identify And Mitigate Risks for First-in-Human Clinical Trials with Investigational Medicinal Products" (http://www.emea.europa.eu/pdfs/human/swp/2836707enfin.pdf), dose calculation should rely additionally on the minimal anticipated biological effect level (MABEL). Even without such known risks, health authorities have requested the calculation of MABEL in some recent examples of therapeutic proteins. The guideline specifies:

> The calculation of MABEL should utilize all *in vitro* and *in vivo* information available from pharmacokinetic–pharmacodynamic (PK–PD) data such as:

- target binding and receptor occupancy studies *in vitro* in target cells from human and the relevant animal species;
- concentration–response curves *in vitro* in target cells from human and the relevant animal species and dose/exposure–response *in vivo* in the relevant animal species;
- exposures at pharmacological doses in the relevant animal species.

Wherever possible, the above data should be integrated in a PK–PD modeling approach for the determination of the MABEL.

Limited practical experience shows that a unique estimate of MABEL is often difficult to achieve due to disparities between, for example, *in vitro* receptor binding, *in vitro* cellular assays, and *in vivo* animal models. Taken to the letter, that is, when the above-mentioned factors of risk have been identified, the lowest of these values is relevant and additional safety factors may be applied. In other cases, these estimates may seem exceedingly low, considering the following limitations: technical (difficulty in providing formulations at very low doses, difficulty in assessing exposure), ethical (if the study is done on patients, many patients are treated without probable benefit), operational (difficulty in recruiting additional cohorts, especially if the study is done on patients), and economical (long duration of trials).

At this stage all available preclinical (*in vitro* and *in vivo*) information is considered to estimate an efficacious dose for humans. If a PK–PD model can be established to relate exposure at the target site and target effects (as inferred from *in vitro* assays) in animal models, this model can be used for translation to humans by adapting such species-specific factors as metabolism, protein binding, and receptor affinity. Ideally, if receptor occupancy calculated from target organ exposure, protein binding, and receptor affinity adequately predicts the outcome of a behavioral test in animal models, there is a certain degree of confidence that a useful prediction of the efficacious dose in humans can be made by predicting receptor occupancy in humans. An obvious premise to do so is that the animal model in question can be considered relevant for the human disease.

The first hurdle is the estimation of exposure at the target site. When the target compartment is in rapid exchange with circulating blood, it is assumed that the effect is driven by the unbound concentration of compound in the blood. This becomes critical in cases where the relevant pharmacological concentrations are impossible or difficult to assess, whether because of low penetration or because the pharmacological activity is driven by an (unknown) fraction of the compound present in the organ. This situation may be present when targeting the brain with small molecules (unknown free fraction) or with therapeutic proteins (unknown penetration), when targeting tumors (limited by binding barrier, interstitial fluid pressure, "mechanical"), and when targeting liver (unknown transport, metabolism, protein binding). Where this information is missing, mechanistic models have been built to estimate relevant exposure, possible delays in drug action, and to identify limiting factors with large differences between species or phenotypes or the influence of co-medication.

At the target level, species differences in binding affinity at the target need to be taken into account. Furthermore, often only unbound compound confers pharmacological activity, and factors such as plasma protein binding have to be considered. These are the rather obvious factors; however, some binding reactions become exceedingly complex and require modeling, as shown in the examples below.

8.8.1. Example: Dimerization and Bell-Shaped Dose Responses

A compound has been reported that dimerizes two serum amyloid protein (SAP) molecules, and it was shown that these dimers are rapidly removed from the body; the reduction of SAP is the primary endpoint of this therapy. Since each SAP entity is itself composed of five identical non-covalently bound subunits, the binding stoichiometry is highly nontrivial, leading to a bell-shaped curve for the formation of dimers and hence for the dose–response. This model was used to predict efficacious doses in humans and was a valuable input to assess the feasibility of the project.

8.8.2. Example: Interactions Between Endogenous and Exogenous Analogs

Fatty acids, hormones, vitamins, and other physiologically crucial entities are bound to specific binding proteins that control their homeostasis. The consequences of pharmacological interference with this system are difficult to grasp by intuition alone and require modeling, in particular for the extrapolation to humans (species differences) or to guide the choice of dosing regimens. Both the endogenous hormone and its analog will drive the response; furthermore, the turnover of both the hormone itself and the binding protein will be changed.

8.8.3. Example: Factors Influencing Antibody-Mediated Responses

Multivalent binding or cross-linking is an important component of some antibody-mediated responses. Obviously, this response is no longer a function of antibody (or antigen) concentration alone, but depends on all system components: the species, the specific tissue, the disease state, and the presence of antigen (Lowe et al., 2007).

8.9. PHASE I AND BEYOND

Whenever the information on efficacy and biomarkers gathered during phase I is not sufficient to build the rationale for a phase II design, preclinical data and mathematical models need to fill the gap. This approach has the advantages that questions of safety are elucidated at that stage and that the PK–PD models can be updated with data-driven models of PK.

8.9.1. Example: Overcoming Adverse Events Observed in Phase I

During phase I of a compound, target-related adverse events were observed at unexpectedly low doses with a steep dose–response relationship. PK–PD-related questions were:

- Is there anything that could have hinted at the steep dose–response relationship?
- Could a slow-release formulation have helped avoid adverse effects by reducing C_{max} with AUC maintained?
- Given the preclinical pharmacology findings, what are the chances that the backup compound has a better safety profile?

By combining dose–response relationships from preclinical models, calculated receptor occupancy, and PBPK modeling, one can begin to address these questions.

8.9.2. Example: Inconclusive Phase I Data

For a compound targeting a neurological disorder, the observations from phase I were considered insufficient to serve as the basis for the phase II design, whereas the safety profile was found to be as expected. The phase II design then relied strongly on a model predicting brain penetration, target binding, and cerebrospinal fluid exposure. The model, in turn, was built using preclinical data and literature from the public domain, and was updated with PK observed during phase I.

8.9.3. Example: Enhancing Dose Selection

There are strong reasons to believe that a given oncology compound in phase I was efficacious. However, there is uncertainty about whether phase II results will make it possible to select an efficacious safe dose. The overriding concern is that given the good safety profile, the doses selected will be higher than optimal. Additional PK–PD studies, together with modeling, were conducted to build a stronger rationale for dose selection.

8.9.4. Example: PK–PD–Disease Model for a Novel Anti-HIV Drug

In this example, a PK–PD–disease model was developed to help design a phase IIa study of a novel anti-HIV drug, maraviroc (a CCR5-receptor antagonist). The model was based on the model published by Bonhoeffer et al. (1997), and was adapted for short-term treatment and for a different mechanism of action. The PK model parameters were derived from published literature, analysis of in-house phase IIa data from other HIV compounds, and from a single-dose study in healthy volunteers. The model was able to capture the complexity of viral dynamics in responding to treatment and was used to simulate a viral load–time profile under different dosage regimens for maraviroc. The model structure includes three components: PK, PD, and a disease model. PD is modeled using a sigmoid maximum effect model (E_{max}) to express the inhibition function (INH) obtained by maraviroc at a given plasma concentration divided by the sum of plasma concentration and EC_{50}. In the disease model, the HIV-1-infected cell compartment is modeled as a function of time, incorporating the viral load (V) and three types of cells: target $CD4^+$ cell (T), actively infected cells (A), and latently infected cells (L). The relationship between infectious virion and each type of cell was described by differential equations. INH is the parameter linking the PD model and the disease model. INH assumes a value of zero in the absence of the drug and a value of 1 when the drug reaches it maximal inhibition. The model was used to simulate different scenarios and to explore the impact of model uncertainty. The simulation and model were able to influence the design of the clinical studies and were used successfully to optimize the phase IIa development program.

8.10. SUPPORT OF EARLY FORMULATION DEVELOPMENT

In response to the high costs associated with discovery and development of a new chemical entity, there has been a paradigm shift, in which the formulation approach has been considered much earlier in drug development as a cost-effective method to eliminate deficiency and to allow development of a molecule to continue (Thombre, 2005). PK–PD modeling has been a basis of many success stories for reengineering old drugs via a controlled-release (CR) approach. One good example is shown by the successful development of an efficacious and compliance-friendly sustained-release formulation of OROS methylphenidate (CONCERTA) for attention-deficit hyperactivity disorder (Swanson et al., 2003). A quantitative characterization of the compound's PK in relationship to its efficacy or side effects via PK–PD modeling enabled selection of an appropriate controlled-release profile in order to achieve the desired PK and PD.

Mechanism-based PK–PD modeling has also been used to support the life-cycle management of a development compound. For example, PK–PD modeling revealed that increasing the circulating half-life of interferon alfa-2a twofold was of limited therapeutic benefit. Model-based predictions, corroborated by clinical trial results, provided a rationale for stopping the development of a new formulation of interferon despite its improved PK (Nieforth et al., 1996).

In another example of CR formulation for a compound under development for gastroesophageal reflux disease, the questions being asked were:

- Could the CR formulation increase 24-hour coverage of pH control, especially during the nighttime, compared to the immediate release (IR) formulation?
- Would the current CR formulation meet the TPP (at least 80% of time with pH > 4, at least 10% better than esomeprazole)?

The calculated dose without PK–PD modeling was estimated to be about three times higher than that for the current IR formulation, and the high-dose requirement projected based on AUC comparison did not support continuing the development program. In parallel, a PK–PD model was developed using available in-house data from the pilot study based on a mechanism-based indirect-response model for lansoprazole (Puchalski et al., 2001). Based on this PK–PD model, the simulated profile and predicted efficacy after multiple dosing was predicted to be consistent with the TPP. In addition, the dosage requirement estimated from the PK–PD modeling was substantially lower than the projected dosage based on AUC calculation. Therefore, in contrast to the AUC estimation, the PK–PD modeling work led to support for continuing the development program. Although there were uncertainties associated with the PK–PD model, the clinical data observed later confirmed the prediction from the PK–PD model—a much lower dose was required to achieve the TPP than that estimated from the AUC calculation. The lesson from this example is that a biological system is often nonlinear in nature and will not necessarily scale proportionately. PK–PD modeling takes into account time-dependent nonlinear changes in PK and PD which could otherwise be difficult to estimate.

The uncertainty associated with any PK–PD model should not hinder its use in decision making. Rather, uncertainty should be spelled out clearly and various scenarios simulated to assist the decision making. PK–PD modeling can provide a critical piece of information for advancing projects efficiently; "timing is everything" is also very true in drug development.

8.11. OUTLOOK AND CONCLUSIONS

In summary, consideration of DMPK and physicochemical properties as part of the drug discovery and development process has substantially improved the quality of drug candidates, especially their pharmacokinetic properties. The main reason for attrition in development is now related to safety and efficacy, and the current challenge is to establish a relationship between pharmacokinetic and pharmacological safety endpoints starting from early discovery stages. Historically, empirical models were used to address these questions. However, we suggest that more mechanistic-based models are needed to support preclinical drug discovery and early development. In this chapter, several PK–PD models were presented that have been employed from drug discovery through phase II. These mathematical models represent an important component of translational research, improving the efficiency of drug discovery and early development stages.

REFERENCES

Agoram, B.M., Martin, S.W., et al. (2007). The role of mechanism–based pharmacokinetic–pharmacodynamic (PK–PD) modelling in translational research of biologics. *Drug Discov Today 12*(23–24), 1018–1024.

Blue, D.R., Daniels, D.V., et al. (2004). Pharmacological characteristics of Ro 115-1240, a selective alpha1a/1L-adrenoceptor partial agonist: a potential therapy for stress urinary incontinence. *Br & Urol Int 93*(1), 162–170.

Bonhoeffer, S., May, R.M., et al. (1997). Virus dynamics and drug therapy. *Proc Natl Acad Sci U S A 94*(13), 6971–6976.

Chan, P.L., Nutt, J.G., et al. (2007). Levodopa slows progression of Parkinson's disease: external validation by clinical trial simulation. *Pharm Res 24*(4), 791–802.

Danhof, M., de Jongh, J., et al. (2007). Mechanism-based pharmacokinetic–pharmacodynamic modeling: biophase distribution, receptor theory, and dynamical systems analysis. *Annu Rev Pharmacol Toxicol 47*, 357–400.

Danhof, M., de Lange, E., et al. (2008). Mechanism-based pharmacokinetic–pharmacodynamic PK–PD modeling in translational drug research. *Trends Pharmacol Sci 29*, 186–191.

de Winter, W., de Jongh, J., et al. (2006). A mechanism-based disease progression model for comparison of long-term effects of pioglitazone, metformin and gliclazide on disease processes underlying type 2 diabetes mellitus. *J Pharmacokinet Pharmacodyn 33*(3), 313–343.

Dixit, N.M., Layden-Almer, J.E., et al. (2004). Modelling how ribavirin improves interferon response rates in hepatitis C virus infection. *Nature 432*(7019), 922–924.

Earp, J.C., Dubois, D.C., et al. (2008a). Modeling corticosteroid effects in a rat model of rheumatoid arthritis: I. Mechanistic disease progression model for the time course of collagen-induced arthritis in Lewis rats. *J Pharmacol Exp Ther 326*(2), 532–545.

Earp, J.C., Dubois, D.C., et al. (2008b). Modeling corticosteroid effects in a rat model of rheumatoid arthritis II: mechanistic pharmacodynamic model for dexamethasone effects in Lewis rats with collagen-induced arthritis. *J Pharmacol Exp Ther 326*(2), 546–554.

Friberg, L.E., Henningsson, A., et al. (2002). Model of chemotherapy-induced myelosuppression with parameter consistency across drugs. *J Clin Oncol 20*(24), 4713–4721.

Jones, H.M., Parrott, N., et al. (2006). A novel strategy for physiologically based predictions of human pharmacokinetics. *Clin Pharmacokinet 45*, 511–542

Khunvichai, A., Chu, H.M., Garg, V., Mchutchison, J.G., Lawitz, E., Rodriguez, M., Kieffer, T., and Alam, J. (2007). Predicting HCV treatment duration with an HCV protease inhibitor co-administered with PEG-IFN/RBV by modeling both wild-type virus and low level resistant variant dynamics. *Gastroenterology, 132*(4), A740–A741.

Krejsa, C.M., Horvath, D., et al. (2003). Predicting ADME properties and side effects: the BioPrint approach. *Curr Opin Drug Discov Dev 6*(4), 470–480.

Lavé, T., Parrott, N., et al. (2007). Challenges and opportunities with modelling and simulation in drug discovery and drug development. *Xenobiotica 37*(10–11), 1295–1310.

Layden, T.J., Layden, J.E., et al. (2003). Mathematical modeling of viral kinetics: a tool to understand and optimize therapy. *Clin Liver Dis 7*(1), 163–178.

Lemmens, H.J., Dyck, J.B., et al. (1994). Pharmacokinetic–pharmacodynamic modeling in drug development: application to the investigational opioid trefentanil. *Clin Pharmacol Ther 56*(3), 261–271.

Lobo, E.D., and Balthasar, J.P. (2002). Pharmacodynamic modeling of chemotherapeutic effects: application of a transit compartment model to characterize methotrexate effects *in vitro*. *AAPS PharmSci 4*(4), E42.

Lockwood, P., Ewy, W., et al. (2006). Application of clinical trial simulation to compare proof-of-concept study designs for drugs with a slow onset of effect; an example in Alzheimer's disease. *Pharm Res 23*(9), 2050–2059.

Lowe, P.J., Hijazi, Y., et al. (2007). On the anticipation of the human dose in first-in-man trials from preclinical and prior clinical information in early drug development. *Xenobiotica 37*, 1331–1354.

Mager, D.E., and Jusko, W.J. (2001). Pharmacodynamic modeling of time-dependent transduction systems. *Clin Pharmacol Ther 70*(3), 210–216.

Mager, D.E., Wyska, E., et al. (2003). Diversity of mechanism-based pharmacodynamic models. *Drug Metab Dispos 31*(5), 510–518.

Miller, R., Ewy, W., et al. (2005). How modeling and simulation have enhanced decision making in new drug development. *J Pharmacokinet Pharmacodyn 32*(2), 185–197.

Musselman, D.M., Ford, A.P., et al. (2004). A randomized crossover study to evaluate Ro 115-1240, a selective alpha1a/1L-adrenoceptor partial agonist in women with stress urinary incontinence. *Br & Urol Int 93*(1), 78–83.

Neumann, A.U., Lam, N.P., et al. (1998). Hepatitis C viral dynamics *in vivo* and the antiviral efficacy of interferon-alpha therapy. *Science 282*(5386), 103–107.

Nieforth, K.A., Nadeau, R., et al. (1996). Use of an indirect pharmacodynamic stimulation model of MX protein induction to compare *in vivo* activity of interferon alfa-2a and a polyethylene glycol–modified derivative in healthy subjects. *Clin Pharmacol Ther 59*(6), 636–646.

Parrott, N., Jones, H., et al. (2005). Application of full physiological models for pharmaceutical drug candidate selection and extrapolation of pharmacokinetics to man. *Basic Clin Pharmacol Toxicol 96*, 193–199.

Poirier, A., Lavé, T., et al. (2008). Design, data analysis and simulation of *in vitro* drug transport kinetic experiments using a mechanistic *in vitro* model. *Drug Metab Dispos*.

Puchalski, T.A., Krzyzanski, W., et al. (2001). Pharmacodynamic modeling of lansoprazole using an indirect irreversible response model. *J Clin Pharmacol 41*(3), 251–258.

Rosario, M.C., Jacqmin, P., et al. (2005). A pharmacokinetic–pharmacodynamic disease model to predict *in vivo* antiviral activity of maraviroc. *Clin Pharmacol Ther 78*(5), 508–519.

Rostami-Hodjegan, A., and Tucker, G.T. (2007). Simulation and prediction of *in vivo* drug metabolism in human populations from *in vitro* data. *Nat Rev Drug Discov 6*(2), 140–148.

Sheiner, L.B., Stanski, D.R., et al. (1979). Simultaneous modeling of pharmacokinetics and pharmacodynamics: application to *d*-tubocurarine. *Clin Pharmacol Ther 25*(3), 358–371.

Sheiner, L.B., and Steimer, J.L. (2000). Pharmacokinetic/pharmacodynamic modeling in drug development. *Annu Rev Pharmacol Toxicol 40*, 67–95.

Sun, Y.N., and Jusko, W.J. (1998). Transit compartments versus gamma distribution function to model signal transduction processes in pharmacodynamics. *J Pharm Sci 87*(6), 732–737.

Swanson, J., Gupta, S., et al. (2003). Development of a new once-a-day formulation of methylphenidate for the treatment of attention-deficit/hyperactivity disorder: proof-of-concept and proof-of-product studies. *Arch Gen Psychiatry 60*(2), 204–211.

Thombre, A.G. (2005). Assessment of the feasibility of oral controlled release in an exploratory development setting. *Drug Discov Today 10*(17), 1159–1166.

Woodcock, J., and Woosley, R. (2008). The FDA critical path initiative and its influence on new drug development. *Annu Rev Med 59*, 1–12.

PART III

APPLICATIONS TO DRUG DEVELOPMENT

CHAPTER 9

Developing Oncology Drugs Using Virtual Patients of Vascular Tumor Diseases

ZVIA AGUR

Institute for Medical Biomathematics, Bene-Ataroth, Israel; Optimata Ltd., Ramat-Gan, Israel

NAAMAH BLOCH, BORIS GORELIK, and MARINA KLEIMAN

Optimata Ltd., Ramat-Gan, Israel

YURI KOGAN

Institute for Medical Biomathematics, Bene-Ataroth, Israel

YAEL SAGI

Optimata Ltd., Ramat-Gan, Israel

D. SIDRANSKY

The Johns Hopkins University School of Medicine, Baltimore, Maryland

YAEL RONEN

Optimata Ltd., Ramat-Gan, Israel

9.1. INTRODUCTION

Despite growing capital investments of pharmaceutical companies in medical research and development, the number of new drugs placed on the market has dropped over the past decade. Moreover, in the wake of problems with Vioxx and other new drugs, the leading national and multinational regulatory agencies have become more cautious about approving new molecular entities (PricewaterhouseCoopers, 2008). The resulting shortage in drugs may have serious consequences on industry, society, and government, and a substantial

Systems Biology in Drug Discovery and Development, First Edition.
Edited by Daniel L. Young, Seth Michelson.
© 2012 John Wiley & Sons, Inc. Published 2012 by John Wiley & Sons, Inc.

crisis is foreseen if drug development becomes too risky and unprofitable. If the pharmaceutical industry is to remain at the forefront of medical research and to continue helping patients, it must become more innovative in reducing the development time and cost of new therapies.

Currently, the physical and toxicological properties of drug candidates are mostly studied *in vitro* by screens to find molecules that "hit" a designated target. The most promising candidates are then selected to be tested in animals. *In silico* methods are used to design new molecules only where the structure of the target is known. The new quantitative structure–activity relationship (QSAR) applications to drug development employed to predict absorption, distribution, metabolism, excretion, toxicity (ADMET) parameters are often more complex to use and are relatively early in their development. The pharmaceutical industry needs a faster and more predictive way of testing molecules before they go into humans.

One strategy is to use *virtual R&D*, R&D aided by computer simulations of the human body, to shorten dramatically the period of development of new drugs and to reduce substantially the chance of clinical failure, thus saving amortized costs across clinical development. Indeed, virtual mice, virtual monkeys, and virtual patients have already been developed and validated preclinically and clinically for accuracy of prediction of both drug efficacy and drug toxicity, as well as for suggesting improved drug regimens. For example, the use of virtual mice and rhesus monkeys accurately simulated mice and individual rhesus thrombopoieis and responses to different thrombopoietin (TPO) regimens, and suggested an improved TPO regimen which maintains drug efficacy but alleviates its immunogenic effects (Skomorovski et al., 2003). This virtual animal–suggested regimen keeps its superiority even following several years of TPO administration (Fatima et al., 2008). In another study, discussed briefly in this chapter, the use of virtual xenografted mice was validated prospectively for precise replication of tumor shrinkage in mice xenografted by biopsied tumors of a mesenchyma chondrosarcoma (MCS) patient treated by various combinations of biological and chemotherapy drugs. Upscaling drug-response parameters and embedding them in a virtual MCS patient resulted in an improved docetaxel regimen, which was administered to the patient, relieving pancytopenia and stabilizing disease (Gorelik et al., 2008b).

In this chapter we discuss the construction and use of the virtual patient technology. We focus on an important module of the virtual patient: tumor vascularization. Recently, tumor vascularization has emerged as an especially important target in drug development. A study by Cancer Research (UK), based on 974 cancer drugs starting initial phase I clinical trials since 1995, calculated that there was an 18% probability that a drug would make it to commercial registration, compared to 5% in 2004. The sharp improvement is due to more targeted drug development, which is based on better knowledge of the biology of cancer. Most notably, kinase inhibitors are almost three times more likely to reach patients than other types of anticancer drugs (Walker and

Newell, 2008). Well-known examples of kinase inhibitors include trastuzumab (Herceptin) and imatinib mesylate (Glivec). Trastuzumab suppresses angiogenesis by both induction of antiangiogenic factors and repression of proangiogenic factors, and imatinib mesylate impairs angiogenic capacity by normalization of vascularity. Understanding the dynamics of the complex angiogenesis-related processes is crucial for predicting long-term efficacy and safety of novel and more traditional drugs.

We will discuss the construction of a multiscale mathematical model for angiogenesis, from the molecular scale through the tissue scale, at various levels of model complexity. Rigorous mathematical analysis of the angiogenesis model is presented, and its role in drug development is discussed. Model validation in a treatment personalization case study is used to illustrate a new theranostic method, which in this case is based on angiogenesis modeling. Finally, we show how the angiogenesis model, embedded in the virtual patient technology, is used to demonstrate that an arrested drug candidate can be efficacious if applied in combination with sunitinib malate (Sutent).

9.2. MODELING ANGIOGENESIS

The first models of tumor angiogenesis appeared as early as the mid-1970s (Deakin, 1976; Liotta et al., 1977; Saidel et al., 1976), following the new J. Folkman paradigm concerning the crucial role of vascularization in tumor development (Folkman, 1971). These works, driven by experimental data on tumor progression in animals, accounted for growth and movement of tumor cells and tumor-supporting blood vessels, and their mutual influence. Since the early 1990s, along with significant advances in the understanding and detailed characterization of biological processes involved in tumor–blood vessel dynamics, a vast body of theoretical work has been developed by a variety of researchers. Several groups have published studies that developed and explored mathematical models describing various aspects of tumor-induced angiogenesis, tumor growth, and blood vessel dynamics. These works also addressed the significance of the foregoing processes for chemotherapeutic, radiological, or antiangiogenic treatments. Naturally, these models differ significantly both in their mathematical underpinnings and in the biological phenomena they represent. In many reviews (e.g., Alarcon et al., 2006; Araujo and McElwain, 2004; Mantzaris et al., 2004) an effort was made to summarize and compare the models. However, at present, no clear classification has been established. When attempting to present such a classification, one can select various criteria for comparison between models. One type of criterion relates to the formal details of the modeling approaches (i.e., type of equations used). In contrast, one can classify the works by their applications: namely, the exact biological phenomena captured by the model or the clinically relevant questions to which the model can be applied.

Below we describe several mathematical models depicting tumor growth and angiogenesis. We focus on models that have already been verified by pre-clinical and clinical studies. From a mathematical point of view, the models we discuss here neglect spatial aspects. Clearly, angiogenesis is a three-dimensional process, as is tumor growth itself. Consequently, most models developed in this field take into account the spatial dimensions of vessels and tumor growth. However, the immense complexity of the process, coupled with the intricacy of a spatial description, renders these models difficult to parameterize and thus almost impossible to investigate analytically and difficult to simulate numerically. All such models at present capture only part of the full and very complex picture (Mantzaris et al., 2004). Yet simpler models (e.g., those discussed herein) can account sufficiently for the tumor–vasculature dynamics observed and are used to explain and predict real experimental and clinical results, even though they overlook spatial aspects. Thus, using the models presented here allows incorporation of experimental data toward clinically meaningful validation and prediction. In addition, these models are both simple enough to allow efficient mathematical investigations and comprehensive enough to represent important components of the tumor angiogenesis.

9.2.1. Simple Two-Dimensional Modeling

The first model we present here was proposed by Hahnfeldt et al. in 1999. This simple model consists of two coupled ordinary differential equations (ODEs) describing tumor mass and vascular support. For the tumor dynamics, the basic hypothesis is that the tumor mass (V) (measured either in volume or cell units) follows the Gompertz growth law:

$$\dot{V} = -\lambda_1 \ln \frac{V}{K} V. \tag{9.1}$$

This equation is accepted as a standard description of saturated tumor growth, supported by experimental evidence (Skehan, 1986; Spratt et al., 1996). The parameter λ_1 is a constant relating the dimensionless expression $\ln(V/K)$ to the growth rate. The parameter K is usually termed the *carrying capacity* of the tumor, to which the tumor mass always converges. From a practical point of view, K is a constant representing the maximal tumor burden the host could support, and when the tumor mass approaches this value, the growth rate is reduced to zero. This may be explained by a limitation on the nutrient supply, as shown both experimentally (Freyer and Sutherland, 1980; Kunz-Schughart, 1999; Sutherland et al., 1971) and theoretically (Byrne, 1999; Greenspan, 1974; Landry et al., 1982; Marusić et al., 1994) for avascular tumors in which growth was limited due to lack of diffusion of exterior nutrients.

The ability of a tumor to recruit a vascular system through angiogenic signaling has an augmenting effect on the tumor carrying capacity, due to better availability of nutrients. This simple concept was considered by

Hahnfeldt et al. (1999) in order to represent the contribution of recruited blood vessels and to describe the dynamics of vascular tumor growth and reaction to antiangiogenic treatment. In this model, K is no longer assumed constant, and its behavior is given by the second ODE in the general form

$$\dot{K} = -\lambda_2 K + bS(V,K) - dI(V,K) - eKg(t). \tag{9.2}$$

Here K is the time-dependent carrying capacity of the tumor, representing the effectiveness of the vascular support; λ_2 represents the intrinsic spontaneous loss of vasculature, resulting in decreased tumor support; $S(V,K)$ and $I(V,K)$ represent, respectively, the stimulatory and inhibitory effects produced by tumor and vasculature together; $g(t)$ is the current concentration of antiangiogenic drug; and b, d, and e are rate constants. To further characterize the functions $S(V,K)$ and $I(V,K)$, the authors refer to the experimental observation that stimulatory factors are local and short-lived, while inhibitory factors act over a longer range and time span (Hahnfeldt et al., 1999). The explicit formulations of these functions are established using the following argumentation. A diffusion–reaction equation for a stimulator or inhibitor concentration, n, is written

$$\frac{\partial n}{\partial t} = D^2 \nabla^2 n - cn + s, \tag{9.3}$$

where D is a diffusion coefficient, c the decay rate, and s a production rate, assumed to be equal to s_0 inside the tumor and zero outside the tumor. To solve this equation it is assumed that the tumor grows relatively slowly, $\partial n/\partial t = 0$, and that the tumor is spherically symmetric of radius r_0. Via these assumptions, one can obtain an explicit expression for the concentration n inside and outside the tumor:

$$n_{\text{inside}}(r) = \frac{s_0}{c}\left[1 - (1 + u_0)e^{-u_0}\frac{\sinh u}{u}\right], \qquad n_{\text{outside}}(r) = \frac{s_0}{c}(u_0 \cosh u_0 - \sinh u_0)\frac{e^{-u}}{u},$$

$$\tag{9.4}$$

where $u_0 = r_0 c^{1/2}/D$ and $u = rc^{1/2}/D$. Assumptions regarding the clearance rates can be applied next. For the inhibitor it is assumed that $c \ll D^2/r_0^2$, leading to

$$n_{\text{inhibitor,inside}}(r) \approx \frac{s_0}{6D^2}(3r_0^2 - r^2), \qquad n_{\text{inhibitor,outside}}(r) \approx \frac{s_0 r_0^2}{3D^2 r}. \tag{9.5}$$

For the stimulator, c is assumed to be large and

$$n_{\text{stimulator,inside}}(r) \approx \frac{s_0}{c}, \qquad n_{\text{stimulator,outside}}(r) \approx 0. \tag{9.6}$$

It is concluded that the overall impact of the inhibitor grows as r_0^2 (i.e., as $V^{2/3}$), while the effect of the stimulator is independent of tumor size and vascularization. Thus, the inhibitor term is taken to be $dV^{2/3}K$ (i.e., the rate of decay of K being defined by r_0^2). Further, for a similar reason it is argued that the ratio between inhibitor and stimulator terms in Eq. (9.2) will be approximately $K^\alpha V^\beta$, with $\alpha + \beta \approx 2/3$. This relation gives the stimulation function in the form $bV^\gamma K^\delta$, where $\gamma + \delta \approx 1$. This term is assumed by Hahnfeldt et al. (1999) to be of the form bV. Equation (9.2) then takes the form

$$\dot{K} = -\lambda_2 K + bV - dV^{2/3}K - eKg(t). \qquad (9.7)$$

The expression for the drug concentration is computed using the standard one-compartment linear PK model:

$$g(t) = \int_0^t C(\tau)e^{-k_e(t-\tau)}d\tau, \qquad (9.8)$$

where $C(\tau)$ is the rate of administration of the antiangiogenic drug and k_e is the elimination rate for this drug.

This model is applied to the control and treatment data for three angiogenesis inhibitors: mouse endostatin, mouse angiostatin, and TNP-470 [see Hahnfeldt et al. (1999) for experimental details]. The model was fitted to the control data and to one dosage experiment for each drug. Subsequently, it successfully predicted the experimental results using different dosages of endostatin and a combination of angiostatin and endostatin. Further, from the simulations it was found that in the absence of treatment, the ratio V/K increases asymptotically to 1 and the tumor size is limited. Simulations also suggested that the vasculature is more responsive to antiangiogenic treatment and that more continuous delivery of the drug may have enhanced efficacy.

In the continuation work (Sachs et al., 2001), the model was modified slightly, removing the linear decay term, $\lambda_2 K$, which has a weak influence on the system dynamics. This model is found to have a single global attractor in the positive V,K quadrant, with the steady-state values $V_0 = K_0 = (b/d)^{3/2}$, supporting the results of the simulations reported by Hahnfeldt et al. (1999).

To summarize, the model presented above illustrates the application of mathematical theory to biological reasoning and practical clinical questions. The model's underlying assumptions are based on two major biological observations: that blood vessels in the tumor microenvironment support tumor growth, and that angiogenesis is stimulated by the tumor. Biological knowledge about the competition between the stimulatory and inhibitory angiogenesis factors is also translated into assumptions for this minimal mathematical model, which is constructed to capture these important postulated properties. This approach allows one to analyze the model and check its validity by comparing its predictions to the experimental data. Furthermore, in this case, the model has a prognostic value, predicting the outcomes of applying a new monotherapy regimen and even drug combination.

9.2.2. Higher-Complexity Models

The models described below include additional details of tumor angiogenesis. Their first key feature is the introduction of one or more signaling molecules, which were discovered to be involved in angiogenic signaling. This progress in understanding the biology of angiogenesis enables formalizing the known properties of these cytokines. An additional key feature is motivated by experimental results reporting more complex dynamics of the tumor–vasculature system: in particular, an oscillatory pattern in the growth of tumor size and vessel density (Gilead et al., 2004; Gilead and Neeman, 1999; Holash et al., 1999). Since the model of Hahnfeldt et al. (1999) does not reflect these two features, more detailed models are required to incorporate the cytokine role in the signaling cascade and allow for nonmonotonic and unstable behavior, even under no anticancer treatment.

First we describe the simplest model that incorporates the mediating role of angiogenic signaling by tumor cells. This model, developed by Agur et al. (2004), consists of three ODEs describing the dynamics of three variables: tumor size, N, amount of protein involved in angiogenic signaling, P, and volume of blood vessels, V.

The tumor growth rate is assumed to depend on nutrient supply, which is proportional to vessel density, defined by $E = V/N$; hence, the first equation:

$$\dot{N} = f_1(E)N. \tag{9.9}$$

Here, the function f_1 is increasing, $f_1(0) < 0$, $\lim_{E \to \infty} f_1(E) > 0$; that is, the tumor will regress for zero vessel density and will grow with bounded rate for high vessel density.

The signaling protein is assumed to be secreted by the tumor as a result of nutrient deficiency:

$$\dot{P} = f_2(E)N - \delta P. \tag{9.10}$$

Here, the function f_2 is decreasing, $f_2(0) > 0$, $\lim_{E \to \infty} f_2(E) = 0$; that is, when the vessel density is large, the secretion of the proangiogenic protein drops, while at small vessel density each tumor cell secretes more protein. The second term accounts for first-order decay of the protein.

The size of the vessels is determined by the protein as follows:

$$\dot{V} = f_3(P)V. \tag{9.11}$$

Here, the function f_3 is increasing, $f_3(0) < 0$, $\lim_{E \to \infty} f_3(E) > 0$; that is, small amount of protein causes vessel regression, while high amounts induce growth of vasculature.

The model given by Eqs. (9.9) to (9.11) was numerically studied by Agur et al. (2004) and Forys et al. (2005) using sigmoidlike functions. It turns out that in contrast to the previous models, here no biologically relevant positive stable steady state exists. Note that the steady state $N = P = E = 0$ is of no interest, since the model describes the dynamics of existing vascular tumors. It was proven analytically by Forys et al. (2005) in this model that both the tumor and the vessel volume always grow monotonically, showing no oscillations. The vessel density can either increase unlimitedly or stabilize at some level, so that the tumor and the vessels grow proportionally, thus resembling the behavior of the previous model. Since these modeled tumor and vascular dynamics fail to capture the full range of the observed real-life cancer growth behavior, such as oscillations, one can consider the introduction of new assumptions that may enrich the model behavior.

The model above was extended by Agur et al. (2004) and Forys et al. (2005) by introducing time delays into the equations. Specifically, it is assumed that the current tumor growth rate and vessel formation rate depend on the prior vessel density and protein concentration some time before. Mathematically, this leads to the following system of delayed differential equations (DDEs):

$$\dot{N} = f_1(E(t - \tau_1))N, \tag{9.12}$$

$$\dot{P} = f_2(E)N - \delta P, \tag{9.13}$$

$$\dot{V} = f_3(P(t - \tau_2))V. \tag{9.14}$$

Here all the functions are the same as in the system of Eqs. (9.9) to (9.11), τ_1 and τ_2 are time delays, so, for example, tumor growth rate depends on vessel density some τ_1 time units ago rather than depending on the current vessel density. Agur et al. (2004) have shown that this model exhibits a specific behavior termed *Hopf bifurcation*: periodic oscillations of tumor size and vessel volume under some specific conditions. Since such behavior is observed in laboratory experiments in untreated animals (Arakelyan et al., 2003), it can thus be concluded that the system of Eqs. (9.12) to (9.14) is a minimal model able to reproduce the experimentally observed nonmonotonic behavior of the angiogenic tumor.

Bodnar and Foryś (2009) modified the models expressed in Eqs. (9.9) to (9.11) and (9.12) to (9.14) by introducing the logistic term into the equation for tumor growth. The addition of this term is justified by the experimentally observed deceleration in tumor growth and the existence of a natural limit for the tumor size, even if no limitations are imposed by the vascular system. Thus, for the system of Eqs. (9.9) to (9.11), the first equation now becomes

$$\dot{N} = \alpha N \left[1 - \frac{N}{1 + f_1(E)} \right], \tag{9.15}$$

and for the system of equations with delay (9.12) to (9.14) the first equation becomes

$$\dot{N} = \alpha N \left[1 - \frac{N}{1 + f_1(E(t - \tau_1))} \right], \tag{9.16}$$

where f_1 is the same as in Eq. (9.9) and α is the maximal tumor growth rate. The analysis by Bodnar and Foryś (2009) shows that these two models always exhibit at least one stable steady state with $N > 0$, thus representing a realistic saturation in tumor growth. The model with delays also exhibits oscillatory behavior, similar to the model given by Eqs. (9.12) to (9.14).

It should be noted that the simple concept of carrying capacity as used by Hahnfeldt et al. (1999) was replaced in the models presented above by the more elaborate notion of vessel density, reflecting the relationship between the vessel volume and tumor size. In fact, the crucial factor governing tumor growth is the efficiency of the vascular support. To account for this, Arakelyan et al. (2002, 2005) introduced the notion of effective vessel density (EVD). It differs from the vessel density used previously in that it takes into consideration that different types of vasculature can contribute differently to nutrient supply. Following this notion, the blood vessels involved in tumor angiogenesis are divided into two groups: mature and immature. The more detailed description of the angiogenic process takes this distinction into account. The new vessels are formed by endothelial cells which proliferate and migrate upon angiogenic signals. These new vessels are immature, being less stable and less efficient in nutrient supply. These vessels may undergo maturation by being covered by pericytes, the smooth muscle cells. This process is governed by a different type of signal, the maturation signal. Mature vessels can also undergo destabilization, due to weakening of maturation signals or appearance of antimaturation signals. Experimental observations (Gilead and Neeman, 1999; Gilead et al., 2004; Holash et al., 1999) suggest that the dynamics of maturation and destabilization may be responsible for the nonmonotonicity in tumor and vasculature growth. Following these hypotheses, an additional model of five DDEs was proposed by Agur et al. (2004). This model describes the growth of immature and mature vessels, V_1 and V_2, respectively, as two interrelated processes. Two types of signaling proteins are considered. The first, P_1, is secreted by tumor cells and is assumed to stimulate immature vessel growth. Its role is equivalent to that of P in the previous models. The second protein, P_2, stimulates maturation. It is also assumed to be secreted by tumor cells. This model takes the following form:

$$\dot{N} = f_1(E(t - \tau_1))N, \tag{9.17}$$

$$\dot{P}_1 = f_2(E)N - \delta_1 P_1, \tag{9.18}$$

$$\dot{P}_2 = aN - \delta_2 P_2, \tag{9.19}$$

$$\dot{V}_1 = f_3(P_1(t - \tau_2))V_1 - f_4(P_2)V_1 + f_5(P_2(t - \tau_3))V_2, \tag{9.20}$$

$$\dot{V}_2 = f_4(P_2)V_1 - f_5(P_2(t - \tau_3))V_2. \tag{9.21}$$

Here Eqs. (9.17), (9.18), and (9.20) are similar to Eqs. (9.12) to (9.14), except for the indices of P_1 and V_1 added here. The function f_4, accounting for the maturation rate, is positive and increasing. The function f_5 computes mature vessels destabilization; it is positive and decreasing to zero. In addition, the computation of E is changed. Now it depends on both types of vessels, $E = (\alpha_1 V_1 + \alpha_2 V_2)/N$, α_1 and α_2 being the relative contribution of immature and mature vessels to the effective vessel density. In this work they were both taken to be 1. This model also exhibits oscillatory behavior, suggesting the possible role of blood vessel maturation and destabilization in tumor growth.

Finally, a more comprehensive model of the processes discussed above has been developed to better represent experiments where human ovary carcinoma spheroid were implanted in mice and tumor growth as well as immature and mature vascular dynamics were monitored *in vivo* (Arakelyan et al., 2002, 2005). This model is formulated in terms of difference equations discrete in time and also by ODE formalism (analyzed in Section 9.3). The model captures the dynamics of the angiogenic tumor, calculating the following variables over time: (1) tumor size, (2) immature vessel density, (3) mature vessel density, (4) number of endothelial cells, (5) number of pericytes, (6) concentration of the angiogenic vascular endothelial growth factor (VEGF), (7) concentration of the maturation platelet-derived growth factor (PDGF), (8) concentration of the pro-maturation factor angiopoietin1 (denoted Ang1), and (9) concentration of its competitor, the antimaturation factor angiopoietin 2 (denoted Ang2). The equations for these variables reflect the biological understanding of the role of the system components, similar to the models described above. We refer the reader to Arakelyan et al. (2002) for a more detailed description.

Arakelyan et al. (2002) show that consistent with the simpler models, if the maturation process is neglected, tumor and vasculature growth become monotonic. In contrast, the introduction of vessel maturation and their destabilization dynamics into the model reduces tumor growth and leads to highly nonmonotonic behavior, including irregular oscillations of tumor and vasculature size. Further, by simulating anti-VEGF and anti-PDGF treatments, it was demonstrated that antiangiogenic treatment alone will not suffice to eliminate the tumor and has to be combined with antimaturation treatment. This prediction has been corroborated in the preclinical setting by showing in pancreatic cancer mouse models that the combination of a VEGFR inhibitor with another distinctive kinase inhibitor targeting PDGFR activity (Gleevec) was able to regress late-stage tumors (Bergers et al., 2003).

Arakelyan et al. (2005) have applied this model to results of animal experiments, in which implanted tumor size and vascularization were measured. The model was able to quantitatively reproduce the experimental data, including nonmonotonic changes of tumor size and mature and immature vessel density. The model predictions of subtle behaviors of mature and immature vessel dynamics were confirmed experimentally.

In summary, a more accurate and detailed description of system dynamics can be obtained using more complex models, which account for known relevant components and processes. Even more important, mathematical modeling allows one to determine the minimal necessary components required to produce the observed phenomena and to understand how the complex behavior emerges from basic system properties. Once validated experimentally, the model can be used to assist researchers to improve and accelerate drug development and help identify the most prominent treatment approaches.

9.3. USE OF RIGOROUS MATHEMATICAL ANALYSIS TO GAIN INSIGHT INTO DRUG DEVELOPMENT

Theoretical and numerical analyses are crucial elements in the development of a mathematical model that aims to mimic any realistic behavior of a biological or physical system. It enables one to take into consideration the types of behavior patterns that the model can reproduce. Typically, one would like to examine the robustness of the model to its initial conditions and check whether chaotic, periodic, or other types of behavior can arise. For example, comparing transfer function rates in dynamic systems can identify key processes, thereby enhancing biological understanding. Under specific conditions, analysis enables dissociation of certain parts of the model from others, and the consequences of decoupling these elements can be examined. When this occurs, one can test whether the model can be reduced to a simpler model. Analysis of the reduced model is frequently easier and can lead to a wider understanding of the system.

At the steady state of a dynamical system, all variables remain constant. Underlying processes may still be active in the steady state, yet the ongoing processes cancel out. An example of such processes is when constant production and elimination are equal in magnitude. Mathematically, the steady state of the system is denoted a *fixed point* of a system at a point where all the time derivatives of the system vanish simultaneously. At the fixed point, the steady-state problem is equivalent to solving a set of equations (in our case, this set of equations is nonlinear). Finding the fixed points of the system and understanding its in- and outflow can provide knowledge on the behavior patterns of the system.

The flow problem is referred to as *stability analysis*. It is addressed by checking how perturbations around the fixed point evolve in time. Fixed points can be characterized in several ways. Among them are (1) *stable fixed points*, where the system tends toward the fixed point; (2) *unstable fixed points*, where the system diverges away from the fixed point; and (3) *limit cycles*, where the system revolves in cycles around the fixed point.

The phase plane is a mathematical representation of the model variables at different time points and their values. The phase-plane analysis reveals the various behavior patterns of the system. To check the stability of the entire system, the Jacobian, a matrix of partial derivatives, is calculated. Often, numerical simulations are performed to create a map of possible points of the system. In this map, arrows indicate flow directions between points. This information is pivotal for comprehension of the model, regardless of our ability to analyze the entire phase plane.

The types of questions that we would like to answer by this stability analysis are the following: How many fixed points exist? Where in the phase plane do these fixed points occur? Are these fixed points stable? Are the fixed points identified biologically reasonable? For example, a trivial example of an unreasonably biological fixed point is when the system variables take negative values. These data regarding the biologically feasible steady-state conditions are of great relevance. In this way, steady-state analysis sheds light on how to stabilize or destabilize a biological system. This insight could be crucial in drug development efforts.

Establishing the existence of one or more fixed points in a solid tumor system, other than the obvious tumor-free one, is not trivial. Clinically, there is no significant evidence of stable untreated cancer patients. The prerequisite clinical success is to eliminate the tumor: that is, to achieve a complete response. However, a more likely possibility may be to transform a progressive disease into a chronic disease by stabilizing tumor progression. It is important to note that introduction of a drug to the system can give rise to additional fixed points. The existence of such additional fixed points will depend on the specific pharmacokinetic–pharmacodynamic (PK–PD) profile of that drug.

The behavior around the fixed points is important. Although, clinically, we are interested in stabilizing or reducing tumor size, model parameters other than tumor size, such as growth factors and vessel density, are of great relevance, as they dictate the behavior of the entire tumor. Thus, mathematical analysis of these factors is instrumental for proper targeting during the drug discovery process, and can serve in the target selection and validation processes. For example, targeting angiogenesis alone, by administering antiangiogenic monotherapy, is known only to delay tumor progression (Quesada et al., 2007). This phenomenon is an example of a system that does not converge to a fixed point (steady state) despite the imposed perturbations (pharmacotherapy). Furthermore, thresholds on variable levels may determine to which stable fixed point the system eventually converges.

In this section we attempt to find fixed points in a complex biological system for a vascular tumor model. The model underlying the work presented here has been described and analyzed previously (Agur et al., 2008; Arakelyan et al., 2002, 2003, 2005). The model in its simplified version is described here by a set of nonlinear ordinary differential equations. We show that this system has a nontrivial fixed point and define the conditions for its existence. For a further explanation of fixed points, see the book by Segel (1984).

9.3.1. Methods

Here we provide an example of a mathematical analysis searching for a fixed point in a biological nonlinear system. The model at hand is an angiogenesis-dependent solid tumor model. This model is a simplified version of an article by Arakelyan et al. (2002). The variables that represent this simplified model may be divided into three main groups.

1. The tumor variables: the number of living tumor cells, L, and the number of necrotic tumor cells, N. Both these variables are measured in volume in units of mm³.

2. The growth factor concentrations: consisting of vascular endothelial growth factor (VEGF), platelet-derived growth factor (PDGF), angiopeitin1 (Ang1), and angiopoeitin2 (Ang2); their amounts are measured in nanograms per milliliter (ng/mL).

3. The vessel-related variables: consisting of volume of immature vessels, V_{im}, mature vessels, V_{mat}, and free perycite cells, Per; their amounts are measured in mm³. The nutrition supply to the tumor is evaluated by the effective vessel density, EVD (Arakelyan et al., 2002), which is dependent on the vessel-related variables and the tumor-related variables.

The main model assumptions are listed below (see also Figure 9.1).

· Living cells, $L(t)$, can proliferate and can undergo necrosis. Both processes are controlled by the transfer function of nutrient supply to the tumor, EVD.

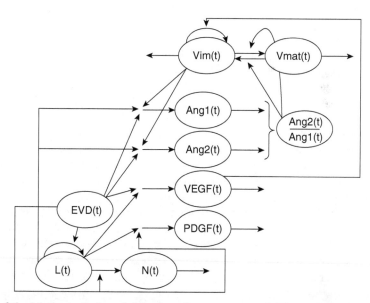

Figure 9.1 Mathematical model for vascular tumor growth. The notation for molecular and cellular entities is defined in the text. [From Arakelyan et al. (2002).]

- The number of necrotic cells grows according to the death of the living cells controlled by EVD.
- VEGF(t) is secreted by the living cells, $L(t)$, and its secretion is controlled by the nutrient supply to the tumor, EVD. VEGF disintegrates with a characteristic disintegration time.
- PDGF(t) is secreted by the living cells, $L(t)$, and its secretion is controlled by the nutrient supply to the tumor, EVD. PDGF also disintegrates.
- Ang1(t) is secreted by the living cells, $L(t)$. Ang1(t) is also produced by immature vessels. Its secretion in both cases is controlled by the nutrient supply to the tumor, EVD. Ang1 also disintegrates.
- Ang2(t) is treated in a manner similar to Ang1(t).
- Immature vessels can form mature vessels. This maturation process is controlled via transfer functions dependent on the amount of Ang1 and by the Ang1/Ang2 ratio. Destabilization of mature vessels occurs when mature vessels shed perycites and again become immature vessels. This is controlled via transfer functions dependent on the amount of Ang1 and Ang2 and on the Ang2/Ang1 ratio, thus enlarging the immature vessels pool. Immature vessels can also disintegrate in characteristic time.
- Mature vessels, $V_{mat}(t)$, are formed when immature vessels mature. These are exactly the same vessels that were subtracted from the immature vessels term. As mentioned above, this process is controlled via transfer functions dependent on the amount of Ang1 and on the Ang1/Ang2 ratio. Destabilization of mature vessels is controlled via transfer functions dependent on the amount of Ang1 and Ang2 and on the Ang2/Ang1 ratio. Mature vessels cannot disintegrate naturally. However, we added this term to the model to allow for a later drug effect on drug-related mature vessel functionality and disintegration.

To analyze the system efficiently, we utilize the fixed-point definition, the point where all time derivatives vanish, to relate a single model variable to all other model variables. In addition to model variables, this mathematical expression also involves model parameter values. As an example of this approach, we consider the volume of immature vessels in the tumor, V_{im}, as the single variable. Other choices would not alter the results.

We survey the model equations to identify their inner relations at the fixed point. First, we analyze the system as a whole, checking for the existence of fixed points. Second, we verify the possibility that this point(s) exists within the biologically realistic parameter space (e.g., positive values of variables such as cell numbers). We also show the existence of biologically relevant constraints on the system parameters. In this case these constrained parameters can be growth factor production rates, replication rates, and so on. Finally, we suggest a numerical method for identifying clinically relevant fixed points based on the mathematical analysis.

9.3.2. Theoretical Analysis of the Angiogenesis Model

Fixed-Point Analysis of the Equation for Living Cells The living cell equation at the fixed point is expressed as follows:

$$\dot{L} = \lambda_L \vec{f}_L(\text{EVD})L - \mu_L \overleftarrow{f}_L(\text{EVD})L \tag{9.22}$$

Here we establish the following definitions and relations:

- $\vec{f}_L(\text{EVD})$ is a monotonically increasing transfer function bounded by two asymptotes at 0 and 1.
- $\overleftarrow{f}_L(\text{EVD})$ is a monotonically decreasing transfer function bounded by two asymptotes at 0 and 1.
- $\text{EVD} = F(V_{\text{im}}, V_{\text{mat}}, L)$.

Demanding that the derivative of the living cell numbers vanish, $\dot{L} = 0$ yields the trivial zero solution and an additional solution:

$$\rightarrow \frac{\overleftarrow{f}_L(\text{EVD})}{\overrightarrow{f}_L(\text{EVD})} = \frac{\lambda_L}{\mu_L} \tag{9.23}$$

The existence of such an EVD, as in Eq. (9.23), depends on an overlap in the effectively nonzero parts of the transfer functions. As the increasing and decreasing functions describe modification of proliferation and death as a function of nutrition supply, it is obvious that the functions overlap to some extent. Equation (9.23) defines a unique value, or values, for EVD, which is used in the analysis for the rest of the equations.

Necrotic Cells The death of cells is described by

$$\dot{N} = \mu_L \overleftarrow{f}_L(\text{EVD})L - \mu_N N \tag{9.24}$$

so

$$\rightarrow N_0 = \frac{\mu_L}{\mu_N} \overleftarrow{f}_L(\text{EVD})L_0 \tag{9.25}$$

Substituting the expression obtained from EVD in Eq. (9.23) in $\overleftarrow{f}_L(\text{EVD})$ above yields a fixed point for N, the number of cells in necrosis, which depend solely on L. Hence, N_0, the number at the fixed point of necrotic cells, is related to L_0, the number of living cells, at the fixed point, and the already determined EVD value at the fixed point.

VEGF Growth Factor Similar to the necrotic cell case, the VEGF-level fixed point, VEGF_0, is obtained as a function of the living cell fixed point and EVD:

$$\dot{VEGF} = \lambda_{VEGF}^{L} \vec{f}_{VEGF}^{L}(EVD)L - \mu_{VEGF} VEGF \qquad (9.26)$$

so

$$\rightarrow VEGF_0 = \frac{\lambda_{VEGF}^{L}}{\mu_{VEGF}} \vec{f}_{VEGF}^{L}(EVD)L_0 \qquad (9.27)$$

The level of VEGF at the fixed point depends on the living cells and the EVD value at the fixed point.

PDGF Growth Factor   The PDGF fixed point is dictated by the living cells, similarly to that described above. In our system, PDGF secretion influences pericyte production.

Ang1 Growth Factor   The growth factors Ang1 and Ang2 are secreted by living cells and by endothelial cells that comprise the immature vessels:

$$\dot{Ang1} = \lambda_{Ang1}^{L} \vec{f}_{Ang1}^{L}(EVD)L + \lambda_{Ang1}^{Vim} \vec{f}_{Ang1}^{Vim}(EVD)V_{im} - \mu_{Ang1} Ang1 \qquad (9.28)$$

Demanding that $\dot{Ang1} = 0$,

$$Ang1_0 = \frac{\lambda_{Ang1}^{L}}{\mu_{Ang1}} \vec{f}_{Ang1}^{L}(EVD)L + \frac{\lambda_{Ang1}^{Vim}}{\mu_{Ang1}} \vec{f}_{Ang1}^{Vim}(EVD)V_{im} \qquad (9.29)$$

Ang2 Growth Factor

$$\dot{Ang2} = \lambda_{Ang2}^{L} \vec{f}_{Ang2}^{L}(EVD)L + \lambda_{Ang2}^{Vim} \vec{f}_{Ang2}^{Vim}(EVD)V_{im} - \mu_{Ang2} Ang2 \qquad (9.30)$$

Demanding that $\dot{Ang2} = 0$, Ang2's fixed point is obtained similarly to Ang1's. The levels of Ang2 and Ang1 at the fixed point depend on the number of living cells and the density of immature vessels at the fixed point, in addition to the EVD determined by Eq. (9.23).

Vessel Fixed Points   Immature vessels can proliferate. They are subtracted from the system when undergoing maturation, and they can be added to the system by mature vessels destabilization. They can also regress. The equation describing the immature vessel dynamics is therefore

$$\dot{V}_{im} = \lambda_{VEGF}^{Vim} \vec{f}_{VEGF}^{Vim}(VEGF)V_{im} + F(V_{mat}) - F(P, V_{im}) - \mu_{V_{mat}} \qquad (9.31)$$

The equations describing the mature vessel dynamics are governed by mature vessel creation by maturation of immature vessels and their destabilization.

$$\dot{V}_{mat} = F(P, V_{im}) - F(V_{mat}) - \mu_{V_{mat}} \qquad (9.32)$$

Adding up these two equations, upon demanding a fixed point $\dot{V}_{im} \equiv 0$ and $\dot{V}_{mat} \equiv 0$, yields a rather simple connection. Note: Some model elements do not appear in the steady-state solution, as they have been canceled out. The following result does not depend on their specific form:

$$\lambda_{VEGF}^{V_{im}} \vec{f}_{VEGF}^{V_{im}}(VEGF)V_{im} - \mu_{V_{im}}V_{im} = \mu_{V_{mat}}V_{mat} \tag{9.33}$$

This equation has important consequences, as detailed below.

1. There are links between V_{mat} and V_{im} at the fixed point by substituting in Eq. (9.33) three connections that have already been described:
   - The volume of living cells, L, in relation to V_{mat} and V_{im}, is defined by the expression of EVD and its value at the fixed point.
   - The living cells are related to the dead cells in Eq. (9.25).
   - VEGF is related to L in Eq. (9.27).

   Furthermore, once V_{mat_0} is related to V_{im_0}, the expression for EVD_0 can relate the living cells L_0 to V_{im_0}.

2. Another important consequence is revealed when we consider a system that lacks mature vessels ($V_{mat} = 0$) (e.g., very early in the tumor progression when mature vessels have not yet been formed, or under medication when mature vessels cannot be formed) in Eq. (9.33):

$$\lambda_{VEGF}^{V_{im}} \vec{f}_{VEGF}^{V_{im}}(VEGF) - \mu_{V_{im}} = 0$$
$$\rightarrow \vec{f}_{VEGF}^{V_{im}}(VEGF) = \frac{\mu_{V_{im}}}{\lambda_{VEGF}^{V_{im}}} \tag{9.34}$$

The transfer function values $\vec{f}_{VEGF}^{V_{im}}(VEGF)$ are limited by two horizontal asymptotes at zero and 1. Clearly, a meaningful result for Eq. (9.34) is obtained only if $\lambda_{VEGF}^{V_{im}} > \mu_{V_{im}}$, so that the transfer function values are smaller than 1. This gives a nontrivial biological constraint in this case ($V_{mat} = 0$) on the proliferation rate of the immature vessels relative to their regression rate.

It is possible to look for other fixed points where mature vessels are present in the model. This can be done only numerically, as the resulting system can be highly nonlinear. For these fixed points, the pericytes that cover vessel walls during the maturation process can be related to the immature vessels' V_{im}. This relationship is added to the connections between the rest of the variables and V_{im} described previously. Thus, a graphical solution to the general problem can be obtained by plotting $\dot{V}_{mat} = F(V_{im})$ and finding the intersection with the abscissa. We note that in this case the existence of such a fixed point can depend on the parameter values. No additional fixed points were found for any specific selection of parameters (not shown).

9.3.3. Discussion of Mathematical Analysis Methods

Solid tumors are an extremely complicated biological system that involves a plethora of internal and external factors. The theoretical analysis of an angiogenesis-dependent vascular tumor model described above was able to identify a nontrivial fixed point in this complex system. We found that there is a constraint on the existence of this fixed point: namely, that it exists when the immature vessel proliferation rate exceeds its death rate. This intriguing result, which may bear important consequences for antiangiogenic therapy, could not have been found without a mathematical examination of a formal, simplified description of the system. Biologically, the fixed point that was identified here was characterized by the absence of mature vessels from the system. This finding implies that targeting vessel maturation and destabilizing already existing mature vessels may force the tumor to a fixed point. The stability of this fixed point is yet to be determined.

Other fixed points may also exist. A complex multidimensional system, such as the one described above, is practically impossible to analyze theoretically. Hence, a numerical analysis is required. The phase plane was investigated numerically for other fixed points by plotting the time derivative of the variables representing mature vessels with respect to the variable representing the immature vessels, as described above. It is important to stress again that in contrast to our general theoretical analysis, this method is numerical and thus depends on the specific choice of parameters. No additional fixed points were found in this numerical analysis.

Numerical stability analysis was also performed. For a specific choice of parameters, calculation of the Jacobian revealed that the system was not stable but, rather, had potentially stable directions. Simulating behavior that results from perturbations around the fixed point (data not shown) supported this finding.

The existence of a fixed point and its stability in such a system can have significant consequences for drug development, by supporting the "go–no go" decision in the early stages of target validation and drug discovery. For example, such an analysis can reveal if targeting certain system components is likely to have clinically desired outcomes. It can also help identify those variables that are robust to perturbations. Moreover, one can analyze combinations of several drugs that have different mechanisms of action in order to assess their stabilizing potentials. This analysis will help in comparing drugs with different mechanisms of action and predicting their degree of synergy.

9.4. USE OF ANGIOGENESIS MODELS IN THERANOSTICS

Theranostics is a collection of diagnostic techniques that guide the choice of individually tuned therapy with the aim of finding the best possible treatment for a given patient. The human genome project (Venter et al., 2001), the

Protein Structure Initiative (Matthews, 2007), and recent identification of many molecular pathways have resulted in the discovery of novel targets for treating inflammatory, infectious, neurological, and oncological diseases.

The relevance of theranostic approaches is higher in multifactor conditions that are characterized by a high interpatient variability. In these cases the amount of biological knowledge and clinical experience does not allow for efficient rationalization of treatment selection and requires a systematic and rational approach. In the context of cancer, theranostic approaches include imaging techniques (e.g., radioimaging/MRI) (Chao, 2007; Kimura et al., 2008; Wieder et al., 2007) and biomarker identification in the blood or at the cellular level (Iwao-Koizumi et al., 2005; Karam et al., 2008; McLeod, 2002; Salter et al., 2008).

9.4.1. Integrating *In Silico* and *In Vivo* Models for Treatment Personalization

Mesenchymal chondrosarcoma (MCS) is a rare malignant disease with as few as 100 new diagnosed patients each year in the United States. One such patient was diagnosed with mediastinal located MCS at age 45. Shortly after resection of the primary tumor, multiple bilateral pulmonary nodules were discovered. The patient underwent aggressive chemotherapy that included ifosphamide, cisplatin, etopside, vincristine, doxorubicin, cyclophosphamide, and dactinomycin and sunitinib. Despite the chemotherapy, additional liver and bone metastases appeared. In addition, the patient developed severe myelosuppression with pancytopenia.

To determine the best possible treatment for this MCS patient, tumor fragments were taken from his lung metastases and implanted in mice. This xenograft model was established and amplified until a sufficient tumor was available to implant in a control and several treatment groups of mice. These animals were then used to compare the various pharmacotherapy regimens. We refer to this model, in which the cells are taken from the patient and never propagated as a cell line, as a *tumor graft*, to distinguish it from cell line xenograft models.

A general mathematical model for angiogenesis-dependent solid tumor, which was described earlier in the chapter, was utilized to perform *in silico* experiments, identical to those performed in the tumor graft model, for predicting the MCS dynamics in control and treated animals. Pharmacokinetic (PK)–pharmacodynamic (PD) models of the relevant drugs were constructed using publicly available data. In addition, qualitative chemosensitivity tests of several cytotoxic drugs were performed on tumor cells from the patient's biopsy. Incorporating the data of these chemosensitivity tests into the calculations allowed a certain level of personalization of otherwise general PK–PD models.

The mathematical model of the MCS tumor grafts was successfully validated with an average accuracy of 81.6% (Ziv et al., 2006) and was later fine-tuned to provide 87.2% accuracy (Gorelik et al., 2008a). After validation of the mathematical model, gene expression analysis of key proteins in the grafted tumors and in the MCS patient was performed in order to adjust the model to describe the tumor dynamics in the human. The resulting mathematical model of the human disease was used to perform patient-specific predictions of various anticancer treatments.

Guided by the results of the personalized *in silico/in vivo* combined model, clinicians administered the MCS patient once-weekly regimen of docetaxel (DOC), a cytotoxic agent that is given routinely every three weeks. Eventually, the patient had a dramatic response to therapy with a marked decrease in serum alkaline phosphatase from bone and an immediate substantial recovery of all three blood elements (hemoglobin, white blood cells, and platelet count). Soft tissue disease in the lungs and liver remained stable and the patient enjoyed a six-month period of good quality of life, ending only after pulmonary progression of his disease, to which he finally succumbed (Gorelik et al., 2008a).

9.4.2. *In Silico* Model's Role in Determining the Optimal Interdose Interval of Cytotoxic Therapy

According to the simulations with the human MCS computer model that compared the efficacy of DOC delivery every 7, 14, 21, or 28 days (maintaining the same average weekly dose), a once-weekly regimen was found to be more efficacious than the alternatives (Figure 9.2). This finding is of interest due to the controversial clinical evidence regarding the relative efficacy of once- versus triweekly DOC regimens. Moreover, once-weekly administration of DOC is problematic due to increased adverse effects and reduced compliance (Chen et al., 2008; Warm et al., 2007). Thus, one would like to identify patients who are more likely to benefit from weekly chemotherapy schedules than from less frequent regimens.

9.4.3. Factors That Determine the Optimal Interdosing Interval

Maximum tumor growth rate occurs when cellular proliferation and angiogenesis work in unison (Agur, 1986, 1998; Agur et al., 1988, 1992, 2004). Cytotoxic agents such as, but not limited to, DOC disturb the dynamic equilibrium between the growing tumor mass and the vessel bed that supports it by direct killing of tumor cells. As a consequence, a cascade of compensating events is triggered.

Tumor recovery time is a crucial factor in determining the interdosing interval. To illustrate this concept, consider a tumor that is exposed to a dose of a cytotoxic compound. If the time period before the administration of the subsequent dose is not big enough for the tumor to recover to its pretreatment size, the net result will be tumor shrinkage. If, however, the second dose is

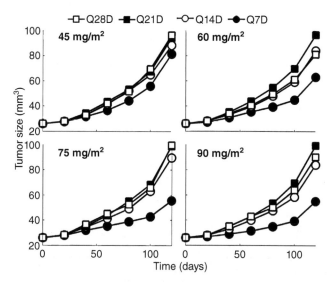

Figure 9.2 Effects of DOC interdosing interval on tumor dynamics as predicted by simulations of the *in vivo* MCS patient's model under 16 BEV and DOC combinations. Schedules include BEV 15 mg/kg given every 21 days, combined with DOC, 1 hour intravenous infusion of 45, 60, 75, and 90 mg/m²; four DOC administration schedules are presented: every 7, 14, 21, and 28 days.

delivered after recovery occurs, the therapy will result in steady growth of the tumor.

To assess tumor recovery from cytotoxic shock, we define the tumor growth inhibition (TGI) factor, TGI_L, in terms of the volume of living cells in the tumor model before and after treatment:

$$TGI_L(\%) = 100 \cdot \left(1 - \frac{T_{L,t} - T_{L,0}}{C_{L,t} - C_{L,0}} \right)$$

(9.35)

where $T_{L,0}$ and $C_{L,0}$ are the initial volumes of the living cells in the treated and control tumor, respectively; $T_{L,t}$ and $C_{L,t}$ are, respectively, the simulated volumes of the living cells in the treated and control tumors at time t. TGI_L has a value of zero if the simulated volume of the living cells in the treated tumor equals that in the control, untreated tumor at the given time point. Larger TGI_L values indicate greater tumor inhibition, and negative TGI_L values indicate the situation where the simulated treated tumor is larger (in terms of living cell volume) than the untreated tumor. In the clinical context, negative TGI_L values mean that the treatment was harmful rather than beneficial.

In human MCS model simulations, the TGI_L value 7 days after a single DOC administration was 46%. As time goes on, this cytotoxic effect decreases to the value of 10% at day 21, a difference of 36% (Figure 9.3). Thus, if the second

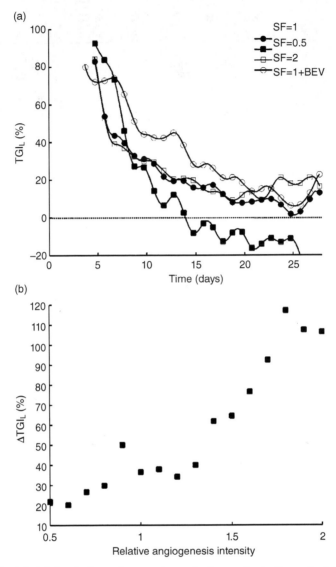

Figure 9.3 Model simulations of tumor dynamics in a patient after a single DOC dose [75 mg/m², 1 hour intravenous (i.v.) infusion]. (A) Smoothed estimated TGI$_L$ after a single DOC dosing for tumors with different levels of angiogenesis intensity. Angiogenesis intensity is determined by scaling the model parameter, which combines VEGF secretion and activity rates. Simulations using two scaling factors are compared to those with estimated angiogenesis intensity of the MCS patient (=1) and in combination with BEV (15 mg/kg i.v.) are presented. Tumor dynamics were smoothed using a moving-average algorithm with a span of 9 days. (B) Predicted decrease in TGI$_L$ from day 7 to day 21 following DOC administration, as a function of angiogenesis intensity relative to efficacy at 7-day intervals.

DOC dose is delivered on day 21, after substantial tumor recovery, the overall efficacy of the treatment would be smaller than that of once-weekly regimens.

As mentioned above, a cytotoxic agent triggers a cascade of tumor recovery events. One would expect that tumor vascularization plays an important role in these processes. Our hypothesis was that increased effective vessel density correlates with faster recovery of the tumor from chemotherapy-induced damage (Gorelik et al., 2008a). Of the many parameters that govern angiogenesis in the *in silico* model, the one that is responsible for vessel endothelial growth factor (VEGF) (Benjamin et al., 1999; Dor et al., 2001; Feng et al., 2007; Shweiki et al., 1992) secretion was chosen for the subsequent screening. The role of this growth factor in angiogenesis processes and its representation inside the computational model were discussed earlier in the chapter.

If the human MCS model is simulated with the VEGF secretion rate reduced by a factor of 2 compared to its original value, the decrease in TGI_L predicted from day 7 to day 21 is only 29% (39 and 10%, respectively), indicating slower recovery from drug-induced tumor inhibition. In contrast, if the rate of new vessel formation is doubled over that calculated for a real MCS patient, the difference in the extent of tumor inhibition by DOC dose between day 7 and day 21 increases to 92%: 69% at day 7 versus a negative value of −22% in day 21 (Figure 9.3). This predicted growth of the tumor beyond that predicted for the untreated model is due to the extensive and rapid formation of blood vessels triggered by the chemotherapy. The impact of the interdosing interval on the treatment efficacy is further amplified by the addition of bevacizumab (BEV), an antiangiogenic drug that binds the VEGF receptor, thus inhibiting its activity. Simulation of DOC–BEV administration to the original MCS model shows that the tumor recovery is slow initially, with a predicted TGI_L value of 76% at day 7 compared to 45% without BEV. As time goes on, BEV is eliminated, which allows rapid angiogenesis and tumor recovery, resulting in 10% TGI_L on day 21 (a difference of 66%).

These results suggest that if the MCS patient had less intensive angiogenesis, less frequent (e.g., triweekly) regimens would have been approximately as efficacious as once weekly, thus providing clinicians with more treatment alternatives. On the other hand, had the patient exhibited more intensive angiogenesis, the weekly DOC schedules would have been the only option to control the tumor growth, even at the cost of intolerable toxicity. Note, though, that our previous results in myelotoxicity modeling show that weekly DOC regimens are generally less toxic than three-weekly regimens (Agur, 2010). Figure 9.3 demonstrates that the dependence of tumor recovery rate on the rate of angiogenesis is almost monotonic over a wide range of kinetic rates, which supports the generality of the conclusions drawn above.

9.4.4. Clinical Relevance of the *In Silico* Predictions

The *in silico* model presented here is composed of a large set of relatively simple mathematical equations that result in a highly complex predictive tool.

The model parameters were estimated by comparison with a single patient suffering from a rare malignant condition, MCS. Of the many alternatives, the impact of one angiogenesis-related model parameter (VEGF secretion rate) was tested, as explained in Section 9.4.3. Nevertheless, the general principle of selecting an interdose interval based on the angiogenesis status stems out of the mechanisms underlying the tumor dynamics. Thus, this hypothesis is not limited to any specific case, but is also expected for other cytotoxic agents and other solid tumors. Once this hypothesis is validated further, clinicians can use the angiogenesis status of their oncologic patients as an aid in the personalization of cytotoxic treatment.

9.5. USE OF ANGIOGENESIS MODELS IN DRUG SALVAGE

Drug development is a challenging, costly, and time-consuming process. Drugs that fail in clinical trials, often due to low efficacy and/or high toxicity levels, are shelved or discontinued altogether (Lievre et al., 2001b). Since increasingly, the pipelines of new compounds seem to be exhausted, it becomes mandatory for pharmaceutical companies to revisit their decision-making process at all stages of drug development.

A new method is proposed here for salvaging prematurely shelved, or discontinued, compounds, whereby virtual clinical trials can be carried out efficiently, accurately, and rapidly to test alternative treatment schedules or alternative patient populations for the discontinued drug. This can be done by computer simulations of synthetic patient populations, which allow for drug–patient dynamic interactions and the characteristic distribution of numerous biological and drug response parameters in the real-life population. To illustrate this approach, we discuss briefly below the case study of a licensed drug, sunitinib malate (Sutent, Pfizer), in combination with a discontinued drug, ISIS-5132 (ISIS Pharmaceuticals), for the treatment of prostate cancer. Results based on virtual patient technology suggest that a new combination treatment will result in more patients reaching a progression-free survival at five years than with either sunitinib malate or ISIS-5132 monotherapy.

Each virtual patient in the synthetic population is constructed using a new biosimulation technology developed to predict drug–patient dynamic interactions. It is based on the integration of the pharmacokinetics and pharmacodynamics of the drug or drugs in question with biomathematical models of the pathological and related physiological processes into one general framework (Arakelyan et al., 2002, 2005). This method allows the prediction not only of the short-term efficacy and toxicity effects of drugs available from conventional PK–PD models, but also of their long-term effects.

9.5.1. Constructing the Disease Model

The angiogenesis-dependent tumor model represents tumor growth and vessel dynamics (formation and maturation). The virtual tumor dynamics are affected by the values of its biological characteristics specified as model parameters. Since measurements of untreated cancer patients are not available, synthetic curves mimicking the growth of untreated tumors may be constructed. These curves are based on initial tumor size measurements and doubling times of untreated cancer patients found in the literature (Feng et al., 2007; Lievre et al., 2001a; Usuda et al., 1994). Accordingly, the size of the untreated tumor at a given moment can then be calculated using the exponential growth model described by Usuda et al. (1994).

Briefly, the following formula calculates the size of an untreated tumor on day t:

$$V_t = V_0 \cdot 2^{t/\mathrm{VDT}} \tag{9.36}$$

where t represents the time of measurement (in days), V_0 represents the initial tumor size (in number of cells), and VDT represents the tumor volume doubling time. The synthetic curves that are generated by this process serve as an input for estimating virtual cancer patients' average vascular tumor parameters ($\vec{P}_{\mathrm{ave}}$).

9.5.2. Constructing Synthetic Human Populations

To predict the effect of a treatment on a population, a virtual patient population must be generated. For each virtual patient the values of the model parameters are set. Patients who belong to this population share most of the model parameters. However, several parameters are selected individually from a predefined distribution. The parameters and their values are selected based on studies indicating that they may have a prognostic value, and given that most of them are measured readily in the lab (Assikis et al., 2004; Caine et al., 2007; Maruyama et al., 2006).

9.5.3. Pharmacokinetics and Pharmacodynamics

For the drugs analyzed here, PK profiles were modeled based on information from the literature, suggesting a linear compartmental model based on the concentrations of the drugs in the plasma (Bello et al., 2006; Britten et al., 2008; O'Farrell et al., 2003; Stevenson et al., 1999; Tolcher et al., 2002). In addition, PD models for both drugs were estimated based on *in vitro* and *in vivo* data (Geiger et al., 1997; Mendel et al., 2003; Monia et al., 1996a,b). The PK–PD effects were then allometrically scaled to human PK–PD (Contrera et al., 2004; FDA, 2005). A combined PK–PD model was created assuming an additive PD relationship with no PK interaction between the two drugs.

9.5.4. Drug Salvage Case Study: Combining Chemotherapeutic and Antiangiogenic Drugs

The compound ISIS-5132 (ISIS Pharmaceuticals) is an antisense oligonucleotide targeted against the c-raf-1 kinase oncogene (Monia et al., 1996b;

Monteith et al., 1998). The c-raf-1 kinase is the direct downstream mediator of the Ras protein, whose oncogene version is associated with more than 30% of human solid tumor types, including lung, colon, and pancreatic cancers (Bos, 1989). ISIS-5132 has been tested in phase I trials in melanoma, pancreas, colorectal, breast, brain, small cell lung, and non-small cell lung cancers (Cunningham et al., 2000; Rudin et al., 2001). Phase II studies were conducted in ovarian, prostate small cell lung, and non-small cell lung cancers (Coudert et al., 2001; Cripps et al., 2002; Oza et al., 2003; Tolcher et al., 2002). However, the phase II trials failed to show significant antitumor activity. The compound has also been tested preclinically in xenograft models of breast, small cell lung, non-small cell lung, prostate, and colorectal cancer (Geiger et al., 1997). Prostate cancer was selected for this investigation given the availability of preclinical pharmacological data. We then ran virtual clinical trials for the ISIS-5132 compound as described briefly below.

The aim of this *in silico* study was to salvage ISIS-5132 for the treatment of prostate cancer by selecting a suitable drug on the market to use in combination with the ISIS drug. This was done by performing virtual "phase II" clinical trials in a synthetic prostate cancer patient population. In the first stage of this study, many drug candidates were screened and analyzed (results not shown). Here we present the virtual clinical trial results of the combination of ISIS-5132 and sunitinib malate. Sunitinib malate is a drug approved by the U.S. Food and Drug Administration for advanced renal cell carcinoma and gastrointestinal stromal cancer.

Model parameters, including drug PK and PD parameters, were based on experimental data reported in the literature. This parameter estimation process was performed for each drug alone and for a combination of the drugs. A concentration–effect function was created to assess the effect of ISIS-5132 on tumor cell proliferation. Similarly, the effects of sunitinib malate on tumor cell proliferation on the number of pericytes and on the formation of new vessels were estimated based on the known drug mechanisms of action.

A synthetic human population was created and simulated under numerous possible regimens of sunitinib malate or ISIS-5132 combinations (Table 9.1). Each of these simulated regimens was evaluated in terms of progression-free survival (PFS). Since the doubling time for untreated prostate cancer is one year and above (Egawa et al., 1997), we examined the efficacy of the drug combinations two and five years post-treatment initiation. The results are presented using Kaplan–Meier curve survival analysis, which describes the probability of PFS at a given moment post-treatment (Figure 9.4). For the purpose of this study, tumor progression is defined as an increase by a factor of 1.75 from the baseline tumor volume.

The simulations (Figures 9.4 and 9.5) predict more than 70% PFS of five years under the best selected regimen, under the accepted dose limiting toxicity (DLT), for the patient population, compared to 40% in patients treated with sunitinib malate alone and to 25% in ISIS-5132. The most effective regimen is ISIS-5132 6 mg/kg every three days + sunitinib malate 50 mg, four

TABLE 9.1   Regimens Simulated for ISIS-5132 and Sunitinib Malate

Drug	Route of Administration	Dose[a]	Regimen[b]
Sunitinib malate	Per os every day	25/37.5/50 mg	1 week on, 1 week off; 4 weeks on, 2 weeks off
ISIS-5132	2 hours intravenous infusion every 3 days	2–10 mg/kg	Every 3 days

[a]All combinations were administered both simultaneously and intermittently (Sunitinib Malate administered one week before ISIS-5132 and ISIS-5132 administered one week before sunitinib malate).
[b]The duration of treatments was about six months.

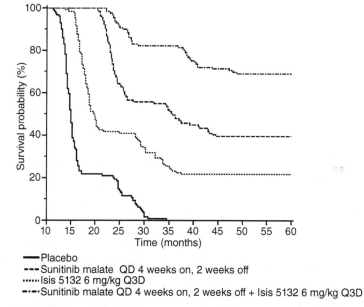

— Placebo
--- Sunitinib malate QD 4 weeks on, 2 weeks off
······ Isis 5132 6 mg/kg Q3D
—·— Sunitinib malate QD 4 weeks on, 2 weeks off + Isis 5132 6 mg/kg Q3D

Figure 9.4 Simulation results of progression-free survival in a synthetic prostate cancer population under ISIS-5132 monotherapy, Sunitinib malate monotherapy, and their combination (ISIS-5132 6 mg/kg every three days + sunitinib malate 50 mg, four weeks on, two weeks off). Simulation results for an untreated synthetic prostate cancer population are provided for comparison.

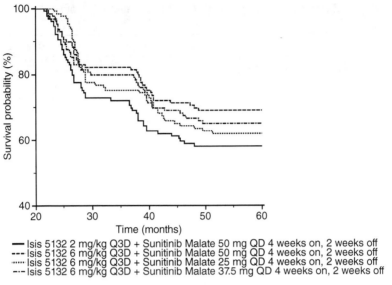

Figure 9.5 Simulation results of progression-free survival in a synthetic prostate cancer populations under different schedules of ISIS-5132 and sunitinib malate combination therapy.

weeks on, two weeks off. Note that the putative toxic effects of the combination studied were neglected in the current study, to simplify the demonstration. Exclusion of toxic effects may explain the visibly overestimated PFS. However, even if overestimated, these results clearly demonstrate the relative improvement of the ISIS-5132/sunitinib malate combination, thus providing an opportunity to salvage ISIS-5132 when administered in combination with sunitinib malate to prostate cancer patients.

9.6. SUMMARY AND CONCLUSIONS

In this chapter we have illustrated how to construct mathematical models for angiogenesis at various levels of biological detail and system complexity. We have shown that a more accurate, detailed, and practical description of system dynamics can be obtained with a more complex model that accounts for more relevant components and processes. Even more important, mathematical modeling allows one to determine the fewest components required to reproduce the phenomena observed and to understand how complex behavior emerges from basic system properties. Uncovered by rigorous mathematical analysis, fixed points and their stability can aid drug development: for example, by supporting "go–no go" decisions in the early stages of target validation and drug discovery.

We described a new method for personalization of solid cancer pharmacotherapy. The method is based on mathematical models for angiogenesis embedded in the *in silico* virtual patient technology used in conjunction with data from tumor xenografts. We described a test case using this technology to suggest an improved treatment schedule for a particular MCS patient. An average accuracy of 87.1% was obtained when comparing *in silico* model predictions to the tumor growth inhibition observed in the xenografted animals. Model predictions suggested that a regimen containing bevacizumab applied intravenously in combination with once-weekly docetaxel is more efficacious in the MCS patient than in other simulated schedules. Weekly docetaxel in the patient resulted in stable metastatic disease and relief of pancytopenia due to tumor infiltration. Based on numerical investigation of the model, we suggest that the advantage of weekly docetaxel versus the tri-weekly regimen is related directly to the tumor's angiogenesis intensity.

Finally, we described a new method for salvaging prematurely shelved, or discontinued, drugs. Virtual clinical trials were simulated efficiently, accurately, and rapidly to test alternative treatment schedules for the discontinued drug. We illustrated this approach by discussing the case study of a licensed drug, sunitinib malate (Sutent, Pfizer), in combination with a discontinued drug, ISIS-5132 (ISIS Pharmaceuticals), for the treatment of prostate cancer. Results based on the virtual patient technology suggest that a novel combination treatment will result in more patients reaching progression-free survival at five years than with either sunitinib malate or ISIS-5132 monotherapy.

REFERENCES

Agur, Z. (1986). The effect of drug schedule on responsiveness to chemotherapy. Ann *NY Acad Sci 504*, 274–277.

Agur, Z. (1998). Resonance and anti-resonance in the design of chemotherapeutic protocols. *J Theor Med 1*, 237–245.

Agur, Z. (2010). From the evolution of toxin resistance to virtual clinical trials: the role of mathematical models in oncology. *Future Oncol 6*, 917–927.

Agur, Z., Arnon, R., and Schechter, B. (1988). Reduction of cytotoxicity to normal tissues by new regimens of cell-cycle phase-specific drugs. *Math Biosci 92*, 1–15.

Agur, Z., Arnon, R., and Schechter, B. (1992). Effect of the dosing interval on myelotoxicity and survival in mice treated by cytarabine. *Eur J Cancer 28A*, 1085–1090.

Agur, Z., Arakelyan, L., Daugulis, P., and Ginosar, Y. (2004). Hopf point analysis for angiogenesis models. *Disc Cont Dyn Syst 4*, 29–38.

Agur, Z., Kogan, Y., Kheiffetz, Y., Ziv, I., Shoham, M., and Vainstein, V. (2008). Mathematical Modeling as a New Approach for Improving the Efficacy/Toxicity Profile of Drugs: The Thrombocytopenia Case Study. Wiley, Hoboken, NJ.

Alarcon, T., Byrne, H., Maini, P., and Panovska, J. (2006). Mathematical modelling of angiogenesis and vascular adaptation. In: *Studies in Multidisciplinarity*, Vol. 3. Elsevier, Amsterdam.

Arakelyan, L., Vainstein, V., and Agur, Z. (2002). A computer algorithm describing the process of vessel formation and maturation, and its use for predicting the effects of anti-angiogenic and anti-maturation therapy on vascular tumor growth. *Angiogenesis* 5, 203–214.

Arakelyan, L., Daugulis, P., Ginosar, Y., Vainstein, V., Selister, V., Kogan, Y., Harpak, H., and Agur, Z. (2003). Multi-scale analysis of angiogenic dynamics and therapy. In: *Cancer Modelling and Simulation* (Preziosi, L., ed.). CRC Press, London.

Arakelyan, L., Merbl, Y., and Agur, Z. (2005). Vessel maturation effects on tumour growth: validation of a computer model in implanted human ovarian carcinoma spheroids. *Eur J Cancer 41*, 159–167.

Araujo, R.P., and McElwain, D.L. (2004). A history of the study of solid tumour growth: the contribution of mathematical modelling. *Bull Math Biol 66*, 1039–1091.

Assikis, V.J., Do, K.A., Wen, S., Wang, X., Cho-Vega, J.H., Brisbay, S., Lopez, R., Logothetis, C.J., Troncoso, P., Papandreou, C.N., et al. (2004). Clinical and biomarker correlates of androgen-independent, locally aggressive prostate cancer with limited metastatic potential. *Clin Cancer Res 10*, 6770–6778.

Bello, C.L., Sherman, L., Zhou, J., Verkh, L., Smeraglia, J., Mount, J., and Klamerus, K.J. (2006). Effect of food on the pharmacokinetics of sunitinib malate (SU11248), a multi-targeted receptor tyrosine kinase inhibitor: results from a phase I study in healthy subjects. *Anticancer Drugs 17*, 353–358.

Benjamin, L.E., Golijanin, D., Itin, A., Pode, D., and Keshet, E. (1999). Selective ablation of immature blood vessels in established human tumors follows vascular endothelial growth factor withdrawal. *J Clin Invest 103*, 159–165.

Bergers, G., Song, S., Meyer-Morse, N., Bergsland, E., and Hanahan, D. (2003). Benefits of targeting both pericytes and endothelial cells in the tumor vasculature with kinase inhibitors. *J Clin Invest 111*, 1287–1295.

Bodnar, M., and Foryś, U. (2009). *Angiogenesis* model with carrying capacity depending on vessel density. *J Biol Syst 17*, 1–15.

Bos, J.L. (1989). ras oncogenes in human cancer: a review. *Cancer Res 49*, 4682–4689.

Britten, C.D., Kabbinavar, F., Hecht, J.R., Bello, C.L., Li, J., Baum, C., and Slamon, D. (2008). A phase I and pharmacokinetic study of sunitinib administered daily for 2 weeks, followed by a 1-week off period. *Cancer Chemother Pharmacol 61*, 515–524.

Byrne, H.M. (1999). A weakly nonlinear analysis of a model of avascular solid tumour growth. *J Math Biol 39*, 59–89.

Caine, G.J., Ryan, P., Lip, G.Y., and Blann, A.D. (2007). Significant decrease in angiopoietin-1 and angiopoietin-2 after radical prostatectomy in prostate cancer patients. *Cancer Lett 251*, 296–301.

Chao, K.S. (2007). 3'-Deoxy-3'-(18)F-fluorothymidine (FLT) positron emission tomography for early prediction of response to chemoradiotherapy: a clinical application model of esophageal cancer. *Semin Oncol 34*, S31–S36.

Chen, J.P., Lo, Y., Yu, C.J., Hsu, C., Shih, J.Y., and Yang, C.H. (2008). Predictors of toxicity of weekly docetaxel in chemotherapy-treated non-small cell lung cancers. *Lung Cancer 60*, 92–97.

Contrera, J.F., Matthews, E.J., Kruhlak, N.L., and Benz, R.D. (2004). Estimating the safe starting dose in phase I clinical trials and no observed effect level based on QSAR modeling of the human maximum recommended daily dose. *Regul Toxicol Pharmacol 40*, 185–206.

Coudert, B., Anthoney, A., Fiedler, W., Droz, J.P., Dieras, V., Borner, M., Smyth, J.F., Morant, R., de Vries, M.J., Roelvink, M., et al. (2001). Phase II trial with ISIS 5132 in patients with small-cell (SCLC) and non-small cell (NSCLC) lung cancer: a European Organization for Research and Treatment of Cancer (EORTC) early clinical studies group report. *Eur J Cancer 37*, 2194–2198.

Cripps, M.C., Figueredo, A.T., Oza, A.M., Taylor, M.J., Fields, A.L., Holmlund, J.T., McIntosh, L.W., Geary, R.S., and Eisenhauer, E.A. (2002). Phase II randomized study of ISIS 3521 and ISIS 5132 in patients with locally advanced or metastatic colorectal cancer: a National Cancer Institute of Canada clinical trials group study. *Clin Cancer Res 8*, 2188–2192.

Cunningham, C.C., Holmlund, J.T., Schiller, J.H., Geary, R.S., Kwoh, T.J., Dorr, A., and Nemunaitis, J. (2000). A phase I trial of c-raf kinase antisense oligonucleotide ISIS 5132 administered as a continuous intravenous infusion in patients with advanced cancer. *Clin Cancer Res 6*, 1626–1631.

Deakin, A.S. (1976). Model for initial vascular patterns in melanoma transplants. *Growth 40*, 191–201.

Dor, Y., Porat, R., and Keshet, E. (2001). Vascular endothelial growth factor and vascular adjustments to perturbations in oxygen homeostasis. *Am J Physiol Cell Physiol 280*, C1367–C1374.

Egawa, S., Matsumoto, K., Iwamura, M., Uchida, T., Kuwao, S., and Koshiba, K. (1997). Impact of life expectancy and tumor doubling time on the clinical significance of prostate cancer in Japan. *Jpn J Clin Oncol 27*, 394–400.

Fatima, S.F., Kaya, A., Visser, T.T.P., Hartong, S.C.C., Agur, Z., and Wagemaker, G. (2008). Efficacy of recombinant human and rhesus thrombopoietin stimulated blood transfusions in comparison to unstimulated whole blood or thrombocyte transfusions in a non-human primate model. Presented at the European Hematology Association 13th Congress, Copenhagen, Denmark.

FDA (2005). Guidance for Industry. Estimating the maximum safe starting dose in initial clinical trials for therapeutics in adult healthy volunteers: in-services, USDHHS, and FDA. Food and Drug Administration Center for Drug Evaluation and Research, Washington, DC.

Feng, Y., vom Hagen, F., Pfister, F., Djokic, S., Hoffmann, S., Back, W., Wagner, P., Lin, J., Deutsch, U., and Hammes, H.P. (2007). Impaired pericyte recruitment and abnormal retinal angiogenesis as a result of angiopoietin-2 overexpression. *Thromb Haemost 97*, 99–108.

Folkman, J. (1971). Tumor angiogenesis: therapeutic implications. *N Engl J Med 285*, 1182–1186.

Forys, U., Kheifetz, Y., and Kogan, Y. (2005). Critical-point analysis for three-variable cancer angiogenesis modeling. *Math Biosci Eng 2*, 511–525.

Freyer, J.P., and Sutherland, R.M. (1980). Selective dissociation and characterization of cells from different regions of multicell tumor spheroids. *Cancer Res 40*, 3956–3965.

Geiger, T., Muller, M., Monia, B.P., and Fabbro, D. (1997). Antitumor activity of a C-raf antisense oligonucleotide in combination with standard chemotherapeutic agents against various human tumors transplanted subcutaneously into nude mice. *Clin Cancer Res 3*, 1179–1185.

Gilead, A., and Neeman, M. (1999). Dynamic remodeling of the vascular bed precedes tumor growth: MLS ovarian carcinoma spheroids implanted in nude mice. *Neoplasia 1*, 226–230.

Gilead, A., Meir, G., and Neeman, M. (2004). The role of angiogenesis, vascular maturation, regression and stroma infiltration in dormancy and growth of implanted MLS ovarian carcinoma spheroids. *Int J Cancer 108*, 524–531.

Gorelik, B., Ziv, I., Shohat, R., Wick, M., Hankins, D., Sidransky, D., and Agur, Z. (2008a). Efficacy of weekly docetaxel and bevacizumab in mesenchymal chondrosarcoma: a new theranostic method combining xenografted biopsies with a mathematical model. *Cancer Res 68*, 9033–9040.

Gorelik, B., Ziv, I., Shohat, R., Wick, M., Hankins, W.D., Sidransky, D., and Agur, Z. (2008b). Efficacy of weekly docetaxel and bevacizumab in mesenchymal chondrosarcoma: a new theranostic method combining xenografted biopsies with a mathematical model. *Cancer Res 68*, 9033–9040.

Greenspan, H.P. (1974). On the self-inhibited growth of cell cultures. *Growth 38*, 81–95.

Hahnfeldt, P., Panigrahy, D., Folkman, J., and Hlatky, L. (1999). Tumor development under angiogenic signaling: a dynamical theory of tumor growth, treatment response, and postvascular dormancy. *Cancer Res 59*, 4770–4775.

Holash, J., Wiegand, S.J., and Yancopoulos, G.D. (1999). New model of tumor angiogenesis: dynamic balance between vessel regression and growth mediated by angiopoietins and VEGF. *Oncogene 18*, 5356–5362.

Iwao-Koizumi, K., Matoba, R., Ueno, N., Kim, S.J., Ando, A., Miyoshi, Y., Maeda, E., Noguchi, S., and Kato, K. (2005). Prediction of docetaxel response in human breast cancer by gene expression profiling. *J Clin Oncol 23*, 422–431.

Karam, J.A., Svatek, R.S., Karakiewicz, P.I., Gallina, A., Roehrborn, C.G., Slawin, K.M., and Shariat, S.F. (2008). Use of preoperative plasma endoglin for prediction of lymph node metastasis in patients with clinically localized prostate cancer. *Clin Cancer Res 14*, 1418–1422.

Kimura, Y., Sumi, M., Sakihama, N., Tanaka, F., Takahashi, H., and Nakamura, T. (2008). MR imaging criteria for the prediction of extranodal spread of metastatic cancer in the neck. *Am J Neuroradiol 29*, 1355–1359.

Kunz-Schughart, L.A. (1999). Multicellular tumor spheroids: intermediates between monolayer culture and *in vivo* tumor. *Cell Biol Int 23*, 157–161.

Landry, J., Freyer, J.P., and Sutherland, R.M. (1982). A model for the growth of multicellular spheroids. *Cell Tissue Kinet 15*, 585–594.

Lievre, M., Menard, J., Bruckert, E., Cogneau, J., Delahaye, F., Giral, P., Leitersdorf, E., Luc, G., Masana, L., Moulin, P., et al. (2001a). Premature discontinuation of clinical trial for reasons not related to efficacy, safety, or feasibility. *Br Med J 322*, 603–605.

Lievre, M., Menard, J., Bruckert, E., Cogneau, J., Delahaye, F., Giral, P., Leitersdorf, E., Luc, G., Masana, L., Moulin, P., et al. (2001b). Premature discontinuation of clinical trial for reasons not related to efficacy, safety, or feasibility. *Br Med J 322*, 603–605.

Liotta, L.A., Saidel, G.M., and Kleinerman, J. (1977). Diffusion model of tumor vascularization and growth. *Bull Math Biol 39*, 117–128.

Mantzaris, N.V., Webb, S., and Othmer, H.G. (2004). Mathematical modeling of tumor-induced angiogenesis. *J Math Biol 49*, 111–187.

Marusić, M., Bajzer, Z., Vuk-Pavlović, S., and Freyer, J.P., (1994). Tumor growth *in vivo* and as multicellular spheroids compared by mathematical models. *Bull Math Biol 56*, 617–631.

Maruyama, Y., Ono, M., Kawahara, A., Yokoyama, T., Basaki, Y., Kage, M., Aoyagi, S., Kinoshita, H., and Kuwano, M. (2006). Tumor growth suppression in pancreatic cancer by a putative metastasis suppressor gene Cap43/NDRG1/Drg-1 through modulation of angiogenesis. *Cancer Res 66*, 6233–6242.

Matthews, B.W. (2007). Protein Structure Initiative: getting into gear. *Nat Struct Mol Biol 14*, 459–460.

McLeod, H.L. (2002). Individualized cancer therapy: molecular approaches to the prediction of tumor response. *Expert Rev Anticancer Ther 2*, 113–119.

Mendel, D.B., Laird, A.D., Xin, X., Louie, S.G., Christensen, J.G., Li, G., Schreck, R.E., Abrams, T.J., Ngai, T.J., Lee, L.B., et al. (2003). *In vivo* antitumor activity of SU11248, a novel tyrosine kinase inhibitor targeting vascular endothelial growth factor and platelet-derived growth factor receptors: determination of a pharmacokinetic/pharmacodynamic relationship. *Clin Cancer Res 9*, 327–337.

Monia, B.P., Johnston, J.F., Geiger, T., Muller, M., and Fabbro, D. (1996a). Antitumor activity of a phosphorothioate antisense oligodeoxynucleotide targeted against C-raf kinase. *Nat Med 2*, 668–675.

Monia, B.P., Sasmor, H., Johnston, J.F., Freier, S.M., Lesnik, E.A., Muller, M., Geiger, T., Altmann, K.H., Moser, H., and Fabbro, D. (1996b). Sequence-specific antitumor activity of a phosphorothioate oligodeoxyribonucleotide targeted to human c-raf kinase supports an antisense mechanism of action *in vivo*. *Proc Natl Acad Sci USA 93*, 15481–15484.

Monteith, D.K., Geary, R.S., Leeds, J.M., Johnston, J., Monia, B.P., and Levin, A.A. (1998). Preclinical evaluation of the effects of a novel antisense compound targeting c-raf kinase in mice and monkeys. *Toxicol Sci 46*, 365–375.

O'Farrell, A.M., Foran, J.M., Fiedler, W., Serve, H., Paquette, R.L., Cooper, M.A., Yuen, H.A., Louie, S.G., Kim, H., Nicholas, S., et al. (2003). An innovative phase I clinical study demonstrates inhibition of FLT3 phosphorylation by SU11248 in acute myeloid leukemia patients. *Clin Cancer Res 9*, 5465–5476.

Oza, A.M., Elit, L., Swenerton, K., Faught, W., Ghatage, P., Carey, M., McIntosh, L., Dorr, A., Holmlund, J.T., and Eisenhauer, E. (2003). Phase II study of CGP 69846A (ISIS 5132) in recurrent epithelial ovarian cancer: an NCIC clinical trials group study (NCIC IND.116). *Gynecol Oncol 89*, 129–133.

PricewaterhouseCoopers (2008). Pharma 2020: Which path will you take? Available at http://www.pwc.com/gx/en/pharma-life-sciences/pharma-2020/pharma2020-virtual-rd-which-path-will-you-take.jhtml (accessed June 16, 2011).

Quesada, A.R., Medina, M.A., and Alba, E. (2007). Playing only one instrument may be not enough: limitations and future of the antiangiogenic treatment of cancer. *Bioessays 29*, 1159–1168.

Rudin, C.M., Holmlund, J., Fleming, G.F., Mani, S., Stadler, W.M., Schumm, P., Monia, B.P., Johnston, J.F., Geary, R., Yu, R.Z., et al. (2001). Phase I trial of ISIS 5132, an antisense oligonucleotide inhibitor of c-raf-1, administered by 24-hour weekly infusion to patients with advanced cancer. *Clin Cancer Res 7*, 1214–1220.

Sachs, R., Hlatky, L., and Hahnfeldt, P. (2001). Simple ODE models of tumor growth and anti-angiogenic or radiation treatment. *Math Comput Model 33*, 1297–1305.

Saidel, G.M., Liotta, L.A., and Kleinerman, J. (1976). System dynamics of metastatic process from an implanted tumor. *J Theor Biol 56*, 417–434.

Salter, K.H., Acharya, C.R., Walters, K.S., Redman, R., Anguiano, A., Garman, K.S., Anders, C.K., Mukherjee, S., Dressman, H.K., Barry, W.T., et al. (2008). An integrated approach to the prediction of chemotherapeutic response in patients with breast cancer. *PLoS ONE 3*, e1908.

Segel, L.A., ed. (1984). *Modeling Dynamic Phenomena in Molecular and Cellular Biology*. Cambridge University Press, New York.

Shweiki, D., Itin, A., Soffer, D., and Keshet, E. (1992). Vascular endothelial growth factor induced by hypoxia may mediate hypoxia-initiated angiogenesis. *Nature 359*, 843–845.

Skehan, P. (1986). On the normality of growth dynamics of neoplasms *in vivo*: a data base analysis. *Growth 50*, 496–515.

Skomorovski, K., Harpak, H., Ianovski, A., Vardi, M., Visser, T.P., Hartong, S.C., van Vliet, H.H., Wagemaker, G., and Agur, Z. (2003). New TPO treatment schedules of increased safety and efficacy: pre-clinical validation of a thrombopoiesis simulation model. *Br J Haematol 123*, 683–691.

Spratt, J.S., Meyer, J.S., and Spratt, J.A. (1996). Rates of growth of human neoplasms: part II. *J Surg Oncol 61*, 68–83.

Stevenson, J.P., Yao, K.S., Gallagher, M., Friedland, D., Mitchell, E.P., Cassella, A., Monia, B., Kwoh, T.J., Yu, R., Holmlund, J., et al. (1999). Phase I clinical/pharmacokinetic and pharmacodynamic trial of the c-raf-1 antisense oligonucleotide ISIS 5132 (CGP 69846A). *J Clin Oncol 17*, 2227–2236.

Sutherland, R.M., McCredie, J.A., and Inch, W.R. (1971). Growth of multicell spheroids in tissue culture as a model of nodular carcinomas. *J Natl Cancer Inst 46*, 113–120.

Tolcher, A.W., Reyno, L., Venner, P.M., Ernst, S.D., Moore, M., Geary, R.S., Chi, K., Hall, S., Walsh, W., Dorr, A., et al. (2002). A randomized phase II and pharmacokinetic study of the antisense oligonucleotides ISIS 3521 and ISIS 5132 in patients with hormone-refractory prostate cancer. *Clin Cancer Res 8*, 2530–2535.

Usuda, K., Saito, Y., Sagawa, M., Sato, M., Kanma, K., Takahashi, S., Endo, C., Chen, Y., Sakurada, A., and Fujimura, S. (1994). Tumor doubling time and prognostic assessment of patients with primary lung cancer. *Cancer 74*, 2239–2244.

Venter, J.C., Adams, M.D., Myers, E.W., Li, P.W., Mural, R.J., Sutton, G.G., Smith, H.O., Yandell, M., Evans, C.A., Holt, R.A., et al. (2001). The sequence of the human genome. *Science 291*, 1304–1351.

Walker, I., Newell, H. (2008). Do molecularly targeted agents in oncology have reduced attrition rates? *Nat Rev Drug Discov 8*, 15–16.

Warm, M., Nawroth, F., Ohlinger, R., Valter, M., Pantke, E., Mallmann, P., Harbeck, N., Kates, R., and Thomas, A. (2007). Improvement of safety profile of docetaxel by weekly administration in patients with metastatic breast cancer. *Onkologie 30*, 436–441.

Wieder, H.A., Geinitz, H., Rosenberg, R., Lordick, F., Becker, K., Stahl, A., Rummeny, E., Siewert, J.R., Schwaiger, M., and Stollfuss, J. (2007). PET imaging with [^{18}F]3'-deoxy-3'-fluorothymidine for prediction of response to neoadjuvant treatment in patients with rectal cancer. *Eur J Nucl Med Mol Imaging 34*, 878–883.

Ziv, I., Shohat, R., Wick, M., Webb, C., Hankins, D., Sidransky, D., and Agur, Z. (2006). Novel Virtual patient technology for predicting response of breast cancer and mesenchymal chondrosarcoma patients to mono- and combination therapy by cytotoxic and targeted drugs. Presented at AACR-NCI-EORTC 18th Symposium: Molecular Targets and Cancer Therapeutics, Prague, Czech Republic.

CHAPTER 10

Systems Modeling Applied to Candidate Biomarker Identification

ANANTH KADAMBI

Entelos Inc., Foster City, California

DANIEL L. YOUNG and KAPIL GADKAR

Theranos Inc., Palo Alto, California

Summary

Multianalyte candidate biomarkers provide feasible means to effectively reduce the time and cost associated with the development of new chemical entities for the treatment of human disease. Traditional data-driven biomarker identification approaches can potentially be accelerated by both systems and statistical modeling approaches. In this chapter we provide an overview of the biomarker discovery process, highlighting areas where modeling approaches provide a unique means of support. Case studies highlighting the utility of mechanistic systems modeling approaches to specific biomarker applications are also reviewed.

10.1. INTRODUCTION

Pharmaceutical drug development is an expensive, time-consuming, and risky process. A newly marketed compound takes an average of 12 to 13 years to develop at a cost of up to $1.7 billion (Gilbert et al., 2003). Most compounds that enter development do not make it to market. Only 8 to 14% of new chemical entities (NCEs) that enter preclinical development are successfully carried forward through human clinical development, achieve regulatory

Systems Biology in Drug Discovery and Development, First Edition.
Edited by Daniel L. Young, Seth Michelson.

approval, and are launched. Recent high-profile failures of promising NCEs for the treatment of cardiovascular disease are illustrative of the major risks associated with current methods for the development of novel therapeutics:

- Despite extensive preclinical testing and success in early human clinical trials, development of the cholesterol ester transfer protein (CETP) inhibitor torcetrapib was halted late in clinical development due to lack of efficacy and a cardiovascular safety risk (Barter et al., 2007).
- The cyclooxygenase-2 inhibitor rofecoxib (Vioxx) was pulled from the market five years following regulatory approval, after two late-stage clinical trials indicated that Vioxx caused an increased incidence of cardiovascular-related deaths (Bombardier et al., 2000; Bresalier et al., 2005).

These cases illustrate the troublesome fact that despite extensive testing, therapeutically ineffective or unsafe NCEs are often advanced late into the development process. Furthermore, NCEs achieve regulatory approval and are marketed despite latent safety issues that are not detected until several years afterward and after significant adverse impact on consumer health. Failures of such NCEs are costly not only to the companies developing the failed NCEs, but also to the clinical trial patients and postmarket consumers, all of which increases overall health care costs. To combat these undesirable outcomes, significant research has focused on approaches that will increase the success rate for the development of NCEs, including an increase in time and resources devoted to the discovery and use of novel biomarkers of both efficacy and safety.

A *biomarker* is defined as "a characteristic (or set of characteristics) that is objectively measured and evaluated as an indicator of normal biologic processes, pathogenic processes, or pharmacologic responses to a therapeutic intervention" (Atkinson et al., 2001). Although biomarkers have been used by physicians for the diagnosis of disease and prediction of prognosis since the dawn of modern clinical practice (e.g., yellowing of the eyes and skin as a biomarker of jaundice), more recently they have been explored as a means to reduce the risks and overall cost associated with NCE development. A summary of possible applications of biomarkers to the clinical development process are shown in Box 10.1.

Biomarkers are typically classified by the following nomenclature:

- *Type 0:* measures obtained prior to an intervention that can be used for stratification of patients according to their expected response to that intervention (lifestyle change or therapeutic)
- *Type 1:* measures obtained following administration of a compound that serve as surrogate indicators of success in modulating a compound's mechanism of action, whether hypothesized or known

---

BOX 10.1: POSSIBLE APPLICATION OF BIOMARKERS TO DRUG DISCOVERY AND DEVELOPMENT

- Translational
  - Bridge animal and human pharmacology
- Early clinical
  - Verify drug–target interaction in humans (proof of mechanism)
  - Establish downstream pharmacological activity (proof of principle)
  - Establish initial proof of efficacy (proof of concept)
- Late clinical and/or postmarketing
  - Predict long-term benefit (surrogate endpoint)
  - Aid identification and selection of responder, nonresponder, and adverse-responder patient subpopulations (patient stratification, safety)
  - Support regulatory claims

BOX 10.2: DESIRED CHARACTERISTICS OF BIOMARKERS

- Measurable
  - Noninvasively or with minimal invasion
  - In a time frame appropriate for a clinical endpoint of interest
- Robust
  - Predictions borne out quantitatively in humans (good *calibration*)
  - Low rate of false positives (high *specificity*) and false negatives (high *sensitivity*)
  - Reproducible success in predictions (*validation*), ideally across multiple subpopulations (e.g., ethnicities, gender, age)
- Cost-effective

- *Type 2:* measures obtained following administration of an intervention that serve as surrogate measures of the efficacy or safety of that intervention

Irrespective of their classification and application, biomarkers useful in clinical trials and in clinical practice share a set of common desired characteristics (Box 10.2). Established biomarkers used routinely for disease diagnosis have been well validated due to the availability of large amounts of human data (e.g., creatinine clearance as an indication of kidney function, elevated diastolic blood pressure as an indicator of arterial stiffness, or AST or ALT elevations as an indication of steatohepatitis). However, candidate biomarkers for NCEs rarely satisfy all of these diverse criteria. Formulating and validating human candidate biomarkers for NCEs is, in part, challenging because human patient populations are both physiologically distinct from preclinical animal models and extremely heterogeneous. These translational problems are compounded by the paucity of available human data for the validation of NCEs. Despite these challenges, even imperfect candidate biomarkers may still be of significant value to decision making related to NCE development. Biomarkers identified in early-stage clinical trials can serve as a starting point for prioritized sample collection and measurements in later-stage clinical trials. Furthermore, data collected from later-stage clinical trials can be used to validate previously identified candidates. Both of these improvements will reduce the time and cost associated with NCE development.

In the last 20 years, genetic and molecular biology methods have provided a wealth of detailed information characterizing the role of genes, their transcription, and the resulting proteins in the regulation of whole organ and organism behaviors. However, connecting the dots between the information provided by these reductionist approaches to fully understand the qualitative and quantitative behavior of these large systems is a challenging task. The term *systems biology* refers to the collection of disciplines that evaluate how components of complex biological systems interact dynamically. In this chapter we provide an overview of the merits and challenges of systems biology approaches for candidate biomarker identification and applications of these methodologies to heterogeneous patient populations. We review several modeling strategies currently in use to aid in the identification of biomarkers, and conclude with two illustrative examples of the application of systems biology approaches to novel candidate biomarker identification.

10.1.1. Biomarkers to Address Challenges Associated with Patient Heterogeneity

Clinical trials designed to demonstrate efficacy and safety of novel therapeutics are faced with the inherent challenge of interpatient heterogeneity in the trial populations recruited and associated variability in clinical response. This interpatient heterogeneity stems from a variety of sources:

- The etiology of many common diseases is multifactorial i.e., single defects in specific biological mechanisms rarely explain a patient's clinical presentation). For example, insulin resistance, characteristic of patients with type 2 diabetes, arises from a combination of defects that lead to decreased pancreatic beta cell function and hepatic and peripheral insulin sensitivity (Harano et al., 2002; Suzuki et al., 2002).

- The multifactorial defects are differentially modulated across patients by combinations of genetic, lifestyle, and environmental factors.
- There is tremendous interpatient heterogeneity in lifestyle, including diet, smoking, and frequency and duration of exercise.
- The absorption, metabolism, and distribution of NCEs [pharmacokinetics (PK)] and effect on target pathways [pharmacodynamics (PD)] vary greatly between patients.

In the clinic, physicians choose the best intervention to treat an individual patient based on firsthand knowledge of their clinical presentation, family history, lifestyle, and in some cases, genetic background. However, in the context of most late-stage clinical trials today, individual patient characteristics are not typically considered, and patient heterogeneity thus becomes a significant impediment. The efficacy of NCEs is typically evaluated by comparison of changes in primary clinical endpoints for a group of patients treated with the NCE to a group of patients treated with placebo or a background standard of care medication. Typically, efficacy and safety can only be demonstrated by enrolling large numbers of patients in a trial to achieve the required statistical power given the inherent variability in response. If late-stage clinical trials do not demonstrate population-level efficacy for the NCE or, worse, demonstrate an adverse safety profile, many patients enrolled in the trial may have been exposed to an unnecessary safety risk. Furthermore, despite the fact that specific subpopulations of patients may have shown improvement in a primary clinical endpoint following NCE administration, if population-level efficacy is not demonstrated, the NCE will not be approved by the U.S. Food and Drug Administration and the subpopulation of patients who responded favorably to such an NCE may not have access to this therapeutic. The consequence is that optimal treatments may never be given to the individual patients who would benefit from them.

Conceptually, systems biology modeling approaches can address in several ways the challenges associated with patient heterogeneity and variability in population-level response to an intervention. First, systems biology approaches predict the response of different "virtual patients" who embody variability in underlying genetics, ethnicity, lifestyle, and diet (Powell et al., 2007) to administration of an NCE. Second, model data can be analyzed to determine candidate biomarkers predictive of NCE efficacy and safety. These analyses can aid in the translation of validated biomarkers from preclinical animal models into humans, enabling earlier detection of potential safety concerns and facilitating patient stratification i.e., segregation of responder subpopulations from non-responder or adverse-responder subpopulations) to enable more focused product labeling postapproval. Although systems-based approaches can be applied to the identification of candidate type 0, type 1, or type 2 biomarkers, the prospect of identifying novel type 0 biomarkers may have the greatest impact on clinical NCE development and public health.

10.1.2. Utility of Type 0 Biomarkers

Type 0 biomarker diagnostics, which consist of either a single measure or a combination of measures sampled at the "baseline" condition (i.e., prior to the administration of a therapeutic under consideration) enable a rigorous, quantitative assessment of the likelihood that a given patient will benefit from or respond adversely to a particular therapy. The availability of such diagnostic tools has several potential benefits for different stakeholders in the drug development life cycle. For pharmaceutical and consumer product companies developing clinical trial designs, type 0 biomarkers can help reduce the time and cost associated with bringing NCEs from bench to bedside by informing critical aspects of the clinical development process:

- In early (phase I or II) clinical development, type 0 biomarkers may inform compound selection and advancement by providing early evidence of safety or toxicology signals and enabling the stratification of patient subgroups.
- In late (phase III) clinical development type 0 biomarkers can be utilized as part of the trial inclusion and exclusion criteria, to improve overall patient safety and reduce the risk of enrolling patients susceptible to safety risks.
- In postmarket and competitive differentiation (phase IV) trials, type 0 biomarkers can be employed to enrich a treatment population for responder patients to improve statistical power.

The cost implications for developing and applying type 0 biomarkers must be evaluated carefully. For pharmaceutical companies, the reduced expense and increased patent life of approved novel therapeutics and the shortened bench-to-bedside time can compensate in part for the possibility that stratification of patients to enrich responders and eliminate adverse responders will reduce the market size and thus the potential revenue generated by an approved NCE.

For physicians and patients themselves, type 0 biomarkers offer the obvious benefit of enhanced personalized medicine. These biomarkers can help increase the probability of prescribing the appropriate medication, at the appropriate dose, to a specific patient, thus reducing the likelihood of prescribing a medication that will pose a safety risk to the particular patient. Thus, from a public health perspective, a broader availability of robust type 0 biomarkers for therapeutics provides the dual benefit of reducing the time and cost associated with the advancement to market of novel therapeutics, and increasing the efficacy and safety of the prescription of therapeutics that have already been approved.

Available systems biology modeling approaches allow the influence of a given intervention on human physiology or pathophysiology to be assessed rapidly *in silico*. Within the last several years, biotechnology, consumer products, and pharmaceutical companies have begun employing systems biology modeling approaches to aid the identification of candidate biomarkers of prognosis, compound efficacy, and safety. There are three main benefits of systems biology-based approaches:

- They enable assessment of the effect of interpatient variability on the efficacy and safety predicted for NCEs (discussed in Section 10.1.1).
- They enable rapid, inexpensive, and high-throughput means of candidate biomarker identification that could otherwise take years of preclinical research.
- A priori candidate biomarker model predictions can enable prioritization of relevant measures to be collected in clinical trials. This information can help reduce trial cost, as well as enabling collection of measurements most relevant to efficacy and safety in later clinical trials, simplifying downstream biomarker analysis.

The key classes of systems biology modeling approaches (hereafter referred to as *systems modeling*) are described below in the context of their potential role in supporting biomarker discovery and validation.

10.2. BIOMARKER DISCOVERY APPROACHES

As discussed in Section 10.1, relatively few biomarkers have been developed sufficiently to enable their reliable, justifiable use in clinical practice. One of the challenges impeding biomarker discovery and validation is the complexity and cost associated with traditional biomarker clinical studies. These challenges must be weighed against the benefits expected for the key stakeholders in the health care system: pharmaceutical companies, patients, and physicians. In this section we discuss traditional, data-driven approaches for biomarker development, highlighting roles for systems modeling approaches to potentially streamline and enhance the biomarker development process.

Traditional data-driven approaches rely solely on preclinical and clinical data to propel the discovery and validation of biomarkers. The process can be described in four main steps (see Figure 10.1):

1. Formulate biomarker hypotheses based on preclinical and clinical data for the target patient population and drug. (Deductive logic)
2. Design clinical trials to test these hypotheses appropriately. The clinical trial should include an appropriate schedule of assessment of noninvasive measures, plasma samples, tissue biopsies, and/or images for patients undergoing specific treatment regimens. (Deductive logic)
3. Based on the initial hypotheses, analyze the clinical samples to quantify relevant biological measures (e.g., serum and tissue protein levels, cell numbers, mRNA and DNA expression, or histological features).

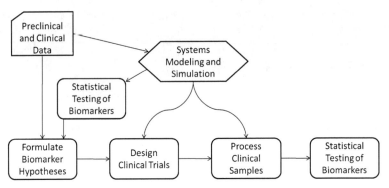

Figure 10.1 The four key steps during biomarker discovery and development: (1) formulate biomarker hypotheses, (2) design clinical trials, (3) process clinical samples, and (4) test biomarkers statistical. Traditional data-driven approaches rely solely on preclinical and clinical data to inform the biomarker development process. Systems modeling and simulation can potentially streamline and enhance multiple aspects of this biomarker development and validation process.

4. Test the original hypotheses relating biomarkers to clinical outcomes and determine the clinical utility by utilizing well-described statistical approaches. (Closing the loop)

Each of these four main steps presents certain challenges and opportunities for refinement. The decision to conduct a biomarker study, as well as the probable overall success of a clinical program, is determined by the ability to complete each of these steps effectively. Enhancements to this biomarker discovery and validation process will improve the ability to demonstrate the clinical value and increase ultimate adoption by physicians and patients.

10.2.1. Hypothesis Generation

Perhaps the most significant challenge to the traditional biomarker approach is the first step of specific hypothesis generation. Sound hypotheses based on a synthesized understanding of available information will greatly improve the likelihood of success of any clinical biomarker program. Conventionally, this knowledge base arises from available nonclinical, preclinical, and clinical data. Hypotheses formulated at early stages of compound development are more likely to be confirmed in future studies if the disease and compound in question have been studied extensively and if the appropriate data are available to the investigators. Unfortunately, the data required to formulate robust hypotheses are often not available, incomplete, or insufficient. For example, biomarker data are not always reported in published clinical trials, especially when results are negative. Furthermore, reported data may be unreliable if the patient sample size is too small, or if only summary statistics are available rather than individual patient records. These challenges can be partially addressed by extrapolating from data available from related diseases, data from the same disease but from a different subpopulation of patients, or data characterizing patient response to treatments with different compounds. Moreover, metaanalyses across studies can increase the power of the data compared to analysis of individual studies, which alone may have insufficient statistical power given the size of the study and variable patient responses. However, these approaches to extract additional knowledge for hypothesis generation may not significantly increase the likelihood of ultimate success of biomarker development and validation, in part due to the inherent limitations of the data available as well as the inability to discern (1) cause-and-effect relationships, (2) key uncertainties, and (3) underlying biological mechanisms affecting disease and treatment response, all of which may significantly affect the hypothesis generation process.

Systems modeling can greatly aid in the hypothesis generation and vetting process, especially during the early stages of biomarker research. The main objectives in such systems modeling approaches are to test alternative hypotheses of disease processes, compound mechanism of action, and interpatient heterogeneity to discover and evaluate candidate biomarkers. Systems modeling can yield a variety of insights, providing support for, or refutation of, data-driven hypotheses, or elucidating novel, unexpected hypotheses.

There are many types of systems models that could be employed to assist in hypothesis generation and evaluation for biomarkers. Relevant model types include qualitative models (including intracellular pathway maps and network maps) and quantitative models (including physiological-based models, mechanistic models, and PK–PD models). The choice of the appropriate model type depends on the specific application, the data available, the biomarkers of interest, and the time scales or dynamics that may affect the analysis. In some cases it is critical to represent disease progression and the dynamic impact of the compound on the disease processes, necessitating a quantitative modeling approach. In other cases, formulation of initial hypotheses may not require dynamic disease models; rather, the key questions may involve differences in gene regulation or expression and their possible impact on cellular responses to a compound, which may be addressed by qualitative intracellular pathway maps.

One advantage of mechanistic models is that they typically include representations of dynamic processes underlying the pathophysiology of a disease in addition to representations of compound mechanisms of action. This juxtaposition enables a more complete simulation of patient-specific responses to specific compounds. Accordingly, given the scope of the model, a range of biomarkers may be tested by exploring patient heterogeneity in both disease processes (such as diversity in disease severity and disease drivers) and compound PK–PD. Models with mechanistic representations could thus provide a prioritized, focused candidate set of biomarkers and enable recommendations for clinical validation. Moreover, mechanistic models can yield important biological insights into why some biomarkers are predicted to be clinically meaningful whereas others are not.

Modeling studies must be designed with the specific aim of assisting the biomarker hypothesis generation process. With this aim in mind, a clear understanding of the specific biomarker objectives will inform the design of the model, including the required level of detail, specific biological components, the time scales of greatest interest, and the relevant patient phenotypes to be represented by the model. These detailed *in silico* efforts thus provide a reasonably stable architecture around which one can eventually build the confirmatory clinical studies of interest.

While univariate biomarkers have been associated with disease diagnoses, outcomes, and adverse events, inclusion of multiple measures may enhance the predictive value of a biomarker. It has been suggested that the incorporation of uncorrelated ("orthogonal") measures into multianalyte biomarkers can enhance their clinical utility (Gerszten et al., 2008). Correlations between physiological measures and their dynamic changes over time are explored readily using systems biology approaches. This deeper understanding of biological measures, including temporal changes and correlations between measures, can provide additional confidence to a clinical research team as it moves forward with a clinical trial for evaluation of a novel therapeutic strategy.

10.2.2. Clinical Studies

After generating biomarker hypotheses, clinical studies must be designed to support adequate validation of these hypotheses. Several guidelines have been developed to improve the quality of such biomarker studies as well as to aid in the subsequent statistical data analysis (McGuire, 1991). The three main types of biomarker studies and their characteristics are described below.

- *Pilot studies* are typically small in size (50 to 100 patients) and are designed to be exploratory rather than definitive. Accordingly, in pilot studies, a diverse patient population may be studied and numerous biomarkers measured at multiple time points, thereby enabling broad-based biomarker hypothesis exploration typical during early stages of compound development.
- *Definitive studies* are designed to test more specific hypotheses and are likely to be more focused on specific patient populations or a refined set of candidate markers based on knowledge gained from prior studies. Trial designs must be powered appropriately by considering the magnitude and variability of the clinical responses and biomarker patterns expected.
- *Confirmatory studies* are carried out to validate candidate biomarkers in a new set of patients and should be powered similarly to definitive

studies. Retrospective studies may be conducted based on archived clinical samples or data sets; however, careful attention must be devoted to account for any potential confounding biases (McGuire, 1991).

Modeling and simulation of clinical trials can be used to help design and optimize potential clinical trial designs for confirming biomarker hypotheses. Such research is designed to consider the interplay between disease processes, compound mechanisms of action, expected biomarker dynamics and variability, and their relationship to clinical outcomes over time. Simulations of such physiological processes are especially applicable for evaluation of a type 1 and type 2 biomarker to assess compound effects on their target and surrogate endpoints, respectively (see Section 10.3 for specific examples). Based on this type of focused research, optimal trial designs can be selected to meet the clinical objectives, acceptable risk profiles, and cost constraints.

10.2.3. Molecular Assay and Imaging Technologies

All biomarker studies require specialized tools to process clinical samples or collect images to support the specific hypothesized biomarker panel. The availability and selection of such tools will have a direct impact on the cost and reliability of clinical studies, and the absence of such tools could render the ideal study impractical or infeasible. Proteomic and genomic studies now benefit from enhanced high-throughput microarray technologies, including multiplex approaches requiring smaller sample volumes (Gerszten et al., 2008). All these molecular assay technologies must be evaluated to assess their reliability, sensitivity, dynamic range, and specificity to assess whether these characteristics meet the study requirements. Medical imaging, such as x-ray, ultrasound, positron emission tomography scans, computed tomography scans, and magnetic resonance imaging, is integral for assessing early functional changes as well as changes in structural features in organs and tissues in the context of certain diseases (Corry et al., 2008; Ramos et al., 2007). Such medical imaging technologies must be evaluated with respect to their resolution, costs, safety, and convenience relative to alternative physiological tests (Graham, 2009).

In addition to central laboratory-based tests, new advancements in point-of-care (POC) tests provide new biomarker opportunities for clinical studies and postmarketing applications. In general, POC tests enable higher sampling rates that allow one to assess more readily physiological changes over time. Such dynamic measurements and patterns could yield more sensitive biomarker signatures compared to static measures. The application and validation of POC tests could expand the types of biomarkers that are feasible for both clinical and commercial uses or increase their ease of assessment. For example, for patients with type 2 diabetes, assessment of blood sugar can be critical. Historically, glucose monitoring required a urine sample, which was replaced by blood draws and finally, "finger-stick" tests available over the counter. POC technology has evolved to eliminate even the need for finger-stick tests, as noninvasive skin-sampling methodologies have been reported (Malchoff et al., 2002) that greatly reduce the delay between testing and treatment. As another example, patients taking anticoagulants typically need rigorous monitoring to maximize efficacy and minimize adverse events (e.g., bleeding). Whereas such monitoring required repeated clinical visits in the past, recent technologies have enabled patients to self-monitor by assessment at home of a validated biomarker, the International Normalized Ratio (Gardiner et al., 2008).

The impact of experimental tests on the biomarker discovery process can be evaluated quantitatively by modeling and simulation. Namely, one may explicitly represent the performance characteristics of experimental tests (e.g., assay analytic sensitivity, specificity, and variability) in a model to provide guidance on the cost/benefit ratio of certain high-performance tests or the need for duplicate assays. For example, a quantitative model that captures dynamic treatment responses could be used to determine the ability of certain assays to capture transient changes in protein levels reliably given the anticipated magnitude of the physiological changes and the assay performance characteristics. Approaches to mitigate assay variability can be simulated, such as the impact of performing multiple pretreatment measurements instead of just one, or focusing the time of data acquisition during the peak response predicted.

10.2.4. Statistical Methods

There is a very rich set of statistical methods available to discover and test biomarker patterns. As detailed above, putative biomarkers can be tested by analysis of both clinical and simulated data from systems models. Both the clinical and model data can be analyzed by the same set of statistical methods, summarized below. In this section we highlight some key approaches and considerations but do not provide an exhaustive review [see Hastie et al. (2009) and Sajda (2006) for more comprehensive reviews].

The basic problem in biomarker discovery is to identify the most discriminating and refined set of explanatory variables to facilitate a predefined patient characterization or to predict subpopulation characteristics. The former problem, typically called *classification*, could involve the use of a type 0 biomarker for predicting patient response or nonresponse. The latter problem, often referred to as *regression*, could entail prediction of changes in blood pressure in, or survival of, patients based on a type 2 biomarker. Applying either method yields a statistical model that captures the relationship between the biomarker (independent variable) and a clinical outcome (dependent variable). The choice of method depends on the dimensionality and character of the independent variable space (i.e., the candidate biomarker components) as well as the type of dependent variable under consideration. For example, different approaches are best suited for continuous independent variables, discrete inputs, or multiple independent variables, which are a combination of continuous and discrete inputs. Continuous variables could include molecular concentrations, such as the serum concentration of C-reactive protein (CRP), tumor necrosis factor-α, or patient age. Examples of discrete variables include genetic variants, patient gender, and treatment history. In addition, some approaches require normally distributed independent variables and appropriate transformations if the independent variables are distributed according to a lognormal or Cauchy distribution as typically exhibited by some biological variables (e.g., serum triglyceride and CRP, respectively).

To build explanatory statistical models solving the problems described above, common techniques include linear regression, Cox proportional hazard regression, logistic regression, linear and quadratic discriminant function analysis, support vector machines, classification and regression (decision) trees, and artificial neural networks. All these methods most generally aim to identify the best model for predicting patient membership in subpopulations or continuous characteristics for a given subpopulation based on a refined set of independent variables with minimal classification error or residuals, respectively. Variable selection, or dimension reduction of the potential explanatory inputs, can be achieved by several techniques, including forward selection, backward elimination, least angle regression, and a wide range of more extensive search strategies (Efron et al., 2004; Hilario and Kalousis, 2008; Kohavi and John, 1997).

Several methods are available to evaluate and increase the robustness of the statistical models. Candidate models can be evaluated by re-substitution, cross-validation, and training or test set validations. These tests enable one to explore the algorithm performance and compute predictive accuracy or error rates. Regression models are often evaluated based on residual plots, while correlation coefficients are useful for comparing alternative models for the same dependent variable. Common statistical measures to describe the performance of classification tests are diagnostic sensitivity, specificity, and accuracy, defined as the proportion of positive cases classified correctly, the proportion of negatives cases classified correctly, and the proportion of total correct classifications in the population, respectively. Positive predictive value is the probability that a predicted positive case is truly positive; negative predictive value is calculated similarly. Receiver operating characteristic (ROC) curves provide a convenient way to optimize and assess biomarkers whereby the trade-offs between sensitivity and specificity can be visualized (see Figure 10.2). Refined thresholds or cutoff points for classification can be evaluated by assessing penalties or costs to certain types of misclassifications, improving the clinical utility of the biomarker. Moreover, the area under the curve of ROC curves (i.e., the C-statistic), provides a method to compare candidate predictive models by assessing the overall discriminating ability of the biomarker. Readers are referred to additional references for further details describing the rich set of approaches and tools to conduct these analyses (Molinaro et al., 2005).

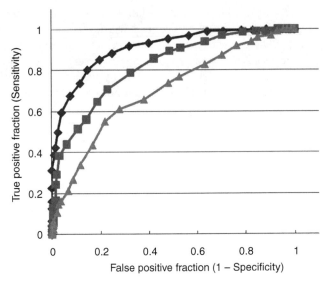

Figure 10.2 Examples of receiver operating characteristic (ROC) curves used to optimize and assess biomarkers. Trade-offs between sensitivity and specificity are easily visualized in an ROC plot for three illustrative candidate biomarkers (A, diamonds; B, squares; C, triangles). For each candidate biomarker, alternative diagnostic thresholds are evaluated and the corresponding sensitivity–specificity pairs are plotted. These results clearly demonstrate that candidate biomarker A is superior to B, which is superior to C, as supported by the calculated area under the curve (AUC) for each candidate biomarker (0.91, 0.82, 0.70, respectively, out of a maximal AUC of 1.0).

10.3. EXAMPLES OF SYSTEMS MODELING APPROACHES FOR IDENTIFICATION OF CANDIDATE BIOMARKERS

Organ- or tissue-level genomic, proteomic, or metabonomic approaches to identifying putative candidate biomarkers predictive of therapeutic response are used to identify candidate biomarkers in indications as diverse as cancer (Lin et al., 2005; Yousef and Diamandis, 2009) to psychiatric disorders (Reckow et al., 2008) to inflammatory bowel disease (Roda et al., 2010). To support discovery and refinement and to facilitate validation of biomarkers identified by these and other traditional methods, systems modeling approaches may be employed, as described in Section 10.2 and discussed in Chapter 9. An example of a systems modeling approach that has been employed for this purpose is embodied in Entelos's PhysioLab platforms, which are large-scale mechanistic computer disease models of the biology and pathophysiology underlying specific diseases [for a representative example, see Shoda et al. (2010)]. Within each PhysioLab platform, virtual patients (VPs) can be created to represent each of multiple hypotheses of disease progression as observed in actual clinical patients. Each hypothesis embodied in a VP is "validated" by ensuring that clinical measures of baseline disease progression and simulated responses to a variety of treatment protocols are within the reported quantitative variability in human clinical populations described in the literature. A large, diverse cohort of VPs can be created to reproduce the heterogeneity in genetic, environmental, and lifestyle factors that are observed in a human clinical population. By assigning prevalence weights to individual VPs, virtual populations can be created to reproduce the clinical population statistics across a wide range of clinical measures (see, e.g., Friedrich and Paterson, 2004). The availability of virtual populations facilitates a diverse set of *in silico* research to support the development of NCEs, ranging from identification, evaluation, and prioritization of novel therapeutic targets in early development, to rapid simulation of human clinical and postapproval trials to predict efficacy and safety endpoints. These capabilities can be especially useful to inform decision making associated with the development of NCEs, markedly reducing time and costs.

10.3.1. Case Studies: Identification of Candidate Biomarkers for Patient Stratification

Cardiovascular disease (CVD) accounts for one-third of all deaths in the United States (American Heart Association, n.d.). Many risk factors for CVD, including dyslipidemia, smoking, and diabetes, have been identified from epidemiological studies and form the basis of current treatment guidelines (Grundy et al., 2004). Despite intense research in the field, there have been notable recent failures of clinical trials that can be attributed to:

- The quality of available standard-of-care medications, such as the statins, which are effective at treating risk factors associated with CVD, including dyslipidemia and inflammation
- The diversity in genetic risk factors, lifestyle choices, and therapy-associated pharmacokinetics in the target patient population

A specific example of these challenges is embodied in the wealth of recent research focused on CETP inhibitors (CETPis), a novel class of NCEs. These compounds have demonstrated increases in "good" cholesterol [high-density lipoproteins (HDLs)] and decreases in "bad" cholesterol [low-density lipoproteins (LDLs)] (Brousseau et al., 2004; Clark et al., 2004; de Grooth et al., 2002; Krishna et al., 2007, 2008; Kuivenhoven et al., 2005) both as a monotherapy and when administered to patients on a background of statins. Although this shift in cholesterol profile is widely considered beneficial for the treatment of CVD, recent late-stage clinical trials of the CETPi torcetrapib showed no statistically significant improvement in atherosclerotic plaque burden (Nissen et al., 2007) and worse, an increase in rate of mortality and incidence of cardiovascular events (Barter et al., 2007). These events led torcetrapib's sponsor,

Pfizer, to terminate the development of torcetrapib. The termination of torcetrapid cast some doubt on the utility of CETPi's as a therapeutic intervention for CVD, despite the fact that torcetrapib trial results were at least partially attributed to an "off-target" effect that caused an increase in patient blood pressure and consequent adverse effects (Vergeer et al., 2008). However, the published data strongly suggested that a subpopulation of patients exists for whom torcetrapib could be a beneficial therapeutic. The key question is whether biomarkers could be developed to identify the patients in this subpopulation a priori, as well as to screen out the subpopulation of adverse-responder patients.

A systems modeling approach using Entelos's Cardiovascular (CV) PhysioLab platform, a large-scale computer model of the biology and pathophysiology of human cardiovascular disease (Powell et al., 2007), was used to identify candidate multianalyte biomarkers predictive of responder and nonresponder patients in the context of CETP inhibition. A schematic of a sample of the relevant biology included in the platform is shown in Figure 10.3. A cohort of 67 VPs that covered a broad diversity in LDL and HDL cholesterol,

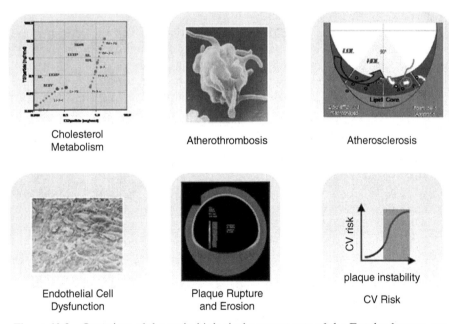

Figure 10.3   Overview of the main biological components of the Entelos human cardiovascular (CV) PhysioLab platform, a large-scale dynamic mechanistic model of cardiovascular disease. The platform enables prediction of the effects of dietary, lifestyle, and therapeutic interventions that modulate circulating lipids, serum inflammatory markers, and local vessel inflammation on relevant CV endpoints, including atherosclerotic plaque burden, stability, and the likelihood of a CV event. (See insert for color representation.)

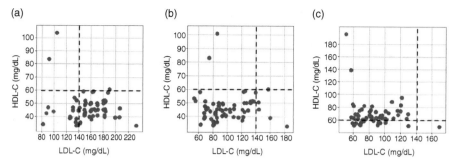

Figure 10.4 Comparison of circulating lipids in the virtual patient cohort developed as the basis to identify candidate biomarkers predictive of responder and adverse-responder subpopulations following addition of CETPi to a background statin. Dashed lines are anchored at LDL-C = 140 mg/dL and HDL-C 60 mg/dL to facilitate comparison. (a) Baseline circulating lipids. The virtual patients exhibit variability in both "good" cholesterol (HDL-C) and "bad" cholesterol (LDL-C). (b) Circulating lipids following two years of simulated statin therapy, which reduces LDL-C. (c) Circulating lipids following two years of simulated CETPi + statin therapy, which both increases HDL-C and decreases LDL-C.

as would be expected in a real clinical population, was developed in the CV PhysioLab platform and used as a basis for research (see Figure 10.4). Each VP was subjected to two distinct simulated treatment arms:

- *Arm 1:* background statin alone
- *Arm 2:* a combination of a pure CETPi and a background statin

In both cases, an eight-week run-in period on a background statin was simulated in the PhysioLab platform, consistent with the torcetrapib clinical protocol (Nissen et al., 2007), in a short period of time. Figure 10.5 displays the simulation predictions of changes in atherosclerotic plaque burden, as quantified by the Entelos CV PhysioLab platform outputs of percent atheroma volume (PAV) for each VP on each simulated treatment arm. As suggested by the published torcetrapib clinical trial data, the VP cohort used in this analysis contains a substantial number of adverse-responder VPs, whose PAV increases upon addition of CETPi to a background statin. However, a reasonable number of responder VPs whose PAV decreases following addition of CETPi to a background statin is also predicted, suggesting that a subpopulation of patients may benefit from addition of the CETPi to their background statin regimen. For the research described below, the change in PAV (ΔPAV) following two years of simulated therapy is used as the primary endpoint of efficacy.

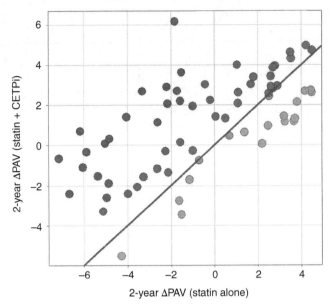

Figure 10.5   Predictions of changes in percent atheroma volume (ΔPAV) for individual VPs following two years of simulated therapy with statin alone (*x*-axis) or statin + CETPi. Each solid circle represents a single virtual patient. VPs below the blue line represent the "responder patients" who show an improved response to the combination therapy compared to atorvastatin alone, while those above the line are "adverse-responder patients," who exhibit exacerbation of atherosclerosis following addition of a CETPi. In this virtual cohort, there are a large number of adverse-responder VPs. (See insert for color representation.)

10.3.2. Identification of Candidate Type 0 and Type 2 Biomarkers

The ability of combinations of analytes measured prior to the start of the treatment to predict patients that exhibit reduced ΔPAV two years following addition of CETPi to a background statin was determined. The pool of candidate analytes included more than 50 outputs from the Entelos CV PhysioLab platform that can be measured clinically, included circulating cholesterol and triglyceride measures at the start and end of the eight-week simulated run-in period. The optimal candidate multianalyte biomarker was determined using discriminant function analysis (McLachlan, 2004). Figure 10.6 shows the predictions of the optimal novel candidate multianalyte biomarker from the Entelos CV PhysioLab platform, which consisted of fewer than 10 circulating measures readily quantified by standard laboratory assays. The candidate biomarker predicted the two-year ΔPAV correctly in 12 of the 18 responder VPs and 46 of the 49 nonresponders, resulting in a sensitivity of 0.61 and specificity of 0.95.

Subsequently, type 2 biomarkers, including both pre- and posttherapy circulating measures, were used to identify a candidate multianalyte biomarker

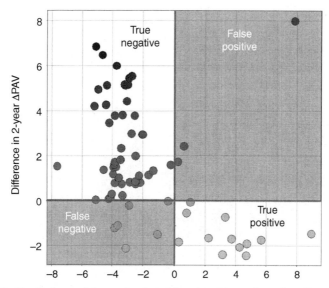

Figure 10.6 Predictions of the optimal multianalyte biomarker of patient response to addition of CETPi to a background statin, including pre-therapy analyte measurements only in the pool of possible analytes. The y-axis indicates the difference in ΔPAV between the combination therapy and the statin monotherapy arm following two years of simulation. The virtual patients with y-axis values greater than zero are the adverse responders; those with values less than zero are the responders. The x-axis indicates the output of the DFA algorithm applied to this analysis: values greater than zero indicate that the virtual patient is predicted to be a responder; values less than zero indicate that the virtual patient is predicted to be a nonresponder. In this case, the candidate biomarker effectively screens out adverse responders, as indicated by a few false positives (upper right quadrant), but is not as effective at identifying responders, as indicated by several false negatives (lower left quadrant). (See insert for color representation.)

predictive of patients who exhibit reduced ΔPAV two years following addition of CETPi to a background statin. In addition to the pre-therapy measurements included in the analysis described earlier, post-therapy measurements taken three months into the simulated clinical trial were included in the pool of potential analytes. Figure 10.7 shows the performance of the novel optimal candidate multianalyte type 2 biomarker. With the inclusion of post-therapy measurements, predictions from the CV PhysioLab platform improved to a sensitivity of 0.85 and a specificity of 0.95.

The candidate biomarkers identified could be validated in upcoming clinical trials of CETPi's. In theory, once validated, the biomarkers could be used either to inform inclusion and exclusion criteria of future CETPi compounds late-stage clinical trials, or as a clinical tool to ensure that CETPi's are prescribed only to those patients expected to benefit from the addition of CETPi to their background statin regimen.

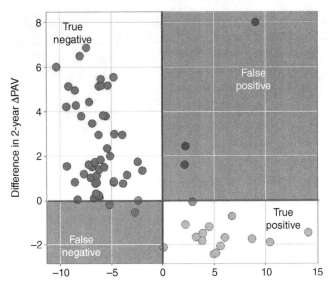

Figure 10.7   Predictions of the optimal multianalyte biomarker of patient response to addition of CETPi to a background statin, including both pre- and post-therapy analyte measurements in the pool of possible analytes. This figure should be interpreted in a manner similar to Figure 10.6. In this case, the candidate biomarker is highly predictive of both responders and adverse responders, as indicated by the presence of both few false negatives (lower left quadrant) and false positives (upper right quadrant). (See insert for color representation.)

10.3.3. Biomarkers to Predict Efficacy of a Novel Strategy for the Treatment of Rheumatoid Arthritis

The Entelos rheumatoid arthritis (RA) PhysioLab platform is a large-scale computer model of the biology and pathophysiology of human rheumatoid arthritis (Defranoux et al., 2005; Rullmann et al., 2005). Different hypotheses of the etiology of RA are represented in the Entelos RA PhysioLab platform as distinct VPs, each of which represents a specific combination of underlying biological mechanisms related to the contribution of local and systemic inflammatory cells (e.g., macrophages, T-cells, B-cells, fibroblast-like synoviocytes, and endothelial cells) and many inflammatory mediators (e.g., IL-6, IL-1, TNF-α, IFN-γ) that play a role in bone erosion, cartilage degradation, and joint space narrowing that occurs during RA disease progression.

Utilizing the Entelos RA PhysioLab platform, a type 0 biomarker predictive of 12-month clinical response (American College of Rheumatology Score, or ACR-N response) following simulated blockade of an inflammatory mediator (referred to here as synovial mediator X) was determined for three different virtual patient populations of clinical relevance. The three virtual patient populations are characterized as follows:

1. A previously untreated virtual population (Vpop1)
2. A virtual population including patients on a background of methotrexate (MTX) therapy but a physiology that renders them nonresponsive to MTX treatment (Vpop2)
3. An anti-TNF-α nonresponder virtual population on a background of MTX therapy (Vpop3)

Sixty-nine analytes, including pretreatment measures of synovial and serum soluble protein and protein complexes in the virtual populations, were included in the analysis. A stepwise multivariate linear regression approach was used to determine the optimal subset of four to five analytes that combined to best predict the 12-month clinical response following complete synovial X blockade. The performance of the candidate multianalyte biomarkers for each of the three populations is shown in Figure 10.8. As the title of each graph in Figure 10.8 suggests, the predictive ability of the candidate biomarker is excellent in each case, with r^2 values above 0.75 for each virtual population of interest. Importantly, for each of the three virtual populations referred to above, the candidate biomarker comprised a different optimal combination of measures. These measures could potentially be used to enrich clinical patient populations for responder patients' synovial mediator X blockade during enrollment of clinical trials. Furthermore, the candidate panels could be validated in future clinical trials of drugs causing synovial X blockade.

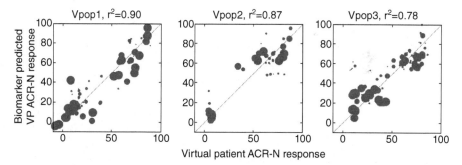

Figure 10.8 Correlation of the simulated and multianalyte biomarker-predicted 12-month ACR-N response to synovial X blockade for untreated patients (Vpop1), MTX nonresponders (Vpop2), and anti-TNF nonresponders (Vpop3) in response to synovial X blockade in the RA PhysioLab platform. Each of the three figures shows the relationship between each virtual patient's ACR-N response (*x*-axis) and the ACR-N response predicted for the candidate biomarker panel (*y*-axis). Each solid circle represents a virtual patient in the population, with the size of the circle corresponding to the prevalence of the virtual patient in that population. The candidate biomarker panel identified for each virtual population is highly predictive of ACR-N response.

10.4. CONCLUSIONS

The modeling and simulation approaches reviewed in this chapter can facilitate progress through the four main steps of data-driven biomarker identification described in Section 10.2 by enabling rapid testing of multiple alternate biomarker hypotheses. Patient variability in the underlying mechanisms of disease pathophysiology, NCE mechanism of action, or changes in clinical measures of disease progression makes the formulation and testing of such hypotheses very difficult using traditional data-driven approaches, which often involve lengthy and costly clinical trials.

The case studies described in Section 10.3 illustrate specific applications of a systems biology modeling and simulation approach to hypothesis evaluation by creating diverse virtual patients and virtual populations and simulating clinical trial protocols and identifying candidate biomarkers of efficacy and safety in response to different therapies. These and similar approaches to identifying biomarkers can reduce the time and costs associated with NCE development.

Acknowledgment

We would like to thank Christina Friedrich for helpful discussion of the concepts presented in this chapter.

REFERENCES

American Heart Association (n.d.). Cardiovascular disease statistics. (http://www.americanheart.org/presenter.jhtml?identifier=4478).

Atkinson, A.J., Colburn, W.A., DeGruttola, V.G., DeMets, D.L., Downing, G.J., Hoth, D.F., Oates, J.A., Peck, C.P., Schooley, R.T., Spilker, B.A., et al. (2001). Biomarkers and surrogate endpoints: preferred definitions and conceptual framework. *Clin Pharmacol Ther 69*, 89–95.

Barter, P.J., Caulfield, M., Eriksson, M., Grundy, S.M., Kastelein, J.J., Komajda, M., Lopez-Sendon, J., Mosca, L., Tardif, J.C., Waters, D.D., et al. (2007). Effects of torcetrapib in patients at high risk for coronary events. *N Engl J Med 357*, 2109–2122.

Bombardier, C., Laine, L., Reicin, A., Shapiro, D., Burgos-Vargas, R., Davis, B., Day, R., Ferraz, M.B., Hawkey, C.J., Hochberg, M.C., et al. (2000). Comparison of upper gastrointestinal toxicity of rofecoxib and naproxen in patients with rheumatoid arthritis. VIGOR Study Group. *N Engl J Med 343*, 1520–1528.

Bresalier, R.S., Sandler, R.S., Quan, H., Bolognese, J.A., Oxenius, B., Horgan, K., Lines, C., Riddell, R., Morton, D., Lanas, A., et al. (2005). Cardiovascular events associated with rofecoxib in a colorectal adenoma chemoprevention trial. *N Engl J Med 352*, 1092–1102.

Brousseau, M.E., Schaefer, E.J., Wolfe, M.L., Bloedon, L.T., Digenio, A.G., Clark, R.W., Mancuso, J.P., and Rader, D.J. (2004). Effects of an inhibitor of cholesteryl ester transfer protein on HDL cholesterol. *N Engl J Med 350*, 1505–1515.

Clark, R.W., Sutfin, T.A., Ruggeri, R.B., Willauer, A.T., Sugarman, E.D., Magnus-Aryitey, G., Cosgrove, P.G., Sand, T.M., Wester, R.T., Williams, J.A., et al. (2004). Raising high-density lipoprotein in humans through inhibition of cholesteryl ester transfer protein: an initial multidose study of torcetrapib. *Arterioscler Thromb Vasc Biol 24*, 490–497.

Corry, J., Rischin, D., Hicks, R.J., and Peters, L.J. (2008). The role of PET-CT in the management of patients with advanced cancer of the head and neck. *Curr Oncol Rep 10*, 149–155.

Defranoux, N.A., Dubnicoff, T.B., Klinke, D.J., Lewis, A.K., Paterson, T.S., Ramanujan, S., Shoda, L.K.M., Soderstrom, K.P., and Struemper, H.K. (2005). Method and apparatus for computer modeling a joint. US Patent No. 6862561.

de Grooth, G.J., Kuivenhoven, J.A., Stalenhoef, A.F., de Graaf, J., Zwinderman, A.H., Posma, J.L., van Tol, A., and Kastelein, J.J. (2002). Efficacy and safety of a novel cholesteryl ester transfer protein inhibitor, JTT-705, in humans: a randomized phase II dose–response study. *Circulation 105*, 2159–2165.

Efron, B., Hastie, T., Johnstone, I., and Tibshirani, R. (2004). Least angle regression. *Ann Statist 32*, 407–451.

Friedrich, C.M., and Paterson, T.S. (2004). *In silico* predictions of target clinical efficacy. *Drug Discov Today: Targets 3*, 216–222.

Gardiner, C., Longair, I., Hills, J., Cohen, H., Mackie, I.J., and Machin, S.J. (2008). Performance evaluation of a new small-volume coagulation monitor: the SmartCheck INR system. *Am J Clin Pathol 129*, 500–504.

Gerszten, R.E., Accurso, F., Bernard, G.R., Caprioli, R.M., Klee, E.W., Klee, G.G., Kullo, I., Laguna, T.A., Roth, F.P., Sabatine, M., et al. (2008). Challenges in translating plasma proteomics from bench to bedside: update from the NHLBI Clinical Proteomics Programs. *Am J Physiol Lung Cell Mol Physiol 295*, L16–L22.

Gilbert, J., Henske, P., and Singh, A. (2003). Rebuilding big pharma's business model. *In Vivo, the Business & Medicine Report 21*(10), 1–10.

Graham, M.M. (2009). Cost-effectiveness of medical imaging. *Lancet Oncol 10*, 744–745.

Grundy, S.M., Cleeman, J.I., Merz, C.N., Brewer, H.B., Jr., Clark, L.T., Hunninghake, D.B., Pasternak, R.C., Smith, S.C., Jr., and Stone, N.J. (2004). Implications of recent clinical trials for the National Cholesterol Education Program Adult Treatment Panel III guidelines. *Circulation 110*, 227–239.

Harano, Y., Suzuki, M., Koyama, Y., Kanda, M., Yasuda, S., Suzuki, K., and Takamizawa, I. (2002). Multifactorial insulin resistance and clinical impact in hypertension and cardiovascular diseases. *J Diabetes Complications 16*, 19–23.

Hastie, T., Tibshirani, R., and Friedman, J. (2009). *The Elements of Statistical Learning: Data Mining, Inference and Prediction*. Springer-Verlag, New York.

Hilario, M., and Kalousis, A. (2008). Approaches to dimensionality reduction in proteomic biomarker studies. *Brief Bioinf 9*, 102–118.

Kohavi, R., and John, G.H. (1997). Wrappers for feature subset selection. *Artif Intel 97*, 273–324.

Krishna, R., Anderson, M.S., Bergman, A.J., Jin, B., Fallon, M., Cote, J., Rosko, K., Chavez-Eng, C., Lutz, R., Bloomfield, D.M., et al. (2007). Effect of the cholesteryl ester transfer protein inhibitor, anacetrapib, on lipoproteins in patients with dyslipidaemia and on 24-h ambulatory blood pressure in healthy individuals: two double-blind, randomised placebo-controlled phase I studies. *Lancet 370*, 1907–1914.

Krishna, R., Bergman, A.J., Jin, B., Fallon, M., Cote, J., Van Hoydonck, P., Laethem, T., Gendrano, I.N., 3rd, Van Dyck, K., Hilliard, D., et al. (2008). Multiple-dose pharmacodynamics and pharmacokinetics of anacetrapib, a potent cholesteryl ester transfer protein (CETP) inhibitor, in healthy subjects. *Clin Pharmacol Ther 84*, 679–683.

Kuivenhoven, J.A., de Grooth, G.J., Kawamura, H., Klerkx, A.H., Wilhelm, F., Trip, M.D., and Kastelein, J.J. (2005). Effectiveness of inhibition of cholesteryl ester transfer protein by JTT-705 in combination with pravastatin in type II dyslipidemia. *Am J Cardiol 95*, 1085–1088.

Lin, B., White, J.T., Lu, W., Xie, T., Utleg, A.G., Yan, X., Yi, E.C., Shannon, P., Khrebtukova, I., Lange, P.H., et al. (2005). Evidence for the presence of disease-perturbed networks in prostate cancer cells by genomic and proteomic analyses: a systems approach to disease. *Cancer Res 65*, 3081–3091.

Malchoff, C.D., Shoukri, K., Landau, J.I., and Buchert, J.M. (2002). A novel noninvasive blood glucose monitor. *Diabetes Care 25*, 2268–2275.

McGuire, W.L. (1991). Breast cancer prognostic factors: evaluation guidelines. *J Natl Cancer Inst 83*, 154–155.

McLachlan, G.J. (2004). *Discriminant Analysis and Statistical Pattern Recognition.* Wiley-Interscience, Hoboken, NJ.

Molinaro, A.M., Simon, R., and Pfeiffer, R.M. (2005). Prediction error estimation: a comparison of resampling methods. *Bioinformatics 21*, 3301–3307.

Nissen, S.E., Tardif, J.C., Nicholls, S.J., Revkin, J.H., Shear, C.L., Duggan, W.T., Ruzyllo, W., Bachinsky, W.B., Lasala, G.P., and Tuzcu, E.M. (2007). Effect of torcetrapib on the progression of coronary atherosclerosis. *N Engl J Med 356*, 1304–1316.

Powell, L.M., Lo, A., Cole, M.S., and Trimmer, J. (2007). Application of predictive biosimulation to the study of atherosclerosis: development of the cardiovascular PhysioLab platform and evaluation of CETP inhibitor therapy. *Proceedings of Foundations of Engineering in Systems Biology*, pp. 295–302.

Ramos, J.J., Williams, M., Synetos, A., and Lerakis, S. (2007). Clinical utility of cardiac computed tomography. *Am J Med Sci 334*, 350–355.

Reckow, S., Gormanns, P., Holsboer, F., and Turck, C.W. (2008). Psychiatric disorders biomarker identification: from proteomics to systems biology. *Pharmacopsychiatry 41*(Suppl. 1), S70–S77.

Roda, G., Caponi, A., Benevento, M., Nanni, P., Mezzanotte, L., Belluzzi, A., Mayer, L., and Roda, A. (2010). New proteomic approaches for biomarker discovery in inflammatory bowel disease. *Inflamm Bowel Dis 16*, 1239–1246.

Rullmann, J.A., Struemper, H., Defranoux, N.A., Ramanujan, S., Meeuwisse, C.M., and van Elsas, A. (2005). Systems biology for battling rheumatoid arthritis: application of the Entelos PhysioLab platform. *Syst Biol (Stevenage) 152*, 256–262.

Sajda, P. (2006). Machine learning for detection and diagnosis of disease. *Annu Rev Biomed Eng 8*, 537–565.

Shoda, L., Kreuwel, H., Gadkar, K., Zheng, Y., Whiting, C., Atkinson, M., Bluestone, J., Mathis, D., Young, D., and Ramanujan, S. (2010). The type 1 diabetes PhysioLab platform: a validated physiologically based mathematical model of pathogenesis in the non-obese diabetic mouse. *Clin Exp Immunol 161*, 250–267.

Suzuki, M., Hattori, Y., Takeuchi, M., Kimura, Y., Yamazaki, Y., Inada, H., Murase, O., Ito, H., Nawata, H., Orimo, H., et al. (2002). Clinical implication of multiple risk factor control in the management of diabetic macrovasucular complications. *J Diabetes Complications 16*, 115–118.

Vergeer, M., Bots, M.L., van Leuven, S.I., Basart, D.C., Sijbrands, E.J., Evans, G.W., Grobbee, D.E., Visseren, F.L., Stalenhoef, A.F., Stroes, E.S., et al. (2008). Cholesteryl ester transfer protein inhibitor torcetrapib and off-target toxicity: a pooled analysis of the rating atherosclerotic disease change by imaging with a new CETP inhibitor (RADIANCE) trials. *Circulation 118*, 2515–2522.

Yousef, G.M., and Diamandis, E.P. (2009). The human kallikrein gene family: new biomarkers for ovarian cancer. *Cancer Treat Res 149*, 165–187.

CHAPTER 11

Simulating Clinical Trials

TOM PARKE

Tessella PLC, Abingdon, UK

Summary

There is more to clinical trials than showing a statistically significant different response to a compound in development compared to placebo; we need to be able to understand the response, to refine models, and to select doses with particular efficacy and safety characteristics. Conventional trial theory provides little help in designing such trials, and our only tool to understanding and refining them is simulation.

11.1. INTRODUCTION

"The objective of the clinical trial simulation paradigm in drug development is to increase the efficiency of drug development, i.e., minimizing the cost and time of the development of a drug while maximizing the informativeness of data generated from a trial or trials" (Duffal and Kimko, 2003). For a compound under development, because of cost, time, and in many cases the scarcity of test subjects, there are limited opportunities to test compounds in humans. Although this pressure is felt most immediately through competitive pressure and patent law implications, it also meets societal requirements for testing, as efficiently as possible, compounds with poorly understood side effects in sick humans, particularly when there are increasingly many compounds to test.

There are thus specific pressures on the experimental design when that experiment is a clinical trial (Piantadosi, 2005). Opportunities to fix the clinical-trial design and rerun it are limited, if not impossible. Accordingly, the ability

Systems Biology in Drug Discovery and Development, First Edition.
Edited by Daniel L. Young, Seth Michelson.
© 2012 John Wiley & Sons, Inc. Published 2012 by John Wiley & Sons, Inc.

to preemptively evaluate and optimize the design via simulation in a reliable and timely manner has been shown to be advantageous to pharmaceutical companies by improving the chance for success while reducing costs.

11.1.1. Types of Clinical Trials

Clinical trials came of age in 1962 in the wake of the thalidomide disaster when the U.S. Congress passed the Kefauver–Harris amendments to the Food, Drug and Cosmetics Act, requiring pharmaceutical companies to demonstrate the efficacy and safety of new compounds before obtaining approval for marketing. For drug development this requirement has given rise to four types of clinical trials, as detailed below (Table 11.1) (Pocock, 1983).

A phase I, or first-in-man, trial is aimed primarily at establishing a safe range of doses of the compound that can be given to humans. These trials are usually very small, using 20 to 30 subjects. The subjects are usually healthy volunteers rather than sick patients, and all the testing is done at one center or a very small number of centers. Usually, the trial tests the subjects in cohorts of fixed size, typically three at a time. The first cohort will be given an amount of the test compound that is well below the maximum safe level that has been predicted from animal testing. These first subjects are monitored, and if all is well, the next cohort is recruited and given the next highest dose, and so on. There are a number of well-established designs, such as "3 plus 3," "up and down," and the "continuous reassessment method," that can be used to govern how the trial should proceed in the light of varying degrees of toxicity. Typically, this trial yields an estimate of the maximum tolerated dose (MTD), which places an upper limit on the dose level that can be used in any of the subsequent trials.[1]

A phase IIa, or proof-of-concept (POC), trial is aimed primarily at establishing whether, at a dose level determined to be safe in phase I, there is sufficient evidence of efficacy, or at least of drug action, to justify continued investment in development of the compound. These trials are somewhat larger, between 60 and 200 subjects. The subjects are patients, although possibly from a particularly easy-to-study subpopulation of the final target patient population. Typically, these trials are randomized and controlled, blinded or double blinded, with two treatment arms. On one treatment arm subjects are given what is believed to be the maximum safe dose [based on the phase I study, pharmacokinetic–pharmacodynamic (PK–PD) models, and animal data], possibly in combination with the standard therapy. On the other treatment arm, subjects are given a placebo or some standard therapy as a comparator.

Of considerable interest in the POC trial is what change in the patients to measure (the endpoint) to determine whether or not the compound is likely

---

[1]It is easily forgotten that it is just an estimate; it is difficult to retain an appropriate degree of uncertainty about what it is we know, or think we know. Simulations can be used to address this when simulating a certain underlying truth by showing just how variable the outcome of the trial can be. This is far from a complete cure, however.

Trial Type	Aims	Measure Type	Size	Simulation Objectives
Phase I: first in man, safety study	To show that there is a usable, tolerable, safe dose of the drug that can be used	Usually, a quick binary outcome: "toxicity yes/no" or "tolerability yes/no"	20–30	
PK–PD study	Parameters of the PK–PD model; the minimum dose required for a given patient to achieve full saturation at the binding site	The drug concentration in the blood stream after a given number of times	20–40	To find the most effective times to take blood samples. To ensure that the sample size is sufficient to establish the PK–PD parameters
Phase IIa: proof of concept	To establish that the drug has some therapeutic effect	Some marker of drug effect usually visible shortly after administration	100–200	Simulation used in adaptive trials that test multiple doses; also used in adaptive seamless phase IIa/IIb designs
Phase IIb: dose finding	To establish a dose of the drug that has sufficient clinical benefit	Where practical, will be the required regulatory endpoint for phase III [when this takes a long time to collect (a year or more) sometimes the risky strategy of using a quicker endpoint is used]	200–400, can be much larger for difficult to measure endpoints such as changes in rates of rare events	Simulation used to evaluate, refine, and validate an adaptive dose-finding trial designs
Phase III: confirmatory	To establish that the drug is safe and has a benefit in a clinical setting	The regulatory clinical endpoint and safety	From several hundred up to thousands, depending on the difficulty of showing a statistically significant difference	Limited adaptation in phase III; simulation used on adaptive seamless phase II and III designs
Phase IV: further safety, marketing	To investigate safety concerns, to research modified uses of the drug; other indications, in combination with other treatments or in new patient populations	The regulatory clinical endpoint and safety	Highly variable	

to be useful. The endpoint will vary widely depending on the disease and the compound's mechanism of action. The ideal change to measure is the endpoint that will have to be used in the final submission to the regulatory authorities in order for the compound to be licensed as a drug (the clinical endpoint). However, in many cases this endpoint either takes a long time to collect (e.g., progression-free survival after two years), has a great deal of variability (e.g., a patient's overall score when answering a set of questions to elicit how depressed they are feeling), or is too blunt an instrument (e.g., change in quality of life). In such cases to keep the time and cost of the POC trial reasonable, an alternative endpoint, a surrogate endpoint or biomarker, is used. These alternatives can avoid these problems, although at the risk that at the end of a successful POC trial, one may have less confidence that the compound will show efficacy in subsequent trials.

An additional type of trial that may be run during development is a PK–PD study aimed at improving the metabolic understanding of the compound. This type of study is sometimes performed as part of, or instead of, the POC trial. The principal aims of a PK–PD study are to learn about some or all of the parameters of the PK–PD model, such as absorption rates, clearance rates, or population covariates, to identify patient subpopulations, or to be able to select the most appropriate PK–PD model from a number of candidate models.

A phase IIb, or dose-ranging study, is aimed primarily at determining the best dose, or dosing regimen for the compound, generating further evidence of efficacy and more safety data. The goal for this trial is to be able to select which dose level of the compound to use in the subsequent confirmatory phase III trial. In particular, there is a desire to use the minimum dosage level at which there is good evidence of efficacy, the minimum effective dose (MED). The MED is chosen to avoid using a dose in phase III that may have safety problems that haven't been noticed up until now simply because, for example, the phase III trial is much larger.

The phase IIb study will typically have a number of different treatment arms, one for control where subjects are given placebo or a standard therapy and several where subjects are given different doses of the compound (again, possibly in combination with a standard therapy). This phase will be a double-blinded randomized clinical trial. If practical, the primary endpoint studied will be the clinical endpoint, which will have to be studied in the phase III trial in order to prove drug effectiveness to the regulators. These trials will be bigger than the POC trials, and range in size from several hundreds of subjects to thousands, depending on the difficulty of showing statistical significance with the endpoint and the problems of comparing multiple treatment arms.

A phase III confirmatory or registration trial is aimed solely at collecting sufficient evidence of efficacy and safety for the compound that the regulatory authorities will grant the compound a license to be used as a drug. The regulators usually require two successful phase III studies before granting a license, although if the phase IIb trial was large enough, or if the disease is particularly difficult to study, the successful phase IIb study may be counted as one of the two successful studies for registration. Typically, this development strategy requires agreement beforehand between the sponsor and the regulatory authorities.

The phase III trial will typically have only two treatment arms, one for control and the other for the dose selected based on the phase IIb trial. This study will be a double-blinded, randomized clinical trial. These studies typically range in size from several hundreds of subjects to thousands, depending on the difficulty of showing statistical significance with the endpoint and the amount of safety data required.

Finally, phase IV trials are conducted on a drug after it has been licensed. The trial, possibly required by the regulatory authority, aims to gather additional safety data in order to detect rare or long-term effects that would have been impractical to study during the phase III trial. Alternatively, the trial may have been instigated by the sponsoring company with the aim of broadening the compound's use or increasing its patent life by establishing its use in new patient populations, different indications, or use in conjunction with other therapies.

The summary above is a "canonical" overview of the sequence of clinical trials during a drug's development. It should not be underestimated how much variation there is in trial design as a result of variability in many factors, in particular the severity of the disease being studied; the rarity of the disease being studied; the availability of treatments; whether the treatment is one-off, short-term, or for the rest of a patient's life; whether the treatment is a prevention, a cure, or is being done simply to alleviate symptoms; whether the drug's effect is immediate or has to be studied over the long term; and the nature and variability in the clinical endpoint.

11.1.2. Distinction Between Learning and Confirming

In a landmark paper, Louis Sheiner (1997) introduced the concepts of learning versus confirming in clinical trials. Sheiner believed that because standard statistical methodology for the analysis of experimental data had been applied to all clinical trials (apart from phase I), drug development had become wasteful and inefficient. The use of standard notions of statistical significance had forced the design of early-phase clinical trials into too rigid a straight jacket. By introducing his dichotomy of learning and confirming, Sheiner wanted to acknowledge the importance of statistical significance in phase III confirming trials, but reduce its hold over the design of the trials earlier in the development process by classifying them as learning trials.

The key goal of a learning trial is to estimate some quantities about the system being tested, parameters of a model being fitted perhaps, whereas a confirming trial answers a dichotomous question such as: Does this compound have an effect comparable to an existing treatment? The learning trial generates hypotheses to test and we use a confirming trial to test them.

The more we want to learn in our learning-phase trials, such as what is the best dose, are there significant subpopulation effects, and what is the course of the treated disease over time, the less useful conventional experimental statistics become. As a consequence of leaving conventional experimental statistics behind, we lose their ability to calculate key quantities analytically. Therefore, the only way to determine if our trial design is sound is to simulate it.

11.1.3. The Clinical Trial Model

To simulate a clinical trial we combine a number of component models (Figure 11.1). The degree of detail and complexity in these models will vary widely between different simulations and will depend on what it is we wish to estimate.

The component models are:

- The *trial protocol*: entry criteria, nature and timing of subject visits and subject monitoring, treatment arms (doses and dosing regimens), nature of endpoints to be studied
- The *population*: population covariates and covariate correlation
- The *responses*: a model of responses observed for a subject given their covariate values and the dosing regimen (also called the input–output model)
- The *trial execution*: recruitment rates, dropout rates, subject compliance
- The *analysis*: an implementation of the analysis plan, other relevant summary statistics, estimation of model parameters
- *Trial adaptation*: trial early stopping, changing inclusion criteria, dropping or adding treatment arms, shifting of randomization probabilities (e.g., the continuous reassessment method, Bayesian dose-finding designs, play-the-winner/biased coin designs)

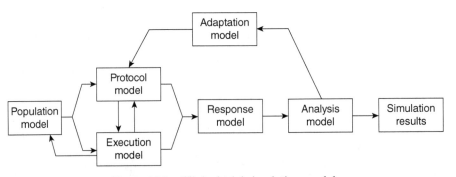

Figure 11.1   Clinical trial simulation model.

The population model creates a population from which the simulator will sample to create the subjects simulated within the trial. These models are dynamic models in which covariates and their correlations either are specified via hypothetical probability distributions or by a fixed set of population data from which samples are taken with replacement.

The protocol model implements inclusion and exclusion criteria, randomization rules, treatment arms, and so on, which govern whether the simulated patient is included in the simulated trial and the treatment received. This model interacts with the trial execution model, which simulates recruitment rates, subjects dropping out, missed visits, and other patient noncompliance. The execution model can interact with the population model to modify the parameters of the population model to simulate changes in the population over time or the opening up of subject recruitment in a different part of the world.

The response, or input–output, model takes the treatment regimen from the protocol model, the patient covariates from the population model, and patient behavior from the execution model and simulates the responses observed for the subject for the different responses and at the different time points at which the subject is being observed.

The analysis model implements the proposed analysis plan on the set of data that should be available at the time, whether at an interim stage or at the end of the trial. If the simulation is of an adaptive trial, the result of an interim analysis is passed to the adaptive model that simulates the preplanned adaptation and updates the appropriate parameters of the protocol: for example, to stop the trial altogether, drop a treatment arm, drop a subpopulation from the trial, or simply vary the probability of randomization to the different treatment arms.

Finally, the results of each simulated trial are compiled in a database of simulation results for analysis of the simulations.

In defining which simulations to run, it is important to note that the parameters that need to be specified for the simulations fall into four distinct groups:

1. Properties of the protocol are fixed parameters over which the clinical team may have some control. These are such properties of the trial as which endpoint will be studied, how many different doses or dosing regimens will be used, and when subjects will be evaluated.

2. The unknown parameters that the trial will be designed to estimate, such as the probability of observing the toxicity at each dose, the between-subject variance in response, the within-subject variance in response, the parameters of a PK–PD model, and the parameters of a dose–response model.

3. The unknown parameters of the trial that cannot be controlled directly by the clinical team. Typically, these include parameters that the trial is not attempting to estimate but that may affect how the trial performs,

such as the rate at which subjects are recruited, the probability of patient noncompliance, and the probability of patients dropping out.

4. The parameters and form of the statistical design: the analysis and (if applicable) the adaptation. These are usually under the control of the trial statistician and need to be set to meet constraints placed on the trial, such as the level of statistical significance, power, and/or trial size. As trial designs become more sophisticated, these statistical parameters are becoming more numerous. For example, parameters to specify include how to perform the analysis (e.g., pairwise comparison, parametric or nonparametric model fitting), the initial values or prior probabilities to use, how to adjust for multiplicity, whether to perform adaptation, and what form of adaptation to use: sample size reassessment, early stopping, dose escalation, arm dropping, or biased randomization.

11.1.4. Analysis of Simulation Results

There are some standard properties of the proposed trial that are important to learn about through simulations, including the probable duration and cost of the trial and the probability of making the correct decision concerning whether or not to continue development of the compound.

One also wants to learn about the probable quality of other decisions made during clinical development, such as the correct identification of the MED or MTD, the correct selection of suitable doses for further development, and the correct identification of patient subpopulations to exclude from treatment. These ancillary decisions can be considered to be just as important as the decision as to whether to continue development of the compound; however, they are not typically planned for during the design of conventional trials.

Finally, there is an assessment of the probable quality of the information that will be learned from the trial, such as the bias and precision in the estimate of the response on different treatment arms, or the precision with which model parameters can be estimated.

11.2. TYPES OF MODELS USED IN CLINICAL TRIAL DESIGN

The models fall into three types:

1. The probabilistic models, which simulate unknowns such as population characteristics, recruitment rates, and subject responses to treatment. These models are the population model, the execution model, and the response model.
2. The control models, including the protocol model and the adaptive model, which implement decisions in the trial.
3. The analysis model, which estimates some of the key parameters that have been simulated.

11.2.1. Population Models

A population model is used to generate the individual characteristics of the simulated subjects that will be used subsequently in the other component models in the simulation. In particular, these will be the characteristics that drive the response model, such as age, weight, gender, baseline score, and membership of genetic subgroups. This form of modeling is particularly a characteristic of trials using PK–PD-driven response models and adaptive trials that are adaptive to patient subgroups.

In some simulations, the population is simply a null model; the response model is simply driven per treatment arm by mean rates of response plus variability using binomial and normal probability distributions.

Population models can simply be probability distributions for each characteristic from which the parameters are sampled or can be more sophisticated models that account for the correlation between values (e.g., age, gender, and weight). Most late-stage trials (phase IIb and later) are international, and for these, regional differences in population characteristics should be included in the model. The population model may interact with the execution model, which determines when and at what rate subjects are recruited in the various regions.

Ideally, population data should be available, even if only for placebo-treated patients, to guide the model. In some cases, the model can be replaced simply by sampling from appropriate available patient-specific data.

11.2.2. Protocol Models

The protocol model implements the trial inclusion–exclusion criteria by filtering the subjects generated by the population model. Such models implement the randomization rules: the proportion of subjects allocated to each treatment arm, the dose titration rules, the subject's visit schedule, and the observations collected at each visit. The protocol model interacts with the response model, as the response simulated for the subject determines whether dose titration occurs and whether the subject should, in fact, remain in the trial. It also interacts with the execution model in order to simulate patient noncompliances.

Moreover, the protocol model is a deterministic model that implements the trial designer's rules applied to the probabilistic data being generated in the other models. It interacts with the adaptation model, implementing the adaptation model decisions, such as to stop the trial, to drop (or add) a treatment arm, to drop a population subgroup, or to modify the randomization probabilities.

11.2.3. Execution Models

The execution model simulates the behaviors and activities in the trial that cannot be controlled directly. The model simulates recruitment rates, possibly with a detailed structure such as when recruitment begins in a region, the rate at which it is expected to ramp up, and the long-term mean recruitment rate. If the population model includes regional differences, the execution model interacts with it to control from which region the next patient is drawn.

Recruitment is usually specified in terms of the mean rate over a period, and variability around the mean rate is typically modeled using a Poisson distribution. Subjects' missing visits and dosing noncompliances (if simulated at all) are usually simulated as random events drawn from a particular probability distribution. Finally, the execution model may include provisions for simulating patient dropouts. This implementation can be simply at random, random per treatment arm, or random per visit. Alternatively, the dropouts can be driven by the response model. For example, patients could drop out due to a perceived lack of efficacy or perceived efficacy, or due to an intolerable level of side effects.

11.2.4. Response (Input–Output) Models

The response model determines the response of a subject given their characteristics (covariates) and the treatment they have been given (the treatment arm to which they have been randomized). It is typically either a PK–PD model or a model that is simply dependent on the treatment arm to which the subject has been randomized.

These models are typically mixed-effect models with fixed and random components. In the treatment arm–driven model, the fixed element is a probability of response per treatment arm or a mean change from baseline per treatment arm. The random component is then provided either by a Bernoulli test with the given probability or by a normally distributed error term. More complexity may be added by including the limits of the range being measured, where the change from baseline can be truncated.

PK–PD models calculate drug exposure from the dose and patient characteristics plus a random effects model that can be additive, proportional, or combined (both additive and proportional). If the endpoint observed is not drug concentration, a model relating the exposure to the endpoint is required.

In some cases, multiple responses need to be simulated: for example, an efficacy endpoint and a toxicity endpoint. These responses can simply be modeled separately, modeled with correlation, or modeled using an underlying exposure in combination with separate exposure response models. Sometimes, to retain simplicity, a composite endpoint is modeled, although simulation (and then analysis) of the separate endpoints should be more powerful.

Additional complexity is introduced when intermediate endpoint observations are made (i.e., the endpoint is also observed at earlier visits) or some other earlier observations (e.g., a biomarker) are observed. In this case the response model must include features such as the proportion of the final change from baseline observed from visit to visit, the intrasubject variability, and the degree of correlation between observations.

In a PK–PD model-driven trial, the intermediate observations will be used to estimate the time component of the model. In an adaptive trial the observations will be used to predict the subjects' final outcomes, in order to increase the information available at early interims.

11.2.5. Analysis Models

The analysis model fits a PK–PD model or statistical model to the simulated data at trial interims in order to drive adaptation or at the end of the trial as part of the trial analysis. The analysis models are used to analyze the responses generated by the response model. Usually, the purpose of the simulations is to see how well the analysis model estimates the simulated "truth." Clearly, the analysis model should have no knowledge of the underlying response model. Rather, it must perform its analysis using only the user-specified parameters to the protocol, analysis and adaptive models, the priors, and the simulated response data.

The analysis model may be completely analytic, or it may use Monte Carlo techniques to fit its models, but it does this only for the purposes of estimating the model parameters. It does not simulate data in the way that the population model, execution model, and response model do. The analysis model carries out the analysis of the key trial data similar to a trial statistician, but it has been automated so that it can be carried out over many simulation runs. Because of the overhead of this automation, only the analysis that is critical to the execution of the trial is automated, not every piece of analysis that the trial statistician will do.

Typically, Bayesian models are used during statistical model fitting, while standard mathematical techniques such as Gibbs sampling and Metropolis–Hastings are employed to estimate the parameters of the model. These techniques use sampling methods to allow complex integrals to be performed that cannot be calculated analytically.

11.2.6. Adaptation Models

Adaptation models are a set of prospectively defined rules for modifying the trial behavior based on the data observed. Common examples of adaptation models include dose escalation rules in phase I trials, such as "3 plus 3," "up and down," and the "continuous reassessment method"; an interim look to judge whether to stop the trial for futility or to calculate the sample size required to finish the trial with the desired power (sample size reassessment); a group sequential design model in which a number of interim looks are used to determine whether the trial can be terminated for efficacy or futility. These designs are sometimes used for phase III trials.

Recently, more adaptive approaches have explored methods such as biasing the randomization toward the more effective treatment arm (e.g., cancer trials comparing different combinations of treatments); adaptively modifying the allocation ratio across a range of different doses of the study drug to best identify a target dose such as the minimum efficacious dose or ED_{90}; over a series of interim looks to identify any treatment arms that are insufficiently likely to be effective or safe and drop them; and modeling the response separately over a number of defined subpopulations and stopping recruitment in subpopulations where the treatment is insufficiently likely to be effective or safe.

To be able to run large numbers of simulations, the adaptation decision cannot be manual but must be coded in a model. In practice, when the trial is run, there may be some manual oversight of the adaptation, and manual override of the adaptation strategy is usually enabled if safety issues need to be taken into account.

11.3. SOURCES OF PRIOR INFORMATION FOR DESIGNING CLINICAL TRIALS

As designs for trials get more complex, we need more information to inform design decisions such as suitable models for analysis, useful endpoints for adaptation, and covariate factors that need to be taken into account. Along with the standard information about the primary endpoint, including the expected placebo response, one must also consider its variability and the best time to collect the data.

For simulated trial design, we also want to know possible values to simulate: parameters for population models, the dose–response curve, dropout rates, and so on. There are many sources of data. For example, published papers may provide theory, accepted parameters, and the behavior of the disease models.

Prior trial or study results can provide data about the endpoint, even if only of placebo-treated patients. However, some care must be taken in how these data are used. For example, studies of the central nervous system exhibit a placebo response that is notoriously variable from trial to trial. For example, see the depression and schizophrenia studies as outlined by Kirsch et al. (2002). Also, care must be taken in the use of data in indications where the standard of care is changing and new treatments are being used. These factors can affect the expected change in endpoint, endpoint variability, and progression of the endpoint over time.

Of particular use are in-house data from animal experiments, PK–PD models, and previous trials, because they are recent and relevant. However, the data are likely to be only mildly informative unless the previous trials were large. This limitation may be due to the risk of applying animal results to humans, the risk of overinterpreting PK–PD models, and because the previous trials are likely to have been small first-in-man studies or may have given equivocal results, and hence need to be repeated. Accordingly, one must not rely too heavily on these data. For example, Bayesian prior probabilities, although not necessarily noninformative, should not be so strong that they dominate the actual study data in the final analysis. One technique to avoid this situation is to incorporate prior data via a hierarchical model and not directly as a prior (Spiegelhalter et al., 2004).

To properly evaluate the design alternatives, cost–benefit analysis should be used, where possible, in a decision-theoretic framework. This requires a different sort of prior data, including the likely time and costs of trials, how those times and costs vary with trial size, requirements for the efficacy and tolerability of the drug for it to be commercially viable, the probable revenue from a commercially viable drug, and how that revenue is affected by trial outcomes, delays, changes in the treatable population, and changes in the treatment regimen. Prior data for this analysis may be difficult to obtain, although in large pharmaceutical companies the commercial division and portfolio management group should be the best sources. Smaller companies may need the help of external bodies such as clinical experts, key investigators, and patient self-help groups.

11.4. ASPECTS OF A TRIAL TO BE DESIGNED AND OPTIMIZED

Simulation has its advantages. As noted by Thall (2001): "I have always considered it more desirable to kill computer generated patients than real ones while calibrating design parameters." Simulation can be used to guide the design and optimize the trial protocol, execution, analysis, and planned adaptation.

- Simulation of different scenarios and the final analysis can help determine if the trial design is consistent with the overall aims of the development program. For example, what should the aim of the trial be? How will new knowledge be used to guide the subsequent steps in drug development? What data would clearly demonstrate that the development of the compound for this indication should be abandoned? What characteristics of the treatment are required if further stages of development are to be undertaken?
- What is the effect of basing the trial on a different endpoint compared to that planned for the phase III trial? For example, one may consider endpoints that are quicker to collect, or more precise but too expensive to use in phase III. Simulation of a phase II trial and analysis of how its endpoint compares to the phase III endpoint can help determine the risk of using an endpoint other than the phase III endpoint for early decision making.
- What is the effect of different patient entry criteria on the probable outcome? For example, if patient improvement is judged as a change from

baseline on some score (e.g., a pain score, HAM-D, ADAS-Cog), what impact does the required baseline score for entry into the trial have on the ability to detect the drug effect? Patients with a severe initial score are more likely to improve on placebo, possibly making it more difficult to demonstrate drug effect, while patients with too mild a score may have less opportunity for improvement. The degree to which patients recover may depend on the baseline score, and it may be possible to allow for this in the trial analysis or by using stratification. With these considerations, simulation of the patient change in endpoint using a disease model can help optimize the trial entry criteria.
- When should tests be performed? For example: when planning PK–PD studies?

Simulation of the trial execution can help with the planning and logistics of the trial. Frequently, the most important aspect of trial execution is the patient recruitment rate. For example, utilizing more centers can expedite a trial; however, this will increase costs, the variability in patient outcomes, and the complexity of the trial logistics. Using more centers may mean using centers in more countries or more continents—further increasing cost, variability, and complexity. If a trial is to be adaptive, faster recruitment usually limits the degree of adaptation possible. Simulation and cost–benefit analysis can help determine a good trade-off between quick recruitment and the cost, variability, and complexity of the trial.

The second most important aspect of trial execution is the number of subject dropouts. Depending on how dropouts are handled in the statistical analysis, a high dropout rate can make achieving a statistically significant result difficult. For example, using the "last observation carried forward" strategy or treating dropouts as nonresponders can significantly reduce the estimate of the drug's response. The likelihood that a patient will drop out will exert its effect on the estimated therapeutic response of the compound and must therefore be accounted for during the design phase to ensure that the trial is not underpowered.

Conventionally, for there to be a reasonable chance of a statistically significant outcome, the project biostatistician has been asked primarily to consider the number of subjects required to be included in the trial. As trials become more complex and the pressure to maximize the information gained from a learning phase trial increases, the analysis plan needs to be more sophisticated. In particular, how should the various options be taken into account, such as possible treatment regimens, endpoints, interim analyses, and patient subpopulations? Frequently, these considerations and the possible designs to cope with them take us outside the range of the simply calculable, and the only way to evaluate them rationally is to use simulation.

The design techniques that are being developed for these problems use various forms of modeling. For example, dose–response modeling, longitudinal modeling (the evolution of a subject's responses over time), and disease and drug modeling with biomarkers and adaptation are all valuable approaches that have shown value to trial design and planning.

The population and response models, however, are essentially given and outside our control. Variations in these models should be tried as part of the sensitivity analysis and robustness testing of the other models.

11.5. TRIAL SIMULATION

Trial simulation makes possible a number of significant technical advances in the design of clinical trials that are discussed below. Perhaps the most profound effect of simulating clinical trials, however, is to engender a deeper understanding of the trial in the clinical team before the trial starts. Trial simulations allow a far wider range of trial characteristics to be evaluated than can be achieved by calculation alone, and a far wider range of possible scenarios to be explored. But in addition to looking at the means and standard deviations of thousands of simulated trials, individual simulations can, and should, be scrutinized by the clinical team. In this way the team gains two particularly profound insights. First, given the underlying "truth" being simulated, one can understand how complex the clinical data might be, perhaps simply because of the variability in the endpoint. Second, the team can better appreciate what they might decide given the data (and how confident they are in that decision) compared to the truth being simulated (Pereira, 2006).

One of the primary reasons for the increased interest in simulation is to explore and evaluate novel trial designs. These designs have been developed to address the difficulties we are facing in drug development: increased concern about the safety, cost, and effectiveness of new drugs, the difficulties of studying the most important diseases that still have no effective treatment (such as Alzheimer's), and increased time pressures on drug development.

To see how effective a novel design is at tackling these problems, simulation is required to generate data on the operating characteristics of the trial designs under different assumptions. The typical operating characteristics considered are:

- How likely is one to make the correct decision at the end of the trial either to terminate or to continue development?
- How likely are the trial data to be inconclusive, leaving the sponsor in the unfortunate position of not knowing whether to stop development of the compound or to press on with its development? Such ambiguity could result in embarking on an expensive subsequent trial with poor confidence of success, or repeating the inconclusive trial, incurring further cost and delay in development.
- How likely are we to choose the correct treatment for further development (e.g., to choose the right dose for phase III)?

- What are the probable bias and error in the estimate of response for the treatment regimen chosen for the next phase?
- How many subjects are we likely to have recruited before we are able to correctly deduce that none of the study treatments are working?
- How many subjects are we likely to have randomized to the treatment chosen for the next phase?

All the operating characteristics will depend on the scenarios being simulated, and simulations can be used to check the robustness of the design over alternative assumptions, such as different recruitment rates, different variability in the endpoint, different dropout rates, different dose–response profiles, and different parameters in the disease and drug-effect models.

An early use of simulation was to integrate disease, drug, and population information with the trial design. These methods used PK and population models to drive the simulation and to explore aspects of the trial design, such as the choice of doses to test, the dosing regimens to use, the time points for patient testing, intra- and intersubject variability, and the impact of changing patient entry criteria. These applications should expand with the growth of translational medicine. Accordingly, one may include features such as disease models, biomarker models, patient subpopulation models, and treatment interaction models in the simulator. These advances provide a mechanism for integrating diverse preclinical information and investigating the expected operating characteristics of the planned design in the light of this information.

By using these underlying models to generate the responses in the simulated trial, we can use this knowledge to guide trial design. The operating characteristics we estimate from these simulations will be based on these models, and the design options will be chosen based on the trade-offs between characteristics that are of most benefit to the business. In the simulated range, it is important to perform a sensitivity analysis on all the unknowns to ensure that the design chosen is robust and not too highly tuned to a very specific set of assumptions.

By simulating very specific scenarios and running many simulations for each, we can get good estimates of how the design performs and the probable error and bias in the values that will be estimated at the end of the trial.

An alternative method of running simulations is to sample randomly from specified distributions for the parameters underlying the given scenario. This method can be used to assess the robustness of the design. Some characteristics, such as the probable trial size and duration, can simply be estimated from the overall simulation results. But other characteristics will require that the analysis be automated, as the results of each simulated trial will need to be analyzed relative to the specific scenario parameters for that run.

Owing to the differences between the two approaches, simulation tools are often built to perform only one or another type of simulation.

11.6. OPTIMIZING DESIGNS

Compared to traditional trial designs, modern designs use multiple looks at the data, along with preplanned adaptation and modeling to address systematically the problems introduced by the large number of unknowns in drug development. This new complexity in modern trial design means that one may have many more free parameters in the designs that need to be chosen for a given trial. For example, one may need to assess the number and nature of the treatment regimens to be tested, the criteria for stopping the trial or dropping treatment arms, the timing of tests on subjects, the effect of varying the recruitment rate, and so on.

In PK–PD studies we can simulate drawing samples from subjects at different intervals and estimate over the range of probable scenarios which test intervals that best allow us to update our PK–PD model. Similarly, by simulating the trial using the PK–PD model to drive the simulated subject responses, one can assess when and how best to evaluate subjects.

For dose-finding trials it is clear that one needs to be concerned about more operating characteristics than simply the probability of making a type 1^2 or type 2^3 error, such as: How often is the right dose selected? How early can one stop the trial if the treatment is ineffective? How best can one maximize the number of subjects allocated to the dose selected? To what degree can one minimize the risk of an inconclusive outcome?

To perform optimization, we need to prioritize the operating characteristics based on their relative importance; optimizing one characteristic will, to differing degrees, be at the expense of the others. Such trade-offs will depend on the parameter being varied. A thorough approach to optimization might entail a utility function for combining the criteria and a decision-theoretic approach. The methodology might, for example, include modeling the remainder of the drug development process and its time, costs, and the likelihood of, and benefit from, a successful registration.

This type of optimization is currently more a research topic than standard practice, and optimization currently follows a more ad hoc approach along the following lines. First, following conventional design, upper limits on the trial size and type 1 and type 2 errors are fixed. The adaptive design in then compared against the conventional design on a small number of conventional scenarios, such as no response, linear response, and perhaps an E_{max} response from the PK–PD model, or some dose–response profile based on data from earlier trials.

The adaptive design usually has to support lower type 1 and type 2 errors for the same maximum study size to be considered as an alternative to the

---

[2] An error where the data from the trial are interpreted as showing that the treatment is successful when in fact it isn't.

[3] An error where the data from the trial are interpreted as showing that the treatment is not successful when in fact it is.

conventional design. Often, the adaptive design is used to test more doses and still match the characteristics of the more basic design. For a proof-of-concept and/or phase II dose-finding study, the next step in optimization is usually to see if an early "stopping for futility" condition can be added in order to save time and cost if the treatment is failing, while keeping the level of type 2 error below the target.

As the adaptive design is explored further, more scenarios for simulation are likely to be added by the clinical team. Examples of these scenarios include conditions where the compound's simulated effectiveness is better than placebo but still insufficiently effective or shows only borderline effectiveness. For these scenarios the target type 1 and/or type 2 error requirements may need to be relaxed.

The next optimization is for scenarios where the compound's simulated effectiveness is clinically better than that of a placebo. Usually, optimization for these scenarios is around the linked characteristics of the probability of identifying the target dose, the probability of identifying a suitable dose for phase III (where the gradient of the response curve is shallow around the target dose, and selection of the target dose is likely to be difficult to achieve, but selection of neighboring doses is acceptable), the proportion of subjects allocated to the dose selected, and the accuracy of the estimate of response at the target dose.

Goals for optimization include saving time and money under futile development scenarios and maximizing information in successful scenarios, while keeping type 1 and type 2 error within acceptable bounds. To modify the design to achieve such optimization, there are a number of design parameters that can be varied (although the clinical team may place restrictions on some of them). These parameters include the rate of recruitment; the number of doses; the duration and allocations used in the initial fixed allocation before adaptation starts; the endpoint(s) used to guide the adaptation; which models are used to fit the response data; the parameters of the models, including initial values and priors; how many subjects must be recruited before early stopping; what conditions and thresholds are used to decide to stop; and the final conditions and thresholds used to evaluate the trial.

Given the combinatorics of the problem, a full exploration of this parameter space is impracticable for all but the simplest designs. For example, the number of simulations required to reduce the sampling error in the estimates of the operating characteristics versus the number of scenarios over which to evaluate will grow multiplicatively. Usually, a starting set of parameters that give close to acceptable levels of type 1 and type 2 error is arrived at by experience and trial and error. Subsequently, each parameter is tuned in turn. Selection parameters such as the choice of the model are usually explored first, with an otherwise simple design (no adaptation) to see which model performs best over the multiple scenarios. Then the scale parameters may be optimized.

For example, optimizing the threshold value for early stopping in the case of futility can reduce the mean trial size for an ineffective scenario. As the stopping criteria become less conservative, there will be a clear and monotonic effect, so that the average study size will reduce. However, adjusting the stopping criteria in this manner will eventually cause an increase in type 2 errors. Accordingly, one must allow for interactions between trial parameters and make adjustments that yield the best trade-offs between reduction in study size and possible increases in type 2 error.

11.7. REAL-WORLD EXAMPLES

The examples discussed below illustrate how prior data, PK–PD models, and simulation can be used to make informed decisions for the design of future trials.

Jumbe et al. (2002) developed a PK–PD model based on data from a previous trial. This model was used in a trial simulator to compare a fixed-dose design with a weight-based dose design. The question posed was: Is a weight-based treatment regimen necessary, or could a simpler fixed-dose regimen be used instead? The indication was chemotherapy-induced anemia. The results showed that by restricting the trial to the central 90% of the patient population by weight, the effect of the simpler regimen on the mean hemoglobin change was negligible.

The design of antidepressant trials was simulated by Gruwez et al. (2007) using a kinetic–pharmacodynamic (K–PD) model. First, using data from a previous trial, the fit of the K–PD model to the data was evaluated. Then using the population model, the investigators simulated and evaluated the use of various statistics to assess the treatment effect and different patient assessment dates.

To optimize the design of HIV lipodystrophy trials, Abbas et al. (2008) built a model for cholesterol levels in HIV patients in addition to their recruitment and dropout rates based on prior clinical data. This study demonstrated that the simulation results were readily understood by clinicians and served as a powerful tool for validating their expert guidance for the trial design. The simulations provided better estimates for the power of a trial design, allowing the total cost of the trial to be minimized.

A detailed description of the simulation process using NONMEM was presented by Gastonguay et al. (2003) for the development of a PK–PD trial in children based on the data from trials in adults. NONMEM, developed at the University of California–San Francisco, is a widely used software package[4] for nonlinear regression analysis of population PK–PD data.

[4]Alternative packages that can be used for analyzing population PK–PD data are WinNonLin; the nlme package in S, S-Plus, and R; and PKBugs, the PK–PD extension to the Bayesian modeling software Bugs.

De Ridder (2004) focused on the design of phase III trials. In particular, in contrast to traditional techniques used in designing phase III trials, the use of clinical trial simulation in this study allowed the uncertainties of the current knowledge to be taken into account, leading to a more conservative, yet more robust phase III design. The phase III design was tested by simulating the drug action and a disease progression model, along with a study execution model. This approach was applied successfully to phase II data and an ongoing phase III study.

The design of the ASTIN stroke study (Krams et al., 2003) exemplifies many of the principles highlighted in this chapter regarding the necessity for trial simulation for adaptive trial designs (Grieve and Krams, 2005). In this study the authors investigated a complex Bayesian design for an adaptive dose-ranging study that would also have been one of the two confirmatory trials had the compound been successful. The design process included a large and time-consuming trial simulation project. Using a factorial design for the simulation experiment, a range of values for different parameters and design choices were assessed over a common set of scenarios. The result not only provided a basis for the final parameter and design choices, but also showed the robustness of the core model and helped validate the software implementation.

11.8. CONCLUSIONS

Drug development is getting more challenging, with longer development times, greater development costs, and fewer successful submissions to regulators. Many causes contribute to this situation: The "low-hanging fruit" has been picked in terms of the diseases for which successful treatments have already been found; also, society is concerned increasingly about the safety of new drugs, about the evidence of clear clinical benefit, and about the increasing speed with which competitors can produce "me too" compounds that can compete directly with a new drug before its patent life has expired.

A significant part of the answer to this problem will be smarter designs for clinical trials that are better aligned to the needs of the development program for that compound, and the only way that we will be able to assess, understand, evaluate, and optimize these designs is by simulating them.

REFERENCES

Abbas, I., Rovira, J., Josep, C., and Greenfield, T. (2008). Optimal design of clinical trials with computer simulation based on results of earlier trials, illustrated with a lipodystrophy trial in HIV patients. *J Biomed Inf 41*(6), 1053–1061.

De Ridder, F. (2004). Predicting the outcome of phase 3 trials using phase 2 data: a case study of clinical trial simulation in late stage development. *Basic Clin Pharmacol Toxicol 96*(3), 235–241.

Duffal, S.B., and Kimko, H.C. (2003). *Simulation for Designing Clinical Trials: A Pharmacokinetic–Pharmacodynamic Modeling Perspective.* Marcel Dekker, New York.

Gastonguay, M.R., Gibiansky, E., Gibiansky, L., and Barrett, J. (2003). Optimizing a Bayesian dose-adjustment scheme for a pediatric trial: a simulation study. In: *Simulation for Designing Clinical Trials* (Duffal, S.B., Kimkp, H.C., eds.). Marcel Dekker, New York.

Grieve, A., and Krams, M. (2005). ASTIN: a bayesian adaptive dose–response trial in acute stroke. *Clin Trials 2*(4), 340–351.

Gruwez, B., Poirier, M.-F., Dauphin, A., Olie, J.-P., and Tod, M. (2007). A kinetic–pharmacodynamic model for clinical trial simulation of antidepressant action: application to clomipramine–lithium interaction. *Contemp Clin Trials 28*(3), 276–287.

Jumbe, N., Yao, B., Rovetti, R., Rossi, G., and Heatherington, A.C. (2002). Clinical trial simulation of a 200-micmog fixed dose of darbepoetin alfa in chemotherapy induced anemia. *Oncology 16*(10, Suppl. 11), 37–44.

Kirsch, I., Moore, T.J., Scoboria, A., and Nicholls, S.S. (2002). The emperor's new drugs: an analysis of antidepressant medication data submitted to the U.S. Food and Drug Administration. *Prev Treat 5*, Art. 23.

Krams, M., Kennedy, R.L., Hacke, W., Grieve, A., Orgogozo, J.-M., and Ford, G.A. (2003). Acute stroke therapy by inhibition of neutrophils (ASTIN), an adaptive dose–response Study of UK-279,2776 in acute ischemic stroke. *Stroke 34*, 2543–2548.

Pereira, L.M. (2006). Critical considerations about clinical trials simulation: current opinion. *Int J Pharm Med 20*(1), 1–15.

Piantadosi, S. (2005). *Clinical Trials: A Methodologic Perspective*, 2nd ed. Wiley Series in Probability and Statistics. Wiley, Hoboken, NJ.

Pocock, S.J. (1983). *Clinical Trials: A Practical Approach.* Wiley, New York.

Sheiner, L.B. (1997). Learning versus confirming in clinical drug development. *Clin Pharamacol Ther 61*, 275–291.

Spiegelhalter, D.J., Abrams, K.R., and Myles, J.P. (2004). *Bayesian Approaches to Clinical Trials and Health Care Evaluation* Wiley Statistics in Practice Series. Wiley, Hoboken, NJ.

Thall, P. (2001). Bayesian clinical trial design in a cancer center. *Chance 15*(3), 23–28.

PART IV

SYNERGIES WITH OTHER TECHNOLOGIES

CHAPTER 12

Pathway Analysis in Drug Discovery

ANTON YURYEV

Ariadne Genomics Inc., Rockville, Maryland

Summary

In this chapter we review pathway analysis and describe the state of the art of this methodology, providing real-life examples of how the methodology is being used in the modern drug development pipeline. We overview available solutions for *in silico* pathway analysis and suggest future directions and applications in drug discovery and personalized medicine.

12.1. INTRODUCTION: PATHWAY ANALYSIS, DYNAMIC MODELING, AND NETWORK ANALYSIS

Computational pathway analysis considers the human organism as a collection of pathways. The analysis focuses on how these pathways interact with each other, how they are altered in disease, and how drugs influence the pathways during therapeutic intervention. The comprehensive pathway collection for the human organism must contain several hundred thousand pathways (Badretdinov and Yuryev, 2006). Such large numbers of pathways are due primarily to the large number of tissues in the human body. At present, however, only a few hundred pathways have been well studied. Therefore, the current focus of pathway analysis is on expanding the pathway collection to enable accurate computerized prediction of drug action and analysis of experimental patient data. The process of pathway building, often called *pathway inference* is currently semiautomatic, utilizing the database of interactions between biological molecules. There are at least 240 different database resources for molecular interactions according to http://www.pathguide.org.

Systems Biology in Drug Discovery and Development, First Edition.
Edited by Daniel L. Young, Seth Michelson.
© 2012 John Wiley & Sons, Inc. Published 2012 by John Wiley & Sons, Inc.

Therefore, the term *database* is used in this chapter to refer to the computational method of storing interactions in a relational database program rather than to any particular data set.

Pathway analysis shares computational tools with network analysis. Both approaches use the database of molecular interactions and graph navigation tools to query the global molecular interactions and network of a cell. Worth emphasizing here is the difference between a biological pathway and a biological network, even though these terms are often used interchangeably. A *biological pathway* is an abstraction that is visualized in the form of a diagram to depict the propagation of information in a biological network. A pathway must have an input signal, terminal target nodes receiving the signal, and directed relations showing how the information is transmitted from one biological molecule to another. The term *biological network* is used to describe the compendium of all possible molecular interactions between all proteins in a cell or between a subset of proteins in the case of disease or signaling networks. A *disease network* consists of biological molecules that have been shown experimentally to be involved in or linked to the disease. A *signaling network* consists of molecules induced by a biological signal such as an increase in hormone concentration. Unlike the pathway that depicts the transient sequence of events, a network, by definition, is a stable community of proteins and other biological molecules persisting in time and space. A biological network serves as the transmission medium for the information propagation depicted by the pathway diagram. If a network distorts normal pathway signaling, it becomes the disease network that enables malignant information flow, causing the disease. A disease network persists in time due to a combination of genetic and/or somatic mutations, environmental factors, patient lifestyle, and medical history. The signaling networks persist in time due to the constant level of hormones that induce them. Such constant levels of hormones exist, for example, in the basal state when these levels are not sufficient to initiate functional cellular response and are used by an organism to enable cell survival in the quiescent state. Constant hormone levels can be altered in a disease and consequently change the corresponding signaling through the network (Saban et al., 2007).

Building a pathway diagram is the first step in the development of a kinetic simulation model for the pathway. A mathematical model can be used for quantitative studies of the information flows and for predicting pathway response to a drug. Currently, dynamic modeling faces challenges that do not allow for wide practical application. The lack of knowledge about conserved molecular pathway mechanisms, about *in vivo* kinetic constants and molecular concentrations, and the small number of available pathway diagrams all slow down the development of reliable kinetic models. The existing models were developed over several years by both biology and mathematics experts. Their development required dedicated molecular biological experiments to measure the quantitative behavior of a pathway to enable model fitting. For example, the elucidation of molecular mechanisms of the cell cycle in yeast began in

1991 by identifying key protein players in this process. This work was preceded by 25 years of yeast cell cycle genetics (Hartwell, 1991) that ultimately yielded one Nobel prize award, hundreds of scientific publications, and finally, the first mathematical model of the yeast cycle, published in 1997 (Novak and Tyson, 1997). A study of the kinetic properties of this model appeared in 2006 (Wang et al., 2006).

The large number of components in the typical biological pathway coupled with the highly sparse and noisy experimental knowledge about system behavior often cause model overfitting, significantly reducing the robustness and reliability of the model (Sun and Zhao, 2004). Therefore, most current models use very few components to explain the most complex behavioral patterns observed in biological objects. For example, oscillation patterns in cell cycle can be modeled using only 11 principal cell cycle proteins (Li et al., 2004; Novak and Tyson, 1997; Wang et al., 2006); the circadian rhythm model contains 12 protein species (Leloup et al., 1999); the model for damped oscillatory activation of NF-κB by an LPS-activated TLR receptor contains seven proteins (Covert et al., 2005); and the threshold mechanism of transition between cell survival and apoptosis is modeled with, at most, nine proteins (Bagci et al., 2006; Bentele et al., 2004; Fussenegger et al., 2000; Hua et al., 2005; Katiyar et al., 2005; Krammer et al., 2007; Legewie et al., 2006; Li and Dou, 2000).

Although mathematical modeling can provide quantitative and qualitative understanding of the dynamics of biological processes, several factors limit its practical application in drug discovery. As mentioned earlier, building a model takes a long time and requires the investment of significant resources. Due to the overfitting problem, the resulting models tend to be relatively small and therefore may have limited scope and predict the behavior of only a small number of proteins.

A comprehensive understanding of drug action ideally requires not only the understanding of the response in a target pathway but also an understanding of the response in all other off-target pathways in the human organism containing the drug targets. By way of example, drug safety has recently become the top concern of the pharmaceutical industry after several block-buster drugs were recalled due to adverse side effects. The side effects typically appear due to drug effects on off-target pathways. They become affected by a drug either because the drug target itself participates in the off-target pathways or because the drug affects additional off-target proteins, which in turn participate in off-target pathways. The ability to predict side effects will require a comprehensive collection of pathways for the human organism. Such a comprehensive collection of pathways and corresponding dynamic models for all processes and signaling events in the human organism will allow not only accurate prediction of drug efficacy but also potential side effects. Hence, the drug discovery community currently focuses on pathway inference and on the development of pathway data management systems aimed at building, maintaining, and querying such pathway collections. Such a collection of pathway diagrams can be used directly for evaluation and prediction of drug performance and later for development of complementary kinetic models for all diagrams.

12.2. SOFTWARE SYSTEMS FOR PATHWAY ANALYSIS

The ultimate goal of computational pathway analysis is to understand and predict how disease networks and drug intervention influence pathways in the human organism. Using this understanding, a pathway analysis should allow for the design of optimal personalized drug therapies based on the individual disease network measured in a patient (Yuryev, 2008). Such rationally designed personalized therapy aims to restore normal pathway signaling while disrupting the disease network and minimizing potential side effects. Two major objectives are involved in achieving this goal. First is the development of a computerized software system for storing, retrieving, and querying the vast collection of human biological pathways. The second objective is the development of algorithms for drug selection and optimization using the pathway collection in the database. Whereas the first problem lies within the domain of computer science, the second is a problem for statistics and mathematics. Computerized systems for storing biological networks have already been developed and even commercialized. The current abundance of such systems reflects the fact that there is no single perfect system. However, a set of functionalities and architectures necessary for the "ideal" software system for pathway analysis becomes clear after reviewing all available technologies. General approaches to software architecture for pathway analysis, including software packages for reader references, have been described in detail (Bokov and Yuryev, 2008; Nikitin et al., 2003). All systems can be classified into freeware made available by academic scientists and in commercial software. Academic packages include *Cytoscape* (http://www.cytoscape.org), *PathCase* (http://nashua.case.edu/PathwaysWeb/), *Pathway Tools* (http://bioinformatics.ai.sri.com/ptools/), *cPath* (http://cbio.mskcc.org/software/cpath/), *GeneMAPP* (http://www.genmapp.org), *Biological-Networks* (http://biologicalnetworks.net/) and *Cell Designer* (http://www.celldesigner.org/). Commercial software products include *Pathway analysis* from Ingenuity (http://www.ingenuity.com), *Pathway Studio* from Ariadne Genomics (http://www.ariadnegenomics.com), and *MetaCore* from GeneGO (http://www.genego.com). All software tools for pathway analysis can store global molecular interaction networks while presenting a pathway to its subnetworks. The software usually includes algorithms for network navigation that make it possible to build subnetworks and semiautomatic pathway inference.

Additionally, most commercial solutions allow import of experimental data that can be analyzed either by comparison with a pathway collection or by building networks from the interactions in the database. Gene set enrichment analysis is the most popular statistical algorithm for comparison of numerical high-throughput experimental data such as a gene expression microarray with a collection of pathways and ontological groups (Sivachenko et al., 2007; Subramanian et al., 2005). In the absence of numerical data the list of responsive genes identified in the experiment can be compared with the pathway collection using Fisher's exact test or other statistical overlap tests (Pavlidis et al., 2002; Sivachenko, 2008). In drug development, identification of pathways affected by the experimental drug treatment using the aforementioned statistical tests is used for drug validation. Indeed, to show drug efficacy, one must demonstrate that the drug treatment influences pathways affected by a disease. Pathway analysis software is also used to build disease networks from experimental data. These networks are used in the early phase of the drug discovery pipeline to understand the disease mechanism and to identify and prioritize drug targets.

A pathway collection for the human organism is estimated to have from 100,000 to 500,000 pathway diagrams (Badretdinov and Yuryev, 2006; Yuryev, 2008). Generating such an enormous number of diagrams requires dedicated computational approaches for accurate automatic pathway reconstruction and data management. Algorithms for automatic inference of a pathway from the molecular interaction data available have been developed for hormone and other biological signaling (Daraselia et al., 2007) and for biological processes (Yuryev et al., 2006). These algorithms which use standard graph navigation tools available in most pathway analysis software, first find the regulatory cascades of proteins in the regulatory network and then connect these proteins with physical interactions to determine how the information propagates through the physical interaction network.

12.3. PATHWAY ANALYSIS IN THE MODERN DRUG DEVELOPMENT PIPELINE

In this section we review current applications of computational pathway analysis and suggest several new applications that do not yet have real-life examples. The review is organized within the context of the modern drug discovery pipeline, which can be described in the following steps:

1. Understanding the disease mechanism
2. Rational selection of drug targets based on the disease mechanism
3. Structure-based drug design to find active molecules for lead compounds
4. Evaluation of drug efficacy and toxicity *in vivo*
5. Personalized rational therapy design

12.3.1. Understanding the Disease Mechanism

The emerging paradigm of modern molecular biology postulates that disease is caused by a self-sustained robust molecular interaction network. Even though the exact mechanisms of the network robustness are still being worked out (Abdollahi et al., 2007; Barabási and Oltvai, 2004; Ideker and Sharan, 2008; Leclerc, 2008), disease networks are currently being built using either experimental data from patients or disease–protein associations extracted from the literature (Abdollahi et al., 2007; Bowick et al., 2007; Chen et al., 2007; Y. Huang et al., 2007; Lim et al., 2006; MacLennan et al., 2006; Tongbai et al., 2008; Witten and Bonchev, 2007; Yang et al., 2007). The theoretical framework for building disease networks was proposed by Loscalzo et al. (2007). The typical approach to network building consists of experimental identification of proteins affected by the disease, followed by connecting these proteins to each other using interactions from the database for pathway analysis. Different types of networks are built, depending on the source of the input proteins. For example, for the proteins expressed differentially in a disease, model builders use either expression regulatory or physical interaction networks (Abdollahi et al., 2007; Lim et al., 2006), and for differentially phosphorylated proteins, they build phosphorylation networks (Chen et al., 2007). High-throughput biological experimental data contain high levels of noise. Although noise due to technological imperfections is constantly being reduced by newer-generation technologies, the intrinsic noise due to natural biological variation between samples will remain unavoidable. Therefore, the ability to form a network by the differentially expressed proteins and/or other types of experimentally determined responsive proteins is often considered as additional validation of the functional importance of these genes. Another reason for building networks for selecting responsive genes is the fact that any biological response always contains nonfunctional or nonspecific components. Such a nonspecific response may be detected from the proteins transcriptionally linked to the responsive genes. Transcriptionally linked proteins are proteins that happen to be regulated by the same transcription factor but are not related functionally.

After a disease network has been built, it is usually validated further by experiments using additional patient samples and then analyzed to determine major network regulators, to select the drug targets, or to find pathways affected by the disease. A fairly recent application of disease networks is the classification of disease. Finding subcategories of major diseases contributes to the advancement of personalized medicine (Ideker and Sharan, 2008; Kuznetsov et al., 2008). Ultimately, every patient has a unique disease network that depends on his or her genetic background, lifestyle, and medical history. All disease networks published to date were built from pools of patient samples and thus represent averaged networks that may not exist in any given patient. Averaged networks may yield important insights into disease mechanism, but individual disease networks may yield a better set of drug targets for a given patient and consequently more efficient drug treatments. Since the uniqueness of an individual disease network necessitates a personalized therapy strategy, the software tools for pathway analysis and network building are likely to become a foundation for personalized medicine. The ability to measure and calculate individual disease networks quickly will lead ultimately to the design of a personalized therapy based on the specific properties of the network in a given patient. Next, we show how disease networks and pathways can be used to prioritize drug targets. Similar approaches can be used to prioritize drug selection for personalized medicine.

12.3.2. Selecting the Drug Targets

In silico target prioritization and selection are necessary because the average disease network may contain several hundred proteins. Due to druggability constraints, it is not possible to have drugs designed for every protein in a network. It is also not possible to try every possible drug on a patient to find the optimal drug therapy using a trial-and-error approach. Therefore, perhaps the most important role of pathway analysis is in the prioritization of potential drug targets. Currently, the selection of drug targets is done by calculating the node centrality in disease networks. The higher the protein centrality in the disease network, the more disruptive its drug inhibition will be. There are several methods to calculate the centrality. The simplest centrality measures the node connectivity (the number of relations the node has in the disease network). This approach to calculating centrality has been validated in several publications (Abdollahi et al., 2007; Miller et al., 2008). More precise, yet more computationally intense approaches for calculating centrality include betweenness centrality, closeness centrality, and eigenvector centrality (Witten and Bonchev, 2007).

Because disease networks are robust and drug response is stochastic, the exact consequence of the network disruption cannot be predicted. Therefore, another method of evaluating the importance of a drug target is the use of dynamic modeling to calculate the impact on information flow in the pathways affected by disease. Since most signaling pathways have redundant information channels, this approach has yielded the recommendation that the best way to alter information flow in a pathway is to target several pathway components simultaneously (Adjei, 2006; Araujo et al., 2005; P.H. Huang et al., 2007; Lehár et al., 2008).

Both network analysis and pathway modeling allow the evaluation of drug target efficacy: predicting the likelihood of the impact on the disease if the protein is targeted by a drug. When the number of pathways predicted for 230 human tissues is compared to the number of proteins in the human genome, it becomes apparent that every protein participates in several pathways in different tissues and even within the same type of cell; therefore, drug side effects are in essence unavoidable (Yuryev, 2008). In addition, the protein hubs in disease networks tend to be the hubs in the global cellular network. Therefore, targeting highly connected proteins in a disease network also increases the risk of affecting multiple pathways and normal signaling networks within one tissue.

Drug target selection and prioritization requires the development of a statistical score for every protein in the disease network. Such a score must reflect the ability of a target to disrupt the disease network, to restore the normal information flow through pathways affected by the disease, and to evaluate the side-effect risks due to drug action in the off-target pathways. In the absence of mathematical models for every pathway in the human organism, the impact of target inhibition or activation on the information flow in every pathway can be estimated from the pathway diagram alone. This simplified approach is explained in Figure 12.1. The approach assumes equal fluxes across every edge and evaluates how upstream a protein is in the diagram and how central the protein is for a pathway. The risk of side effects can be estimated as the sum of impacts of the target in all pathways in the human organism. The potential to disrupt a disease network is proportional to the centrality of the protein in the network (Albert et al., 2000).

12.3.3. Stucture-Based Drug Design

Structure-based drug design may appear to have no relation to pathway analysis, yet the druggability constraint may force one to consider less optimal drug targets from the point of view of pathway analysis and network biology. Also, the choice of designing a protein agonist versus an antagonist depends on the function of the protein in the pathways affected by a disease.

12.3.4. Evaluation of Drug Efficacy and Toxicity *In Vivo*

Evaluation of drug efficacy and toxicity *in vivo* is currently the most popular application of pathway analysis. This assessment is usually done by analyzing the drug-treated cell lines (Hanifi-Moghaddam et al., 2005; Mulvey et al., 2007), then by moving to validation of drug action in animal models and patient samples (Gielen et al., 2005; Lee et al., 2008). In most cases researchers analyze gene expression and proteomics data to show that genes affected by the drug treatment can be linked to the disease network or to pathways affected by the disease.

12.3.5. Personalized and Combinatorial Therapy Design

The realization that every druggable target is involved in several pathways, coupled with the necessity to target network hubs to disrupt disease networks and the necessity of targeting multiple pathway components to effectively change information flow, all lead to the conclusion that the best strategy for treatment of complex disease is combinatorial therapy (Yuryev, 2008). Combining selective drugs to create drug mixtures allows almost infinite flexibility to make personalized medicine effective. Indeed, targeting multiple pathway components with a rationally designed drug mixture should reduce the risk of side effects and increase specificity toward target pathway(s). Increased specificity is achieved due to the combination of selective drugs that act uniquely against the components of one target pathway. Even though every

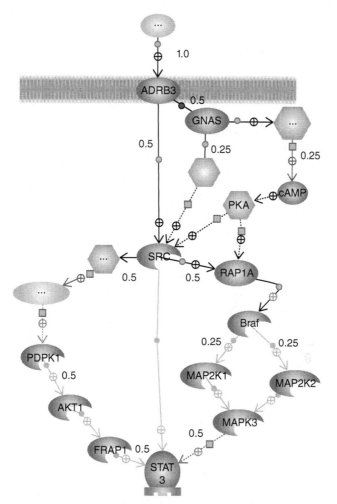

Figure 12.1 The efficacy of a drug target toward restoring the normal information flow in the pathway can be estimated from the pathway diagram itself as long as it contains the major channels for information flow in the pathway. The principal information channels can be determined using mathematical modeling, experimental measurements, and/or by sequence homology with proteins in the well-studied pathways from model organisms or other human tissues.

Drug molecules usually target a protein in all possible molecular states, such as different protein modification states or protein localization states. Therefore, up to a certain point, the diagram for estimation of drug efficacy does not need to be overcomplicated by detailed information about different molecular species for every protein component. However, the information on molecular species is necessary in the diagram for accurate mathematical modeling.

The drug efficacy estimation can be based on the simple assumption of equal fluxes between principal pathway components. The statistical score for every protein component in the pathway can be calculated as the amount of flux conducted by a protein in the pathway. It is obvious from the diagram in this figure that ADRB3, SRC, and STAT3 are the best targets for drug intervention because they conduct the biggest fluxes in the pathway. This approach can be viewed as a simplified version of the flux balance analysis for regulatory pathways (Min Lee et al., 2008; Papin and Palsson, 2004). While looking at one diagram, such simplistic flux calculations may seem unnecessary, since the conclusions are quite self-evident. One has to keep in mind, however, that these simple calculations have to be done by computer algorithms for more than 100,000 pathways in the human body to calculate the risk of side effects for a drug.

individual selective drug affects the off-target pathway(s), the combination of selective drugs will have increased potency against the target pathway only. The toxicity risk associated with multiple drugs applied to a patient can be offset by using a suboptimal concentration for each drug. Even though the suboptimal concentration of one drug reduces its efficacy toward the target pathway, this is mitigated by adding additional drug components against the target pathway. Additional components can also be added in suboptimal concentrations to avoid, in turn, their own off-target effects. Similar to the disease networks, drug toxicity depends on the individual genotype (Hamilton, 2008; Tang, 2007). Therefore, the combinatorial therapy can allow the development of drug mixtures optimized both for efficacy toward individual disease networks and for toxicity due to individual genetic backgrounds. Additional alleviation of potential toxicity can be achieved by adding into the drug mixture compounds that directly counteract the side effects.

Strategies for rational development of drug mixtures have been proposed (Sivachenko et al., 2006). Two major examples of successful *combinatorial therapy* (also called *drug cocktails*) are treatment of cancer and HIV (Daskivich et al., 2007). An HIV drug cocktail contains viral protease and reverse transcriptase inhibitors (Henkel, 1999). It has been developed to block viral replication and capsid assembly simultaneously, but also to overcome finite individual inhibitor's affinity, which does not allow 100% inhibition of the target protein. In cancer it has been shown that inhibition of a pro-survival PI3K/AKT pathway considerably lowers resistance to other anticancer drugs (Martelli et al., 2003; O'Gorman et al., 2000). Other cancer examples include drug cocktails with rituximab for head and neck cancer (Held et al., 2006), combinations of drugs with epidermal growth factor receptor inhibitors (Adjei, 2006), and combinations of sulfonylureas and biguanides for diabetes treatment (Monami et al., 2006). Promiscuous drugs targeting several proteins simultaneously provide one more example of combinatorial therapy. The best known example is aspirin, which targets both COX1 and COX2 enzymes. This strategy allows this popular drug to avoid the side effects caused by COX1 inhibitors (coxibs) such as Bextra, Celebrex, and Vioxx (Yuryev, 2008).

12.4. CONCLUSIONS

Pathway analysis is an integral component to modern drug development with applications in drug discovery and personalized medicine. Among many applications reviewed in this chapter, the most important role of pathway analysis is in the prioritization of potential drug targets. Pathway analysis results in target priorities that reflect the ability of a target to disrupt the disease network, restore normal information flow through pathways affected by the disease, and induce limited side effects due to drug action in the off-target pathways. Integrated software applications allow for efficient data and powerful pathway analyses, enhancing complex drug development decisions and patient treatment.

REFERENCES

Abdollahi, A., Schwager, C., Kleeff, J., et al. (2007). Transcriptional network governing the angiogenic switch in human pancreatic cancer. *Proc Natl Acad Sci USA 104*, 12890–12895.

Adjei, A.A. (2006). Novel combinations based on epidermal growth factor receptor inhibition. *Clin Cancer Res. 12*(14, Pt. 2), 4446s–4450s.

Albert, R., Jeong, H., and Barabasi, A.L. (2000). Error and attack tolerance of complex networks. *Nature 406*(6794), 378–382.

Araujo, R.P., Petricoin, E.F., and Liotta, L.A. (2005). A mathematical model of combination therapy using the EGFR signaling network. *Biosystems 80*(1), 57–69.

Badretdinov, A., and Yuryev, A. (2006). Pathway analysis in drug development. Published online in Pharma and Bioingredients. http://www.pharmabioingredients.com/articles/2006/03/pathway-analysis-in-drug-development.

Bagci, E.Z., Vodovotz, Y., Billiar, T.R., Ermentrout, G.B., and Bahar, I. (2006). Bistability in apoptosis: roles of bax, bcl-2, and mitochondrial permeability transition pores. *Biophys J 90*(5), 1546–1559.

Barabási, A.-L., and Oltvai, Z. (2004). Network biology: understanding the cell's functional organization. *Nat Rev 5*, 101.

Bentele, M., Lavrik, I., Ulrich, M., et al. (2004). Mathematical modeling reveals threshold mechanism in CD95-induced apoptosis. *J Cell Biol 166*(6), 839–851.

Bokov, F., and Yuryev, A. (2008). Software infrastructure and data model for pathway analysis. In: *Pathway Analysis for Drug Discovery*, Wiley, Hoboken, NJ.

Bowick, G.C., Fennewald, S.M., Scott, E.P., et al. (2007). Identification of differentially activated cell-signaling networks associated with pichinde virus pathogenesis by using systems kinomics. *J Virol 81*, 1923–1933.

Chen, Y., Choong, L.Y., Lin, Q., et al. (2007). Differential expression of novel tyrosine kinase substrates during breast cancer development. *Mol Cell Proteom 6*, 2072–2087.

Covert, M.W., Leung, T.H., Gaston, J.E., and Baltimore, D. (2005). Achieving stability of lipopolysaccharide-induced NF-kappaB activation. *Science 309*(5742), 1854–1857.

Daraselia, N., Yuryev, A., Egorov, S., Mazo, I., and Ispolatov, I. (2007). Automatic extraction of gene ontology annotation and its correlation with clusters in protein networks. *BMC Bioinf 8*, 243.

Daskivich, T.J., Regan, M.M., and Oh, W.K. (2007). Distinct prognostic role of prostate-specific antigen doubling time and velocity at emergence of androgen independence in patients treated with chemotherapy. *Urology 70*(3), 527–531.

Fussenegger, M., Bailey, J.E., and Varner, J. (2000). A mathematical model of caspase function in apoptosis. *Nat Biotechnol 18*(7), 768–774.

Gielen, S.C., Kühne, L.C., Ewing, P.C., et al. (2005). Tamoxifen treatment for breast cancer enforces a distinct gene-expression profile on the human endometrium: an exploratory study. *Endocr Relat Cancer 4*, 1037–1049.

Hamilton, S.R. (2008). Targeted therapy of cancer: new roles for pathologists in colorectal cancer. *Mod Pathol 21*(Suppl. 2), S23–S30.

Hanifi-Moghaddam, P., Gielen, S.C., Kloosterboer, H.J., et al. (2005). Molecular portrait of the progestagenic and estrogenic actions of tibolone: behavior of cellular networks in response to tibolone. *J Clin Endocrinol Metab 90*, 973–983.

Hartwell, L.H. (1991). Twenty-five years of cell cycle genetics. *Genetics 129*(4), 975–980.

Held, G., Poschel, V., and Pfreundschuh, M. (2006). Rituximab for the treatment of diffuse large B-cell lymphomas. *Expert Rev Anticancer Ther 6*(8), 1175.

Henkel, J. (1999). Attacking AIDS with a "cocktail" therapy. FDA Consumer Magazine. http://www.fda.gov/fdac/features/1999/499_aids.html.

Hua, F., Cornejo, M.G., Cardone, M.H., Stokes, C.L., Lauffenburger, D.A. (2005). Effects of Bcl-2 levels on Fas signaling-induced caspase-3 activation: molecular genetic tests of computational model predictions. *J Immunol 175*(2), 985–995.

Huang, P.H., Mukasa, A., Bonavia, R., et al. (2007). Quantitative analysis of EGFRvIII cellular signaling networks reveals a combinatorial therapeutic strategy for glioblastoma. *Proc Natl Acal Sci USA 104*(31), 12867–12872.

Huang, Y., Fernandez, S.V., et al. (2007). Epithelial to mesenchymal transition in human breast epithelial cells transformed by 17β-estradiol. *Cancer Res 67*, 11147–11157.

Ideker, T., and Sharan, R. (2008). Protein networks in disease. *Genome Res 18*(4), 644–652.

Katiyar, S.K., Roy, A.M., and Baliga, M.S. (2005). Silymarin induces apoptosis primarily through a p53-dependent pathway involving Bcl-2/Bax, cytochrome *c* release, and caspase activation. *Mol Cancer Ther 4*(2), 207–216.

Krammer, P.H., Kaminski, M., Kiessling, M., and Gulow, K. (2007). No life without death. *Adv Cancer Res 97C*, 111–138.

Kuznetsov, V., Thomas, S., and Bonchev, D. (2008). Data-driven networking reveals 5-genes signature for early detection of lung cancer. *Biomed Eng Inf 2*, 413–417.

Leclerc, R.D. (2008). Survival of the sparsest: robust gene networks are parsimonious. *Mol Syst Biol 4*, 213.

Lee, J.I., Dominy, J.E., and Sikalidis, A.K. (2008). HepG2/C3A cells respond to cysteine-deprivation by induction of the amino acid deprivation/integrated stress response pathway. *Physiol Genom*, doi: 10.152/physiolgenomics.00263.2007.

Legewie, S., Bluthgen, N., and Herzel, H. (2006). Mathematical modeling identifies inhibitors of apoptosis as mediators of positive feedback and bistability. *PLoS Comput Biol 2*(9), e120.

Lehár, J., Krueger, A., Zimmermann, G., and Borisy, A. (2008). High-order combination effects and biological robustness. *Mol Syst Biol 4*, 215.

Leloup, J.C., Gonze, D., and Goldbeter, A. (1999). Limit cycle models for circadian rhythms based on transcriptional regulation in *Drosophila* and *Neurospora*. *J Biol Rhythms 14*(6), 433–448.

Li, B., and Dou, Q.P. (2000). Bax degradation by the ubiquitin/proteasome-dependent pathway: involvement in tumor survival and progression. *Proc Natl Acad Sci USA* 97(8), 3850–3855.

Li, F., Long, T., Lu, Y., Ouyang, Q., and Tang, C. (2004). The yeast cell-cycle network is robustly designed. *Proc Natl Acad Sci USA 101*(14), 4781–4786.

Lim, J., Hao, T., Shaw, C., et al. (2006). A protein–protein interaction network for human inherited ataxias and disorders of Purkinje cell degeneration. *Cell 125*, 801–814.

Loscalzo, J., Kohane, I., and Barabási, A.L. (2007). Human disease classification in the postgenomic era: a complex systems approach to human pathobiology. *Mol Syst Biol 3*, 124.

MacLennan, N.K., Rahib, L., Shin, C., et al. (2006). Targeted disruption of glycerol kinase gene in mice: expression analysis in liver shows alterations in network partners related to glycerol kinase activity. *Hum Mol Genet 15*, 405–415.

Martelli, A.M., Tazzari, P.L., Tabellini, G., et al. (2003). A new selective AKT pharmacological inhibitor reduces resistance to chemotherapeutic drugs, TRAIL, all-trans-retinoic acid, and ionizing radiation of human leukemia cells. *Leukemia 17*(9), 1794.

Miller, J.A., Oldham, M.C., and Geschwind, D.H. (2008). A systems level analysis of transcriptional changes in Alzheimer's disease and normal aging. *J Neurosci 28*, 1410–1420.

Min Lee, J., Gianchandani, E.P., Eddy, J.A., and Papin, J.A. (2008). Dynamic analysis of integrated signaling, metabolic, and regulatory networks. *PLoS Comput Biol 4*(5), e1000086.

Monami, M., Luzzi, C., Lamanna, C., et al. (2006). Three-year mortality in diabetic patients treated with different combinations of insulin secretagogues and metformin. *Diabetes/Metab Research Rev 22*(6), 477.

Mulvey, L., Chandrasekaran, A., Liu, K., et al. (2007). Interplay of genes regulated by estrogen and diindolylmethane in breast cancer cell lines. *Mol Med 13*, 69–78.

Nikitin, A., Egorov, S., Daraselia, N., and Mazo, I. (2003). Pathway studio the analysis and navigation of molecular networks. *Bioinformatics 19*(16), 2155–2157.

Novak, B., and Tyson, J.J. (1997). Modeling the control of DNA replication in fission yeast. *Proc Natl Acad Sci USA 94*(17), 9147–9152.

O'Gorman, D.M., McKenna, S.L., McGahon, A.J., et al. (2000). Sensitisation of HL60 human leukaemic cells to cytotoxic drug-induced apoptosis by inhibition of PI3-kinase survival signals. *Leukemia 14*(4), 602.

Papin, J.A., and Palsson, B.O. (2004). The JAK–STAT signaling network in the human B-cell: an extreme signaling pathway analysis. *Biophys J 87*(1), 37–46.

Pavlidis, P., Lewis, D.P., and Noble, W.S. (2002). Exploring gene expression data with class scores. *Pac Symp Biocomput 7*, 474–485.

Saban, R., D'Andrea, M.R., Andrade-Gordon, P., et al. (2007). Regulatory network of inflammation downstream of proteinase-activated receptors. *BMC Physiol 7*, 3.

Sivachenko, A.Y. (2008). *Pathway Analysis of High-Throughput Experimental Data.* Wiley, Hoboken, NJ.

Sivachenko, A., Kalinin, A., and Yuryev, A. (2006). Pathway analysis for design of promiscuous drugs and selective drug mixtures. *Curr Drug Discov Technol 3*(4), 269–267.

Sivachenko, A.Y., Yuryev, A., Daraselia, N., and Mazo, I. (2007). Molecular networks in microarray analysis. *J Bioinf Comput Biol 5*(2B), 429–456.

Subramanian, A., Tamayo, P., Mootha, V.K., et al. (2005). Gene set enrichment analysis: a knowledge-based approach for interpreting genome-wide expression profiles. *Proc Natl Acad Sci USA 102*(43), 15545–15550.

Sun, N. and Zhao, H. (2004). Genomic approaches in dissecting complex biological pathways. *Pharmacogenomics 5*(2), 163–179.

Tang, W. (2007). Drug metabolite profiling and elucidation of drug-induced hepatotoxicity. *Expert Opin Drug Metab Toxicol 3*(3), 407–420.

Tongbai, R., Idelman, G., Nordgard, S.H., et al. (2008). Transcriptional networks inferred from molecular signatures of breast cancer. *Am J Pathol 172*, 495–509.

Wang, J., Huang, B., Xia, X., and Sun, Z. (2006). Funneled landscape leads to robustness of cell networks: yeast cell cycle. *PLoS Comput Biol 2*(11), e147.

Witten, T.M., and Bonchev, D. (2007). Predicting aging/longevity-related genes in the nematode *Caenorhabditis elegans*. *Chem Biodivers 4*(11), 2639–2655.

Yang, Z., Quigley, H.A., Pease, M.E. et al. (2007). Changes in gene expression in experimental glaucoma and optic nerve transection: the equilibrium between protective and detrimental mechanisms. *Invest Ophthalmol Vis Sci 48*, 5539–5548.

Yuryev, A. (2008). *In silico* pathway analysis: the final frontier towards completely rational drug design. *Expert Opin Drug Discov 3*(8), 867–876.

Yuryev, A., Mulyukov, Z., Kotelnikova, E., et al. (2006). Automatic pathway building in biological association networks. *BMC Bioinf 7*, 171.

CHAPTER 13

Functional Mapping for Predicting Drug Response and Enabling Personalized Medicine

YAO LI

Quantitative Genetic Epidemiology, Fred Hutchinson Cancer Research Center, Seattle, Washington

WEI HOU

University of Florida, Gainesville, Florida

WEI ZHAO

St. Jude Children's Research Hospital, Memphis, Tennessee

KWANGMI AHN

Pennsylvania State College of Medicine, Hershey, Pennsylvania

RONGLING WU

Center for Statistical Genetics, Pennsylvania State University, Hershey, Pennsylvania

Summary

Accurate prediction of a person's response to a drug is an important prerequisite of personalized medicine. Recent pharmacogenomic research has inspired our hope to predict drug response based on DNA information extracted from the human genome. However, many genetic experiments do not incorporate biochemical principles of host–drug interactions, limiting the derivation of predictive models. We argue that functional mapping, aimed to map genes and genetic networks for dynamic traits, will provide a useful analytical tool for determining the detailed genetic architecture of drug response explained by pharmacokinetic and pharmacodynamic processes. Functional

Systems Biology in Drug Discovery and Development, First Edition.
Edited by Daniel L. Young, Seth Michelson.

mapping is particularly powerful for testing the genetic commonality and differences of drug efficacy versus drug toxicity and drug sensitivity versus drug resistance. We pinpoint several future directions where functional mapping can be married with systems biology to unravel the genetic and metabolic machinery of drug response.

13.1. INTRODUCTION

Substantial interpersonal variation is observed in pharmacological response to medications. Although such variability in drug effects may be attributed to many biochemical, developmental, and environmental factors, increasing recognition has been given to genetic influences (reviewed by Evans and Johnson, 2001; Evans and McLeod, 2003; Johnson, 2003; Weinshilboum, 2003; Wang and Weinshilboum, 2008). For example, genes are observed to affect drug transport (e.g., polymorphisms in the gene encoding P-glycoprotein 1 and the plasma concentration of digoxin), drug metabolism (e.g., polymorphisms in the gene encoding thiopurine S-methyltransferase and thiopurine toxicity), and drug targets (e.g., polymorphisms in the gene encoding the β_2-adrenoceptor and response to β_2-adrenoceptor agonists) (Johnson, 2003). It is likely that drug response involves a network of multiple genes in which the expression of one gene depends not only on that of other genes but also on developmental and environmental stimuli. Thus, to predict the pattern of how individual patients respond to a specific drug, there is a pressing need to fully understand the organization and function of a genetic network for drug reactions and effects. Genetic mapping combining Mendelian genetics and statistics (Kao et al., 1999; Lander and Botstein, 1989; Zeng, 1994) has proved to be powerful for dissecting interpersonal variability in individual genetic components at the quantitative trait locus (QTL) or quantitative trait nucleotide (QTN) level (Watters and McLeod, 2003; Watters et al., 2004), although such a combination does not produce mechanistic results about trait formation and dynamics.

More recently, a new statistical framework called *functional mapping* has been proposed by R. Wu and group, aimed to map and identify dynamic QTLs or QTNs that are responsible for the change of trait development in time (Ma et al., 2002; Wu and Lin, 2006; Wu et al., 2004a–c). A general principle of functional mapping is to embed the mechanistic aspects of biological processes into the framework for genetic mapping, thus realizing the integration of classic genetics, statistics, and biology. Functional mapping models the dynamic trajectories of trait development by biologically meaningful nonlinear mathematical equations and allows the formulation of various hypotheses about the interplay between genetic actions or interactions and the pattern, plan, and program of trait development. In statistics, by modeling the mean–covariance structures of longitudinal traits, functional mapping estimates fewer parameters compared to traditional multivariate treatments, thus increasing the precision of parameter estimation and the power of gene detection (Ma et al., 2002).

Functional mapping, originally proposed for stem growth in a forest tree (Ma et al., 2002), has been expanded successfully to study the genetic architecture of other dynamic traits, such as programmed cell death (Cui et al., 2006, 2008), allometric scaling (R. Wu et al., 2002; Long et al., 2006), reaction norm (J. Wu et al., 2007), biological clock (Liu et al., 2007), HIV-1 dynamics (Wang and Wu, 2004; Wang et al., 2005), human growth trajectories (Li et al., 2009), periodic gene expression profile (Berg et al., 2011), and proteomic dynamics. In these studies, functional mapping provides an organizing framework to understand the coherent behavior of an entire biological system through integration and coordination of its parts. The significant implication of functional mapping was also exemplified in the pharmacogenetic study of drug response (Gong et al., 2004; Lin et al., 2005, 2007). A drug acts in a patient's body through two different but related biochemical processes characterized by what the body does to the drug [pharmacokinetics (PK)] and what the drug does to the body [pharmacodynamics (PD)], respectively. Functional mapping models the dynamic nature of pharmacological interactions, which determine the manner in which drugs affect the body over time.

Figure 13.1 can be used to illustrate the results for functional mapping of drug response. The genetic variation in drug metabolism and degradation (expressed as PK reactions) is due to one hypothesized gene with three genotypes, homozygote for the wild-type allele (*WT/WT*), heterozygote for the wild-type and variant (*V*) allele (*WT/V*), and homozygote for the variant allele (*V/V*), displaying marked differences in drug concentration–time curves (top, Figure 13.1). By estimating and testing the parameters that define PK curves, functional mapping can quantify the contribution of this gene. The same gene

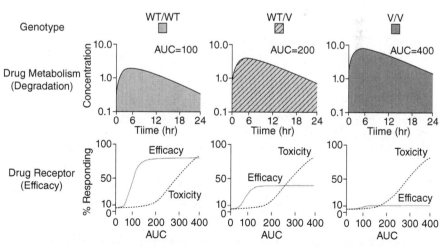

Figure 13.1 Genetic control of drug response as a longitudinal characteristic. AUC is the area under the plasma concentration–time curve. [Adapted from Evans and McLeod (2003).]

can be tested for whether it affects drug targets and receptors (expressed as PD reactions). A comparative analysis of response–concentration curves among the three genotypes shows that this gene also affects the efficacy (favorable effect) of the drug, but has no effect on drug toxicity (adverse effect) (bottom, Figure 13.1). Results such as those from the hypothetical example above, will help survey the pattern of how genes from the entire human genome affect different aspects of drug response and, ultimately, tailor a personalized medication to improve drug efficacy and reduce the number and severity of drug toxicities based on individual patients' genetic makeup.

In this chapter we provide a brief overview of functional mapping, followed by a description of its applications to study the genetic basis of drug response. We show how functional mapping can address many biological questions related to drug response, such as the pattern of genetic control in time or across different doses, the duration of genetic effects, as well as the mechanistic causes of change or no change in drug response. Examples are presented to illustrate how to apply functional mapping to advance pharmacogenetic and pharmacogenomic research. Finally, a systems approach for integrating functional mapping in pharmacogenetic studies is discussed.

13.2. FUNCTIONAL MAPPING

13.2.1. Theory and Framework

The statistical foundation of functional mapping is based on a finite mixture model, a type of density model comprising a number of component functions that are usually Gaussian. These component functions contribute to a multimodal density function which can be used to model genotypic segregation of genes that control dynamic traits. According to this model, each observation of drug response (y) in a mapping population corresponds to a curve fitted by a finite set of measurements with L time points or dose levels for subject i, arrayed by $\mathbf{y}_i = (y_i(C_1), \ldots, y_i(C_L))$. Each observation is assumed to have arisen from one (and only one) of a total of J possible components (i.e., genotypes for a set of genes for drug response), with each component being modeled by a multivariate normal distribution density. Consequently, the density function of $\mathbf{y}_i$ is expressed as the sum of component-specific densities weighted by the proportions of each component:

$$\mathbf{y}_i \sim p(\mathbf{y}_i \mid \boldsymbol{\omega}, \mathbf{u}, \boldsymbol{\Sigma}) = \sum_{j=1}^{J} \omega_j f_j(\mathbf{y}_i; \mathbf{u}_j, \boldsymbol{\Sigma}) \tag{13.1}$$

where $\boldsymbol{\omega} = (\omega_1, \ldots, \omega_J)$ are the mixture proportions (i.e., genotype frequencies), which add up to unity; $\mathbf{u} = (\mathbf{u}_1, \ldots, \mathbf{u}_J)$ are the component (or genotype)-specific parameters; $\boldsymbol{\Sigma}$ are the parameters that are common to all components; and $f_j(\mathbf{y}_i; \mathbf{u}_j, \boldsymbol{\Sigma})$ is a parametric density function.

The likelihood of longitudinal data $\mathbf{y}$ for a mapping population of size n will be constructed in terms of the mixture model (13.1), expressed as

$$L(\omega, \mathbf{u}, \boldsymbol{\Sigma} \mid \mathbf{y}, \mathbf{M}) = \prod_{i=1}^{n} \sum_{j=1}^{J} \omega_{j|i} f_j(\mathbf{y}_i; \mathbf{u}_j, \boldsymbol{\Sigma}) \tag{13.2}$$

where $\omega_{j|i}$ is the probability with which subject i belongs to genotype j for a set of functional mapping for drug response. Although functional genes cannot be observed directly, their genotypes can be inferred from the marker genotypes observed. For subject i, $\omega_{j|i}$ is described as the conditional probability of functional genotype j given the marker genotype of the subject (R. Wu et al., 2007). For a mating population, $\omega_{j|i}$ is described by the recombination fraction, whereas for a natural population it is described by the linkage disequilibrium.

If genotype-specific densities are assumed to be normally distributed, we have

$$f_j(\mathbf{y}_i; \mathbf{u}_j, \boldsymbol{\Sigma}) = \frac{1}{(2\pi)|\boldsymbol{\Sigma}|^{1/2}} \exp\left[-\frac{1}{2}(\mathbf{y}_i - \mathbf{u}_j)\boldsymbol{\Sigma}^{-1}(\mathbf{y}_i - \mathbf{u}_j)^{\mathrm{T}} \right]$$

specified by time- or dose-dependent mean vectors for different genotypes,

$$\mathbf{u}_j = (u_j(C_1) \ldots, u_j(C_L)) \tag{13.3}$$

and residual covariance matrix,

$$\boldsymbol{\Sigma} = \phi\boldsymbol{\Sigma}_e + (1-\phi)\boldsymbol{\Sigma}_\varepsilon \tag{13.4}$$

where $\boldsymbol{\Sigma}_e$ is the covariance matrix due to permanent errors of longitudinal measures over time points or dose levels, $\boldsymbol{\Sigma}_\varepsilon$ the covariance matrix due to random or innovation errors at specific time points or dose levels, and ϕ the relative proportion of the permanent and random variances.

Functional mapping uses a mathematical equation to model the structure of the mean vector in Eq. (13.3). If drug response is expressed as the PD process, one can capitalize on a commonly used $E_{\max}$ model (Giraldo, 2003) to describe the response–concentration curve:

$$E = E_0 + \frac{E_{\max}C^H}{EC_{50}^H + C^H}$$

where C is the concentration of a drug, E_0 the baseline value for the drug response parameter, $E_{\max}$ the asymptotic (limiting) effect, EC_{50} the drug concentration that results in 50% of the maximal effect, and H the slope

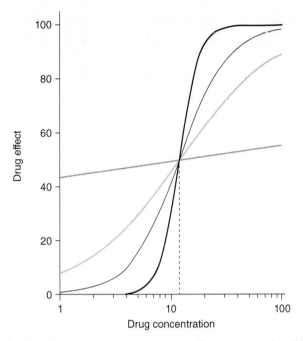

Figure 13.2   Varying shapes of response–concentration curves under different combinations of PD parameters. [Adapted from Lin et al. (2005).]

parameter that determines the slope of the response–concentration curve. The larger H is, the steeper is the linear phase of the log(response–concentration) curve. Thus, different combinations of parameters $(E_0, \mathrm{EC}_{50}, E_{max}, H)$ will produce different shapes of drug response curves (Figure 13.2).

For a specific genotype j, an array of parameters $(E_{0j}, E_{maxj}, \mathrm{EC}_{50j}, H_j)$ will be needed to define its PD curve. Thus, a genotype-specific mean vector (13.3) is modeled as

$$\mathbf{u}_j = E_{0j} + \frac{E_{maxj}C_1^{H_j}}{\mathrm{EC}_{50j}^{H_j} + C_1^{H_j}}, \dots, E_{0j} + \frac{E_{maxj}C_L^{H_j}}{\mathrm{EC}_{50j}^{H_j} + C_L^{H_j}} \tag{13.5}$$

If the combination of these parameters is different among different genotypes, this suggests that the drug response is controlled by genes. Functional mapping not only detects the overall differences in curve shape among genotypes based on the null hypothesis, H_0: $(E_{0j}, E_{maxj}, \mathrm{EC}_{50j}, H_j) \equiv (E_0, E_{max}, \mathrm{EC}_{50}, H)$, but also provides a quantitative framework for testing the genotypic differences in the pattern of drug response.

Similarly, functional mapping of the PK process can be incorporated by a biexponential equation for specifying the change of drug concentration with time. Thus, by estimating and testing genotype-specific parameters for the PK curves, the genetic control of drug response can be examined.

Because of the autocorrelation pattern, the covariance matrix of a longitudinal trait can be structured. The structured covariance matrix reduces the noise level of measurements and the number of parameters that need to be estimated; this property increases the flexibility, stability, and power of functional mapping. The first-order autoregressive [AR(1)] model is among the simplest choices to model the autocorrelation structure of Σ_e, expressed as

$$\sigma_e^2(C_1) = \cdots = \sigma_e^2(C_L) = \sigma_e^2$$

for the variance, and

$$\text{cov}_e(C_l, C_{l'}) = \sigma_e^2 \rho^{|C_{l'} - C_l|}$$

for the covariance between any two time points or dose levels C_l and $C_{l'}$, where $0 < \rho < 1$ is the proportion parameter with which the correlation decays with time or dose lag.

It is reasonable to assume that innovation errors at different time points or dose levels are independent and thus Σ_e contains only variances on its diagonal. We further assume that the innovation variances are constant [i.e., $\sigma_\varepsilon^2(C_1) = \cdots = \sigma_\varepsilon^2(C_L) = \sigma_\varepsilon^2$]. In sum, the residual covariance matrix (13.4) can be structured by an array of parameters: $(\sigma_e^2, \sigma_\varepsilon^2, \rho, \phi)$.

Various computational algorithms, such as expectation maximization (EM) (Ma et al., 2002), Newton–Raphson (Li et al., 2007), Markov chain Monte Carlo (MCMC) (Liu and Wu, 2009), and simplex (Zhao et al., 2004a), have been used to estimate the parameters that define the structures of time-dependent mean vectors for different genotypes and covariance matrices. Hypothesis tests can be formulated about the existence of QTLs and their effects on the patterns of PD or PK processes.

13.2.2. Example: Use of Dobutamine for Cardiovascular Disease

Cardiovascular disease, including heart disease and stroke, is the leading killer for both men and women in all racial and ethnic populations (Yu et al., 2003). The drug dobutamine is designed to treat congestive heart failure. Dobutamine can increase heart rate and cardiac contractility, with actions on the heart similar to the effect of exercise. Dobutamine is a synthetic catecholamine that stimulates primarily β-adrenergic receptors (βARs) that regulate cardiovascular function and responses to drugs (Johnson and Terra, 2002; Nabel, 2003). Two receptor genes, β_1AR and β_2AR, each have several polymorphisms that are common in the population (Genet, 2002). The β_1AR gene has two common polymorphisms located at codons 49 (Ser49Gly) and 389 (Arg389Gly), whereas the β_2AR gene has two common polymorphisms at codons 16 (Arg16Gly) and 27 (Gln27Glu) (Nabel, 2003).

A group of patients who are unable to perform an exercise stress test received dobutamine, aimed to screen for heart disease. These patients had a wide range of untreated heart rates. Dobutamine was injected into these patients to investigate their response in heart rate to this drug. The patients received increasing doses of dobutamine until they achieved the target heart rate response or the predetermined maximum dose. There are six dosage levels—0 (baseline), 5, 10, 20, 30, and 40 µg/min—at which the heart rate was measured. An interval of 3 minutes is allowed between two successive doses for patients to reach a plateau in response to that dose. Finally, there were 107 patients whose heart rate data included all six dosage levels.

The study was designed to investigate the association between haplotypes constructed by different single-nucleotide polymorphisms (SNPs) and the response curves of heart rate to different doses of dobutamine. All the patients were genotyped for SNP markers at codons 49 (with alleles T and G) and 389 (with alleles A and G) within the β_1AR gene and at codons 16 (with alleles A and G) and 27 (with alleles G and C) within the β_2AR gene. Liu et al. (2004) developed a statistical model for detecting and estimating haplotype effects on a complex trait with unphased genetic marker data. This model was integrated with functional mapping to study the effects of haplotypes on drug response (Lin et al., 2005). The results from functional mapping are derived from Lin et al.'s work.

The raw heart rate data were adjusted to remove the baseline effect and thus only E_{maxj}, EC_{50j}, and H_j are estimated for different genotypes from the adjusted data. Also, Lin et al.'s (2005) analysis assumed that the residual variance was due purely to the permanent error (i.e., $\phi = 1$). It was found that haplotypes within the β_1AR gene have no significant effect on heart rate curves. Our analysis focuses on the significant β_2AR gene. Two SNPs typed within the β_2AR gene produce four haplotypes: AG, AC, GG, and GC. By assuming that one of them is the risk haplotype and the rest are the nonrisk haplotype, functional mapping estimates the curve parameters of the heart rate for three different composite diplotypes. Combinatory analysis suggests that GG is an optimal risk haplotype, producing a much higher likelihood than those when any other haplotype is assumed as a risk haplotype.

Figure 13.3 illustrates the profiles of the heart rate response to increasing dose levels of dobutamine for three composite diplotypes comprising haplotypes GG and non-GG (symbolized by $\overline{GG}$). The composite homozygote [GG][GG] displayed a consistently higher heart rate across all dose levels, especially at higher dose levels than the composite homozygote [$\overline{GG}$][$\overline{GG}$]. But the composite heterozygote [GG][$\overline{GG}$] consistently had the lowest curve at all dosage levels tested. Lin et al. (2005) used the area under the curve (AUC) to test how haplotypes affect drug response curves for heart rate. The testing results suggest that both additive and dominant effects are important in determining heart rate response curves, together accounting for about 14% of the variation observed in drug response.

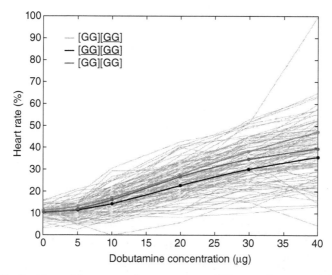

Figure 13.3 Profiles of heart rate in response to different dosages of dobutamine (indicated by dots) for three composite genotypes (thick curves) identified at two SNPs within the β_2AR gene. The profiles of 107 subjects studied from which the three composite genotypes were detected are also shown (thin curves). (See insert for color representation.)

13.3. PREDICTIVE MODEL

13.3.1. Dissecting Drug Response

Functional mapping can identify specific genes that contribute to interpersonal variation in drug response, but the prediction of drug response from these genes should be deployed with other factors, such as biochemical, developmental, environmental, and residual error, because the final outcome of drug response is the consequence of the mutual coordination of all these factors (Evans and Johnson, 2001; Evans and McLeod, 2003; Johnson, 2003; Weinshilboum, 2003; Wang and Weinshilboum, 2008). Figure 13.4 is a general model for dissecting drug response into its various components. The formulation of a model for predicting whether subjects will respond to a particular drug or treatment regimen will need a comprehensive understanding of the interactions between these components. The predictive measurement is then used with biochemical, developmental, and environmental parameters obtained from a subject to predict whether that subject will respond to the particular drug or treatment regimen.

Traditional genetic mapping detects genes for drug response based on a direct genotype–phenotype relationship, whereas functional mapping does so through linking biochemical influences to the outcome of drug response in pharmacokinetic and pharmacodynamic pathways. Functional mapping has

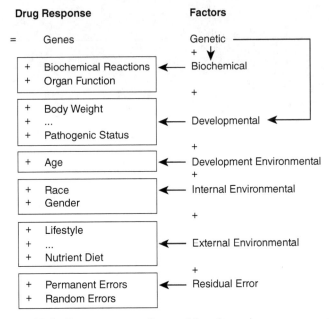

Figure 13.4   Drug response dissected into its various components.

been extended to incorporate environmental signals into the model, testing genotype × environment interaction effects on biological processes (Zhao et al., 2004b,c). In pharmacological research, environmental influences can be sorted into three different types: developmental (due to different ages), internal (due to different genders and races), and external (due to different lifestyle, nutrients, and so on). Each of these environmental types may affect the drug response in different ways, so that it is necessary to characterize and quantify their respective roles to derive a precise predictive model for drug response. Furthermore, some environmental types are discrete, such as gender and race, whereas others are continuous, such as age and nutritional level. The statistical derivations of functional mapping need to consider these differences since they require different statistical foundations.

The pattern of how patients respond to a particular drug or treatment regimen may also be affected by developmental factors. Functional mapping should incorporate these factors into the model for predicting drug response. Different from other environmental factors, some developmental factors, such as body weight and pathogenic status, may also be controlled by genes, the same as or different from those for drug response. Such uniqueness should be reflected in the derivations of functional mapping. As an example, we describe the procedure of how to incorporate body weight into functional mapping of drug response.

13.3.2. Allometric Functional Mapping

Allometric scaling is a good predictor of a variety of biological variables, including metabolic rate, lifespan, growth rate, heart rate, DNA nucleotide substitution rates, and length of aortas (Schmidt-Nielsen, 1984; West and Brown, 2004, 2005; West et al., 1997, 1999a,b). Allometric scaling principles can also be used for scaling preclinical evaluation of drug metabolism and response (Boxenbaum, 1982; Gronert et al., 1995; Hu and Hayton, 2001; Lepist and Jusko, 2004; Zuideveld et al., 2007). Allometric scaling has been assembled into functional mapping (Li et al., 2007; Long et al., 2006; Wu et al., 2002). Here we show how allometric scaling can enhance understanding of the genetic regulation of pharmacokinetic and pharmacodynamic reactions, and ultimately predict the time courses of drug concentrations and drug effects.

The allometric equations for scaling PD parameters with body mass (M) have been established (Khor et al., 2000) and are expressed as

$$
\begin{aligned}
E_0 &= \alpha_0 M^{\beta_0} \\
EC_{50} &= \alpha_{50} M^{\beta_{50}} \\
E_{max} &= \alpha_{max} M^{\beta_{max}} \\
H &= \alpha_H M^{\beta_H}
\end{aligned}
\tag{13.6}
$$

Each of these expressions is integrated into specifying genotype-specific mean vectors in Eq. (13.5). Because the body mass of subject i ($i = 1, \ldots, n$) is included, the mean vector for genotype j ($j = 1, \ldots, J$) will be expressed as $\mathbf{u}_{j|i}$. This model will allow a test not only for the existence of genes affecting drug response directly, but also for whether the genes affect drug response through allometric scaling. The null hypothesis of testing the existence of genes is expressed as

$$
\begin{aligned}
H_0 : (\alpha_{0j}, \beta_{0j}) &\equiv (\alpha_0, \beta_0), \ (\alpha_{50j}, \beta_{50j}) \equiv (\alpha_{50}, \beta_{50}), \\
(\alpha_{maxj}, \beta_{maxj}) &\equiv (\alpha_{max}, \beta_{max}), \ \text{and} \ (\alpha_{Hj}, \beta_{Hj}) \equiv (\alpha_H, \beta_H)
\end{aligned}
\tag{13.7}
$$

If significant genes are detected, the tests of individual equalities above can be made to show how the genes affect different aspects of drug response through allometric scaling.

An alternative model for implementing allometric scaling into functional mapping is to express pharmacological variables as a function of genotype-specific body mass (μ_{M_j}). Specifically, this can be written

$$
\begin{aligned}
E_{0j} &= \alpha_{0j} \mu_{M_j}^{\beta_{0j}} \\
EC_{50j} &= \alpha_{50j} \mu_{M_j}^{\beta_{50j}} \\
E_{maxj} &= \alpha_{maxj} \mu_{M_j}^{\beta_{maxj}} \\
H_j &= \alpha_{Hj} \mu_{M_j}^{\beta_{Hj}}
\end{aligned}
\tag{13.8}
$$

This model needs to estimate genotype-specific body mass in the mean vector and the residual variance of body mass and its covariances with pharmacological variables at different time points or dose levels. It is not unreasonable to assume that these covariances are constant over time points or dose levels.

If there are different genes for drug response and body mass, we will remodel the allometric scaling of Eq. (13.8):

$$
\begin{aligned}
E_{0j_1j_2} &= \alpha_{0j_1}\mu_{M_{j_2}}^{\beta_{0j_1}} \\
EC_{50j_1j_2} &= \alpha_{50j_1}\mu_{M_{j_2}}^{\beta_{50j_1}} \\
E_{\max j_1j_2} &= \alpha_{\max j_1}\mu_{M_{j_2}}^{\beta_{\max j_1}} \\
H_{j_1j_2} &= \alpha_{Hj_1}\mu_{M_{j_2}}^{\beta_{Hj_1}}
\end{aligned}
\tag{13.9}
$$

where $j_1 = 1, \ldots, J_1$ and $j_2 = 1, \ldots, J_2$ indicates different genotypes at genes for drug response and body mass, respectively.

The comparison between models (13.8) and (13.9) can test whether the same gene pleiotropically affects drug response and body mass, or whether the correlation between these two variables is due to the linkage between their underlying genes. If both the pleiotropy and linkage are important for trait correlation, the test based on model selection criteria will permit us to examine which mechanism is a relatively more important contributor to the correlation between drug response and body mass.

13.3.3. Example: Response to Various Dopamine Doses

This example is derived from the study used in Section 13.2.2. The study genotyped a group of patients ($n = 107$) for different SNPs within the β_1AR and β_2AR receptor genes and measured their heart rates in a response to different doses of dobutamine: 0 (baseline), 5, 10, 20, 30, and 40 µg/min. Body mass was measured for each patient. The analysis in this example will be based on the two SNPs within the β_2AR gene.

In theory, each PD parameter can be modeled by a power equation. However, because of a limited sample size, only $E_{\max}$ is modeled in this manner, which changes Eq. (13.5) to

$$
\mathbf{u}_{ji} = E_{0j} + \frac{\alpha_{\max j}M_i^{\beta_{\max j}}C_1^{H_j}}{EC_{50j}^{H_j} + C_1^{H_j}}, \ldots, E_{0j} + \frac{\alpha_{\max j}M_i^{\beta_{\max j}}C_L^{H_j}}{EC_{50j}^{H_j} + C_L^{H_j}}
\tag{13.10}
$$

where the mean vectors are subject specific because the subject's body mass is embedded.

Before data analysis by allometric functional mapping, the raw data were adjusted to remove the baseline effect so that ($\alpha_{\max j}$, $\beta_{\max j}$, EC_{50j}, H_j) are estimated. Allometric functional mapping has the power to estimate and test

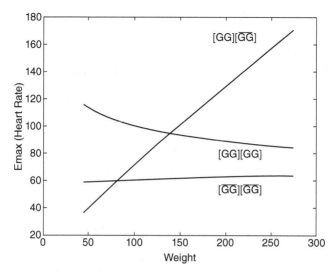

Figure 13.5 Different patterns of allometric scaling between the asymptotic effect of dobutamine (E_{max}), measured in heart rate and body mass for different composite diplotypes constituted by risk haplotype [GG] and nonrisk haplotype [$\overline{GG}$]. [Adapted from Wu and Lin (2008).]

haplotype effects on drug response and scaling law. The choice of GG as a risk haplotype produces the best fit to the data. It is found that the power curves of the E_{max} scaling with body mass are remarkably different among the three composite diplotypes: [GG][GG], [GG][$\overline{GG}$], and [$\overline{GG}$][$\overline{GG}$] (Figure 13.5). The heterozygote displays much greater sensitivity to body mass in heart rate than do the two homozygotes. With lighter body mass, the three composite diplotypes respond to the dose of dobutamine in a similar manner, but the slope of the responsiveness is much larger for the heterozygote than for the two homozygotes when body mass increases (Figure 13.6). It is also interesting to note that the significance level to detect the haplotype effect on drug response is increased from pure functional mapping of drug response ($p = 0.021$) to functional mapping with allometric scaling ($p = 0.002$).

13.4. FUTURE DIRECTIONS

Typically, when prescribing therapies one does not consider the biological and genetic characteristics of individual patients, resulting in similar regimen and administration dosage for all patients. Functional mapping provides an unprecedented opportunity to detect and map individual genes and genetic interactions for drug response. The major advantage of functional mapping is that it combines information about biochemical and developmental pathways of

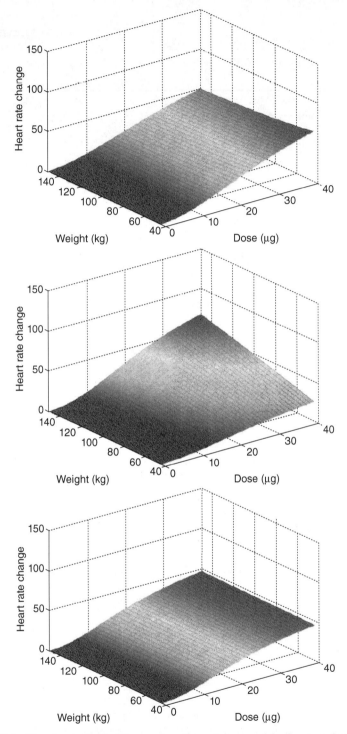

Figure 13.6 Heart rate (μg/min) as a function of dose and body mass for different composite diplotypes—[GG][GG] (top), [GG] $[\overline{GG}]$ (middle), and $[\overline{GG}][\overline{GG}]$ (bottom)—constituted by risk haplotype [GG] and nonrisk haplotype $[\overline{GG}]$. [Adapted from Wu and Lin (2008).]

drug response with statistical models for genetic mapping, whose results will be biologically more relevant than those from traditional mapping approaches. With the complete sequencing of the human genome and the development of DNA analysis techniques, functional mapping can be integrated with genome-wide association studies (GWAS) to characterize a detailed atlas of genetic variation across the entire human genome for drug response.

To tailor it for predicting drug response, functional mapping has been expanded to model the genetic control of drug efficacy and toxicity (Lin and Wu, 2005). Stated simply, the administration of a drug to a patient can produce two different types of responses: beneficial therapeutic effects (efficacy) and adverse drug reactions (toxicity). The considerable variability that occurs in the pattern of drug response within a group of people can be categorized into four types: (1) there is a benefit and toxicity, (2) there is a benefit but no toxicity; (3) there is no benefit, but there is toxicity; and (4) there is neither benefit nor toxicity. Lin and Wu's model allows the identification of genetic machineries specific for drug efficacy and drug toxicity and the ability to test whether or not these two machineries have a shared basis. The deployment of the results from such models will help to personalize medicines based on individual patients' genetic makeup, helping to maximize beneficial therapeutic effects and minimize adverse drug reactions.

Elucidating the molecular basis of drug sensitivity and resistance is of paramount importance for the choice of optimal medication and its optimal administration dose and schedule. It is now believed that drug resistance may occur at all different stages of drug action, including a pre-target event, drug–target interaction, and a post-target event. Functional mapping has the flexibility to incorporate each of these drug resistance mechanisms into the model, allowing physicians to detect the genetic variants underlying different aspects of drug response.

Although many studies on predicting drug response are based on gene–drug correlations, a growing body of evidence shows that transcriptional and proteomic profiling will more directly solve current functional and pharmacological problems (Ma et al., 2006; Nagasaki and Miki, 2008; Shimizu et al., 2004; Staunton et al., 2001). It has been recognized that the integrative gene expression and proteomic signatures of untreated cells may be more accurate for the prediction of chemosensitivity in cancer than may gene expression or proteomic expression alone (Ma et al., 2009). A rapidly emerging science—systems biology—integrates various "omics" technologies to model the behavior and relationships of all units of information in a biological system from a functional perspective rather than focusing on individual information bits (Butcher et al., 2004). Although systems biology is in its infancy, its integration with GWAS-based functional mapping will accelerate the pace of modeling network genetics of physiology related to drug response and target validation and predicting reaction patterns of drugs from the perspectives of pharmacokinetics versus pharmacodynamics, efficacy versus toxicity, and sensitivity versus resistance.

Acknowledgments

The preparation of this manuscript was partially supported by joint National Science Foundation–National Institutes of Health grant DMS/NIGMS-0540745 and Florida Center for AIDS Research incentive award 2008.

REFERENCES

Berg, A., Li, N., Tong, C.F., Wang, Z., Berceli, S.A., and Wu, R. L. (2011). Functional mapping of expression quantitative trait loci that regulate oscillatory gene expression. *Methods Mol Biol 734*, 241–255.

Boxenbaum, H. (1982). Interspecies scaling, allometry, physiological time, and the ground plan of pharmacokinetics. *J Pharmacokinet Pharmacodyn 10*, 201–227.

Butcher, E.C., Berg, E.L., and Kunkel, E.J. (2004). Systems biology in drug discovery. *Nat Biotechnol 22*, 1253–1259.

Cui, Y. H., Zhu, J., and Wu, R.L. (2006). Functional mapping for genetic control of programmed cell death. *Physiol Genom 25*, 458–469.

Cui, Y.H., Wu, R.L., Casella, G., and Zhu, J. (2008). Nonparametric functional mapping quantitative trait loci underlying programmed cell death. *Statist Appl Genet Mol Biol 7*, 1, Art. 4.

Evans, W.E., and Johnson, J.A. (2001). Pharmacogenomics: the inherited basis for interindividual differences in drug response. *Annu Rev Genom Hum Genet 2*, 9–39.

Evans, W.E., and McLeod, H.L. (2003). Pharmacogenomics: drug disposition, drug targets, and side effects. *N Engl J Med 348*, 538–549.

Genet, A.J.H. (2002). A polymorphism in the β_1-adrenergic receptor is associated with resting heart rate. *Am J Hum Genet 70*, 935–942.

Giraldo, J. (2003). Empirical models and Hill coefficients. *Trends Pharmacol Sci 24*, 63–65.

Gong, Y., Wang, Z., Liu, T., Zhao, W., Zhu, Y., Johnson, J.A., and Wu, R.L. (2004). A statistical model for functional mapping of quantitative trait loci regulating drug response. *Pharmacogenom J 4*, 315–321.

Gronert, G.A., Fung, D.L., Jones, J.H., Shafer, S.L., Hildebrand, S.V., and Disbrow, E.A. (1995). Allometry of pharmacokinetics and pharmacodynamics of the muscle relaxant metocurine in mammals. *Am J Physiol Regul, Integr Comp Physiol 268*, 85–91.

Hu, T.M., and Hayton, W.L. (2001). Allometric scaling of xenobiotic clearance: uncertainty versus universality. *AAPS PharmSci 3*, E29.

Johnson, J.A. (2003). Pharmacogenetics: potential for individualized drug therapy through genetics. *Trends Genet 19*, 660–666.

Johnson, J.A., and Terra, S.G. (2002). β-Adrenergic receptor polymorphisms: cardiovascular disease associations and pharmacogenetics. *Pharm Res 19*, 1779–1787.

Kao, C.H., Zeng, Z.B., and Teasdale, R.D. (1999). Multiple interval mapping for quantitative trait loci. *Genetics 152*, 1203–1216.

Khor, S.P., McCarthy, K., Dupont, M., Murray, K., and Timony, G. (2000). Pharmacokinetics, pharmacodynamics, allometry, and dose selection of rPSGL-lg for phase I trial. *J Pharm Exp Ther 293*, 618–624.

Lander, E.S., and Botstein, D. (1989). Mapping Mendelian factors underlying quantitative traits using RFLP linkage maps. *Genetics 121*, 185–199.

Lepist, E.I., and Jusko, W.J. (2004). Anti-inflammatory drugs modeling and allometric scaling of S(+)-ketoprofen pharmacokinetics and pharmacodynamics: a retrospective analysis. *J Vet Pharmacol Ther 27*, 211–218.

Li, N., Das, K., and Wu, R.L. (2009). Functional mapping of human growth trajectories. *J Theor Biol 261*, 33–42.

Li, H., Huang, Z., Gai, J., Wu, S., Zeng, Y., Li, Q., and Wu, R.L. (2007). A conceptual framework for mapping quantitative trait loci regulating ontogenetic allometry. *PLoS ONE 2*, doi: 10.1371/journal.pone.0001245.

Lin, M. and Wu, R.L. (2005). Theoretical basis for the identification of allelic variants that encode drug efficacy and toxicity. *Genetics 170*, 919–928.

Lin, M., Aquilante, C., Johnson, J.A., and Wu, R.L. (2005). Sequencing drug response with HapMap. *Pharmacogenom J 5*, 149–156.

Lin, M., Li, H., Hou, W., Johnson, J.A., and Wu, R.L. (2007). Modeling sequence–sequence interactions for drug response. *Bioinformatics 23*, 1251–1257.

Liu, T., and Wu, R.L. (2009). A Bayesian algorithm for functional mapping of dynamic traits. *Algorithms 2*, 667–691.

Liu, T., Johnson, J.A., Casella, G., and Wu, R.L. (2004). Sequencing complex diseases with HapMap. *Genetics 168*, 503–511.

Liu, T., Liu, X.L., Chen, Y.M., and Wu, R.L. (2007). A computational model for functional mapping of genes that regulate intra-cellular circadian rhythms. *Theor Biol Med Model 4*, doi: 10.1186/1742-4682-4-5.

Long, F., Chen, Y.Q., Cheverud, J.M., and Wu, R.L. (2006). Genetic mapping of allometric scaling laws. *Genet Res 87*, 207–216.

Ma, C.X., Casella, G., and Wu, R.L. (2002). Functional mapping of quantitative trait loci underlying the character process: a theoretical framework. *Genetics 161*, 1751–1762.

Ma, Y., Ding, Z., Qian, Y., Shi, X., Castranova, V., Harner, E.J., and Guo, N.L. (2006). Predicting cancer drug response by proteomic profiling. *Clin Cancer Res 12*, 4583–4589.

Ma, Y., Ding, Z., Qian, Y., Wan, Y.W., Tosun, K., Shi, X., Castranova, V., Harner, E.J., and Guo, N.L. (2009) An integrative genomic and proteomic approach to chemosensitivity prediction. *Int J Oncol 34*, 107–115.

Nabel, E.G. (2003). Cardiovascular disease. *N Engl J Med 349*, 60–72.

Nagasaki, K., and Miki, Y. (2008). Molecular prediction of the therapeutic response to neoadjuvant chemotherapy in breast cancer. *Breast Cancer 15*, 117–120.

Schmidt-Nielsen, K. (1984). *Scaling: Why Is Animal Size So Important?* Cambridge University Press, Cambridge, UK.

Shimizu D., Ishikawa, T., Ichikawa, Y., Togo, S., Hayasizaki, Y., Okazaki, Y., and Shimada, H. (2004). Current progress in the prediction of chemosensitivity for breast cancer. *Breast Cancer 11*, 42–48.

Staunton J.E., Slonim, D.K., Coller, H.A., Tamayo, P., Angelo, M.J., Park, J., Scherf, U., Lee, J.K., Reinhold, W.O., Weinstein, J.N., et al. (2001). Chemosensitivity prediction by transcriptional profiling. *Proc Natl Acad Sci USA 98*, 10787–10792.

Wang, L.W., and Weinshilboum, R.M. (2008). Pharmacogenomics: candidate gene identification, functional validation and mechanisms. *Hum Mol Genet 17*, R174–R179.

Wang, Z.H., and Wu, R.L. (2004). A statistical model for high-resolution mapping of quantitative trait loci determining HIV dynamics. *Statist Med 23*, 3033–3051.

Wang, Z.H., Hou, W., and Wu, R.L. (2005). A statistical model to analyze quantitative trait locus interactions for HIV dynamics from the virus and human genomes. *Statist Med 25*, 495–511.

Watters, J.W., and McLeod, H.L. (2003). Using genome-wide mapping in the mouse to identify genes that influence drug response. *Trends Pharmacol Sci 24*, 55–58.

Watters, J.W., Kraja, A., Meucci, M.A., Province, M.A., and McLeod, H.L. (2004). Genome-wide discovery of loci influencing chemotherapy cytotoxicity. *Proc Natl Acad Sci USA 101*, 11809–11814.

Weinshilboum, R. (2003). Inheritance and drug response. *N Engl J Med 348*, 529–537.

West, G.B., and Brown, J.H. (2004). Life's universal scaling laws. *Phys Today 57*, 36–42.

West, G.B., and Brown, J.H. (2005). The origin of allometric scaling laws in biology from genomes to ecosystems: towards a quantitative unifying theory of biological structure and organization. *J Exp Biol 208*, 1575–1592.

West, G.B., Brown, J.H., and Enquist, B.J. (1997). A general model for the origin of allometric scaling laws in biology. *Science 276*, 122–126.

West, G.B., Brown, J.H., and Enquist, B.J. (1999a). A general model for the structure and allometry of plant vascular systems. *Nature 400*, 664–667.

West, G.B., Brown, J.H., and Enquist, B.J. (1999b). The fourth dimension of life: fractal geometry and allometric scaling of organisms. *Science 284*, 1677–1679.

Wu, J.S, Zhu, J., Zeng, Y.R., and Wu, R.L. (2007). Functional mapping of norm reactions to environmental signals. *Genet Res 89*, 27–38.

Wu, R.L., and Lin, M. (2006). Functional mapping: how to map and study the genetic architecture of dynamic complex traits. *Nat Rev Genet 7*, 229–237.

Wu, R.L., and Lin, M. (2008). *Statistical and Computational Pharmacogenomics*. Chapman & Hall/CRC, London.

Wu, R.L., Ma, C.X., Littell, R.C., and Casella, G. (2002). A statistical model for the genetic origin of allometric scaling laws in biology. *J Theor Biol 219*, 121–135.

Wu, R.L., Ma, C.X., and Casella, G. (2007). *Statistical Genetics of Quantitative Traits: Linkage, Maps, and QTL*. Springer-Verlag, New York.

Wu, R.L., Ma, C.X., Lin, M., and Casella, G. (2004a). A general framework for analyzing the genetic architecture of developmental characteristics. *Genetics 166*, 1541–1551.

Wu, R.L., Wang, Z., Zhao, W., and Cheverud, J.M. (2004b). A mechanistic model for genetic machinery of ontogenetic growth. *Genetics 168*, 2383–2394.

Wu, R.L., Ma, C.X., Lin, M., Wang, Z., and Casella G., (2004c). Functional mapping of quantitative trait loci underlying growth trajectories using a transform-both-sides logistic model. *Biometrics 60*, 729–738.

Yu, S., Yarnell, J.W., Sweetnam, P.M., and Murray, L. (2003). What level of physical activity protects against premature cardiovascular death? The Caerphilly study. *Heart 89*, 502–506.

Zeng, Z.B. (1994). Precision mapping of quantitative trait loci. *Genetics 136*, 1457–1468.

Zhao, W., Ma, C.X., Cheverud, J.M., and Wu, R.L. (2004a). A unifying statistical model for QTL mapping of genotype–sex interaction for developmental trajectories. *Physiol Genomics 19*, 218–227.

Zhao, W., Wu, R.L., Ma, C.X., and Casella, G. (2004b). A fast algorithm for functional mapping of complex traits. *Genetics 167*, 2133–2137.

Zhao, W., Zhu, J., Gallo-Meagher, M., and Wu, R.L. (2004c). A unified statistical model for functional mapping of genotype × environment interactions for ontogenetic development. *Genetics 168*, 1751–1762.

Zuideveld, K.P., Van der Graaf, P.H., Peletier, L.A., and Danhof, M. (2007). Allometric scaling of pharmacodynamic responses: application to 5-Ht1A receptor mediated responses from rat to man. *Pharm Res 24*, 2031–2039.

CHAPTER 14

Future Outlook for Systems Biology

DANIEL L. YOUNG

Theranos Inc., Palo Alto, California

SETH MICHELSON

Genomic Health Inc., Redwood City, California

Summary

Biological research has shown enormous growth recently as new technologies provide incredible windows into the underlying machinery of living systems. With the growth of such tools, the breadth and complexity of biological data have also grown. We suggest that successful drug discovery and development requires enhanced integration of preclinical data with patient data to more fully understand factors affecting both health and disease. Systems biology aims to enhance the analysis and understanding of such data broadly and boldly via the systemic integration of the information into a unified, quantitative whole. As we review in this chapter, extending current methodologies as well as developing new approaches to tackle these hurdles will further enhance the productivity of drug discovery and development.

14.1. INTRODUCTION

The discovery and commercialization of new and effective medicines is a challenging and rewarding endeavor for those involved in its many facets. The approach, however, is not a static formula or set of procedures. Rather, the methodologies of drug discovery and development are continuing to advance by the integration of sophisticated technologies, growing biological knowledge, and more flexible business practices. Such continual refinement is necessary

Systems Biology in Drug Discovery and Development, First Edition.
Edited by Daniel L. Young, Seth Michelson.
© 2012 John Wiley & Sons, Inc. Published 2012 by John Wiley & Sons, Inc.

to adapt to the changing landscapes in the competitive environment, medical costs and practice, and new challenging disease indications.

In an effort to reduce costs and enhance the productivity of drug discovery and development, the U.S. Food and Drug Administration (FDA) in its Critical Path Initiative has called for establishing novel approaches to drug discovery and development, including scientific and technical methods such as animal- or computer-based predictive models, safety and efficacy biomarkers, and new clinical evaluation techniques (http://www.fda.gov/oc/initiatives/criticalpath/whitepaper.pdf). The aim of this book is to illustrate with concrete approaches and examples how systems biology can enhance the critical path by targeting these key areas. In this chapter we look ahead to upcoming challenges and opportunities for the field of systems biology in improving productivity, reducing costs, and enhancing new and current therapeutics. We review concepts of system complexity, discuss ongoing opportunities for the systems approach throughout the development pipeline, look ahead to personalized medicine, and finally, consider challenges and solutions for effective communications and training of systems biologists.

14.2. SYSTEM COMPLEXITY IN BIOLOGICAL SYSTEMS

Health is conventionally considered a physical state of well-being that may be assessed at a given moment in time. However, this basic notion neglects time-varying behaviors that are characteristic of health and may even be central for establishing and maintaining healthy conditions. Ahn et al. (2006a, b) note that "it is the *behavior* of a system rather than the *state* of a system that remains consistent" in well-functioning biological systems. Therefore, it is necessary to consider dynamic, biological responses to completely characterize system-level behaviors. A more complete understanding of health would naturally aid in diagnosis by assessing the differences between time-dependent healthy behaviors and disease-specific behaviors. Although this strategy necessitates more complex experimental investigations and analyses, it is an opportunity to exploit the benefits provided by systems biology, a discipline whose foundation is the quantitative assessment of complex dynamic biological interactions.

Accepting that biological systems need to be understood more fully with respect to dynamic behaviors rather than simply discrete states or measures, one must consider more complex methods for describing and assessing their behavior over time. This notion invokes various system-level concepts, such as stability, robustness, modularity, and adaptability—concepts that when applied to biological systems have led to new and deeper understandings (Carlson and Doyle, 2002; Csete and Doyle, 2004; Kitano, 2004; Lauffenburger, 2000; Stelling et al., 2004). These properties of biological systems are central in establishing and maintaining healthy behaviors over time despite changes in environmental conditions and stresses—however, they are not unique to healthy systems.

For example, diseased organisms can also exhibit system-level properties similar to those exhibited by healthy organisms. For example, robustness is a system-level characteristic evident in both healthy and diseased systems and, in fact, may be one factor that can impede treatment of diseases. Therefore, complete assessment of biological systems requires in-depth systems analysis and is critical for diagnosis, prevention, and the design and administration of effective treatments.

The foundations of general systems theory were laid down by von Bertalanffy (1968) and have been applied extensively across many disciplines. Notably, Wiener (1965) elegantly applied these types of systems concepts to biological systems, leading to a discipline termed *cybernetics*. Cybernetics is focused on understanding the organization and function of regulatory systems (Wiener, 1965). Over the last several decades, systems analyses have been used extensively to better understand complex biological regulatory networks and are well suited for understanding behaviors emerging from the interactions of many subelements. These approaches are invaluable for understanding the nature of stability and robustness in biological systems (Araujo et al., 2007). For example, robustness has been shown to depend on characteristics ubiquitous in biological systems, including modularity, redundancy, and feedback (Kitano, 2004). Due to the increasing understanding of these biological system–level properties, many efforts have now been made to replicate these biological system features in manmade devices, a practice commonly referred to as *synthetic biology*. Opportunities abound for synthetic biological approaches: for example, in the design of circuits, energy production, drug production, diagnostics, mechanical systems, and information processing and controllers (Chopra and Kamma, 2006; Csete and Doyle, 2002; Endy, 2005; Kaznessis, 2007).

System-level properties of living organisms are of paramount importance for a complete understanding of health, disease, and the transition between them. A systems-level perspective and analysis are especially suited to a study of the continuum between healthy and disease behaviors. Appreciation of this continuous behavioral space affords the opportunity to assess not just current conditions but also the direction in which a person's state is progressing based on prior history and current conditions. This more complete temporal knowledge is fundamental for developing more effective and early preventive approaches as well as potent curative interventions (Kitano, 2007). For example, the metabolic syndrome is a pervasive, progressive condition for which temporal biological knowledge across multiple disease modalities (e.g., endocrine, inflammatory, cardiovascular, and environmental conditions), and analysis thereof could improve patient diagnosis, management, and treatment.

14.3. MODELS FOR QUANTITATIVE INTEGRATION OF DATA

As with all scientific research, the interpretation and integration of biological data requires careful consideration of its context in order to yield robust

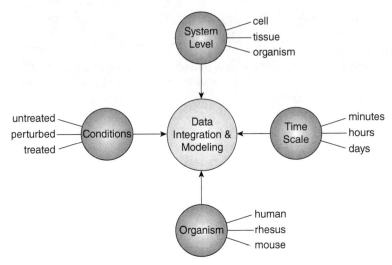

Figure 14.1 System biology enables the integration of biological information into a unified context in order to generate relevant, context-dependent insights from the data available. Numerous factors affect the interpretation and relevance of biological data, including the system level of the experiment (e.g., molecular, intracellular, interacting cells, intact organs, whole body), the time scale of the investigation (e.g., minutes, hours, days), the environmental conditions and perturbations made to the system (e.g., specific assay conditions, drug exposures), the organism being studied (e.g., mouse, rat, primate, human), and the health and/or genotype of the system (e.g., disease specific, genetic knockout, inbred strain, other covariates).

insights and conclusions. As illustrated in Figure 14.1, numerous factors can affect the interpretation and relevance of biological data, including the system level of the experiment (e.g., molecular, intracellular, interacting cells, intact organs, whole body), the time scale of the investigation (e.g., minutes, hours, days), the environmental conditions and perturbations made to the system (e.g., specific assay conditions, drug exposures), the organism being studied (e.g., mouse, rat, primate, human), and the health and/or genotype of the system (e.g., disease specific, genetic knockout, inbred strain, other covariates). The growing complexity of such data represents a major hurdle for drug discovery and development. A paramount challenge and opportunity for systems biology is therefore to facilitate the integration of biological information into a unified intelligible context. Namely, the systems approach enables one to utilize a family of methodologies to account for the multitude of factors affecting complex biological systems in order to generate relevant, context-dependent insights from the available, often disparate, data.

The investigation of cell cycle regulation is an example in which insight generation is hampered by data integration challenges. Because of its fundamental importance in development, aging, and many disease states, the cell cycle has been studied extensively over many decades. The cell cycle (including proliferation and apoptosis) is regulated by both intracellular mediators, such as cyclins and cyclin-dependent kinases (CDKs), and extracellular stimuli. Numerous nonlinear interactions between these molecules and regulated gene expression give rise to complex behaviors whose understanding can shed light on certain pathophysiological conditions, such as disease initiation, disease progression, and response to therapy, especially in the realm of cancer and anemia. However, it is increasingly evident that numerous factors complicate data interpretation and therefore impede our understanding of these important cellular phenomena. For example, key cell cycle behaviors and dependencies are known to differ across various tumor types and tumor cell lines (Yang et al., 2006). Moreover, results can vary based on the duration of experiments, the measurement sampling times, stimuli types, and the relationship between exposure times and cellular states. Often, the relevance of these confounding factors becomes lost during data integration, possibly leading to incorrect conclusions and obviating important insights that could otherwise have been discerned.

Systems analysis can help mitigate some of the concerns related to experimental conditions by employing quantitative methods that simultaneously explicitly account for and probe the affect of many confounding variables. A prerequisite for quantitative modeling is experimental data collection and, typically, development of biochemical interaction maps. Extensive intracellular maps have been developed for the mammalian cell cycle (Kohn, 1999). Following such molecular mappings, computational modeling of the cell cycle, including the dynamic interplay of multiple intracellular molecular pathways, can be carried out and serves as a powerful tool for discriminating the nature of these complex processes. For example, this methodology can be used to probe the factors that most affect cell fate, such as the restriction point at which cells enter the proliferative phase from the resting state (Novak and Tyson, 2004). Such quantitative models can also be used to investigate the impact of combining stimuli that activate interacting intracellular pathways, possibly leading to novel combination therapies (Araujo et al., 2007; Chassagnole et al., 2006; Fitzgerald et al., 2006). The utilization of such computational test beds affords extensive, rapid exploration of treatment approaches that may be infeasible and/or too costly to conduct in the laboratory. These analyses can highlight possible synergistic effects of drugs, temporal dependencies such as the role of drug exposure times, and time-varying or adaptive cellular responses. The identification of such complex responses via modeling and simulation can lead to further laboratory investigations for confirmation, refinement, and extension.

An elegant example of the application of modeling and simulation to understanding emergent biological behaviors was shown in Chapter 7. In this study, the investigators developed a series of models to understand and predict dose–response profiles for drugs and xenobiotics. The power of this approach was that it allowed the integration of fundamental *in vitro* data into a quantitative model to gain valuable insights that would otherwise have required extensive and complex laboratory investigations. Moreover, their results showed that single-cell behaviors are not necessarily indicative of whole-organism responses. To come to these insights, the authors first identified, via modeling and simulation, emergent cellular behaviors of bistability and hysteresis that resulted from the input–output properties of a ligand-mediated molecular network for gene autoregulation. Taking into account sources of biological fluctuation, including cell-to-cell variation in dose and the stochastic nature of the reaction steps involved in the switching of an individual cell, the authors were able to extend the results from a single cell to a population of cells. They also showed that the time of measurement, an experimental factor often overlooked, affected the apparent dose–response profile. This application of systems biology provides a powerful example of how data integration through the formalism of quantitative models can lead to key insights affecting biological responses, whether toxic or efficacious. Such applications of systems biological modeling can greatly enhance the value of preclinical data via data integration, modeling, and evaluation of compound safety and efficacy.

Another example shows the power of the systems approach in connecting cellular molecular interactions to tissue-level outcomes through the integration and modeling of diverse experimental data. In this case, the investigators developed a data-driven model of a human cancer cell to explore multiple perturbations, such as gene knockdown/knockout and drug responses (Christopher et al., 2004). The focus of the quantitative dynamic model was to understand the molecular and gene expression network controlling the proliferative and apoptotic behaviors of human cancer cells. The authors developed a graphical model to describe the network of over 1000 genes and proteins as well as a dynamic simulation model, including several hundred molecules controlling the cell's fate. The rational development of the model was dependent on a systematic and expansive mining of the literature to determine the relevance and quality of the data available. Via a network inference engine, novel connections were integrated into the model, leading to the identification of novel interactions between genes, proteins, and metabolites. This powerful inference approach illustrates the efficient integration of data into a quantitative look-forward simulation architecture that can be used for pathway discovery, the evaluation of novel targets, and the investigation of drug mechanisms of action. Future extension of this and similar modeling architectures to patient-specific data could lead to tailored treatment approaches based on DNA, RNA, and proteomic assessments.

14.4. CHANGING REQUIREMENTS FOR SYSTEMS APPROACHES DURING DRUG DISCOVERY AND DEVELOPMENT

A fundamental tenant of drug discovery and development is that the available biological data must be assessed at every stage of development in the context of well-defined drug development objectives. These objectives in combination with contextual biological knowledge should therefore determine which data are most relevant and how those data should be evaluated. Therefore, the relevant questions, and hence data requirements, during drug discovery are naturally very different than those during drug development. For example, during discovery, one aim may be to differentiate and prioritize possible drug targets and compounds *in vitro* for specific indications. In some instances, data derived from murine cell lines may be invaluable to meet such objectives. However, as discovery progresses, the relevance of such early insights based on *in vitro* animal data must be confirmed in more realistic biological settings. In situ and *in vivo* animal models would be a natural progression.

To remain aligned with research goals, the aims of the systems biologist must progress in concert with the advancement of drugs through the pharmaceutical pipeline (Figure 14.2). The changing objectives of systems biology throughout preclinical and clinical phases of research are reflected in the scope and organization of this book. For example, early discovery efforts are likely to focus on models of intracellular pathways. As development progresses, experiments advance to systems of cells and more complex biological

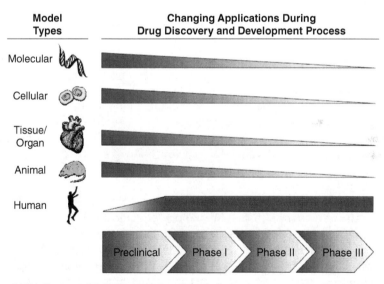

Figure 14.2 Systems biologists must tailor their analyses to meet changing requirements as drugs advance through the pharmaceutical pipeline. For example, early discovery efforts typically focus on models of molecular and intracellular pathways. As development progresses, experiments and modeling advance together to systems of cells and more complex biological networks, including *in vivo* animal studies. Analyses during clinical development phases typically focus on optimizing trial designs and discovery of biomarkers by integrating models of drugs, human physiology, and pathophysiology.

networks across space and time. Subsequent efforts focus on translational questions as well as issues of toxicity. Clinical phases focus on questions of optimizing trial designs and discovery of biomarkers. Accordingly, pharmaceutical companies that choose to adopt systems approaches must recognize the variety and scope of systems biology methodologies at their disposal, and then apply them appropriately. Although empowering, this flexibility also represents a challenge to the pharmaceutical industry in adopting and integrating new methodologies throughout their organizations, and doing so in a manner consistent with their changing objectives at each discovery and development stage.

We argue that there is much to be gained by applying systems approaches as early as possible during drug discovery. Such early application allows the progressive advancement and enrichment of knowledge to be incorporated into a quantitative, and hence interpretable, systems framework. It also affords ample time for feedback between experimentalists and systems biologists, as insights from each domain are iteratively tested and refined in a cooperative manner.

14.5. BETTER MODELS FOR BETTER DECISIONS

Pharmaceutical drug discovery and development has always been faced with the challenge of making rapid, rational decisions in the face of incomplete or limited data. Key decisions, such as whether to advance a compound into a phase III trial, are not based solely on scientific and medical considerations, but also incorporate business and market factors, such as the competitive landscape and other, internal potential development opportunities. Accordingly, systematic quantitative methods to assess each candidate compound in an unbiased fashion will enable more rapid and better decisions. Continuous risk assessment is required to evaluate the current state of knowledge and to assess the cost and value of collecting additional data that may reduce material uncertainties.

The rational evaluation of biological data necessitates the realistic assessment of their relevance to human biology. Significant concerns have been raised regarding the current dependence of medical research on reductionist cell-based approaches as well on nonvalidated animal models of the human condition (Horrobin, 2003). Advancements in *in vitro* methodologies have been made to improve their relevance to disease states by combining multiple cells and stimuli so as to better reflect *in vivo* disease conditions (Kunkel et al., 2004). The predictive nature of such cellular systems still requires careful and costly validation. Moreover, further work is required to understand the differences between healthy and diseaselike behaviors at the cell-culture level by utilizing cells with multiple phenotypes. In addition, such cell-based assays typically are not geared toward investigating the diversity inherent in human disease conditions. A recent analysis suggests that greater ethnic diversity in the library of laboratory cell lines available is required for more broadly relevant research and drug development (Laurent et al., 2010).

At the *in vivo* level, most animal models have not been adequately validated with respect to their relevance to human disease, yet are still critical hurdles for advancing drug development programs. Each animal model, whether spontaneous or induced, has its unique characteristics which make it more or less comparable to human disease. There is undoubtedly much to be learned from animal disease models with respect to basic biological functions and disease development. However, such animal-specific insights are not necessarily relevant to human disease conditions and, we suggest, require extensive validation in order to be considered trustworthy by the research organization as well as regulatory agencies.

For example, a comparison of *in vivo* cancer models against human clinical phase II trials revealed that *in vivo* activity in particular tumor models did not closely correlate with human cancer histologies (Johnson et al., 2001). In this study, for preclinical animal survival models, "positive" response levels were defined as 25 and 50% increased life spans, while for subcutaneous xenograft models, 40 and 10% tumor weight ratios for treated and controls groups were defined as a positive response. A positive phase II trial result was defined as a 50% reduction in tumor size in at least 20% of patients treated. However, more encouraging, the analysis did reveal that for compounds with *in vivo* activity in at least one-third of xenograft models, there was an increased correlation with some phase II trial results.

Similar to preclinical cancer models, the relevance of the nonobese diabetic (NOD) mouse for the study of type 1 diabetes (T1D) has been debated by researchers within the diabetes research community (Leiter and von Herrath, 2004; Roep, 2007; Roep and Atkinson, 2004; Roep et al., 2004). The study of T1D in human patients has been hampered by several factors, including its largely asymptomatic progression before clinical manifestation and the difficulties of assessing immunologic processes occurring in the target tissue based on peripheral measures alone. The NOD mouse model is considered the preferred model for human T1D and has been studied extensively to gain insight in autoimmune disease initiation and progression (Atkinson and Leiter, 1999). Interestingly, as of 2005, over 460 treatments had been tested in the NOD mouse, and 60 to 70% of these treatments were discovered to suppress development of diabetes or to induce remission in the NOD mouse (Shoda et al., 2005). However, thus far, none of these treatments that have been tested in humans have been approved for the treatment of human T1D (Shoda et al., 2005). There are many possible reasons for such discrepancies. For example, it is possible that the NOD mouse model is generally a poor model for human T1D, due to underlying biological differences such as the predominant disease-driving cell types and mediators, initiating disease events, and the disease time course. However, a more complete comparative assessment might find that specific types of treatments could be tested more reliably in the NOD mouse based on the drug's mechanisms of action and the conservation of key pathways between the NOD mouse and human T1D patients. For example, drugs directly targeting immunological pathways associated with B cells may be more or less predictive of the human response than drugs targeting certain metabolic pathways. In addition, there are fundamental challenges associated with translating drugs from the preclinical setting to the human setting, which may be related to species differences in the drug's pharmacokinetics (PK) and pharmacodynamics (PD) (Mahmood, 1999; Singh, 2006).

Significant efforts are under way to discover and develop more relevant animal models of human disease (Beckers et al., 2009). Spontaneous as well as induced models of disease are typically evaluated to consider the natural history of the animal disease in order to assess pathophysiologic comparability between the animal model and human etiology. Aspects taken into account include time to onset of a disease or condition, the time course of progression of the disease or condition, and signs and symptoms. Genetic engineering approaches enable the powerful ability to develop knockout (loss of function) or knock-in (gain of function) animal models using one or more genes. Conditional genetic modifications allow tissue-specific and time-dependent changes in gene expression, avoiding complications such as developmental lethality. Although such approaches are powerful tools and yield scientifically interesting results, human diseases rarely result from one or a few polymorphisms. Moreover, the diversity of human disease has been well established, raising concerns regarding the relevance of genetically engineered animal models in which a limited number of genes are modified.

Applying the tenets of systems biology throughout the drug discovery and development pipeline can help address some of these challenges, and aid critical decision analysis in several ways. First, a novel application of systems biology is to aid in the unbiased evaluation and development of animal models of human disease. For example, quantitative models of both animal physiology and human physiology could be used to identify key biological processes held in common that affect disease progression and response to therapy. One approach for comparing models of different species is to conduct parameter sensitivity analyses to assess whether the various systems have comparable disease drivers. Such quantitative comparisons can aid in an evaluation of the concordance between different species. By identifying specific, targeted, genetically altered characteristics in animal models, such analyses could improve the development of more predictive animal models for specific human conditions and intervention modalities. In addition to *in vivo* model analysis, the simulation and analysis of cell-based assays could help assess their predictive nature as well as the identification of methods for improving their clinical relevance.

Second, systems biology approaches provide a systematic platform for effectively identifying biological uncertainties that can affect key clinical outcomes. This information is extremely valuable for research organizations, as it crystallizes how gaps and uncertainties in current information may or may not affect efficacy and/or toxicity (Michelson and Cole, 2007). If predictions are not affected significantly by uncertainties or biological variability, the assessed risks are low. In contrast, risks are high when predicted outcomes are highly sensitive to biological uncertainties. In such high-risk scenarios, additional focused laboratory experiments and/or additional clinical studies should be conducted. Naturally, all uncertainties cannot be resolved (due to numerous factors, such as limited resources, time, and technologies), but the systems biology approach can be used to highlight the most important uncertainties, enabling more informed rational decisions. Techniques for model sensitivity analyses are invaluable tools that address how simulated outcomes are affected by biological uncertainties (Gutenkunst et al., 2007). In summary, the integration of such quantitative, model-sensitivity analyses into critical decision processes should improve risk assessment, enhance strategies for reducing risks, and optimize pharmaceutical resource allocation.

14.5.1. Model Validation

Proposed applications such as enhancing the evaluation and utilization of animal models using quantitative models of biological systems naturally raise the question of *in silico* model validation. A common question asks whether mathematical models of human disease can be any more reliable or predictive than animal models of human conditions. This issue is of great importance and is a basic issue facing systems biological research and its widespread adoption. More fundamentally, given the prior discussion, the trusted extrapolation of results from any "model" of human biology, whether *in silico* or biological, necessitates a level of trusted validation. With this perspective, mathematical models could be assessed, in some respects, using approaches similar to those of biological models of human conditions. Hence, one could begin by asking questions of *in silico* models similar to those asked of physical biological models, such as: What is the comparability of the simulated time to onset of disease or condition, time course of progression of disease or condition, and signs and symptoms?

However, the evaluation of *in silico* models can extend beyond the largely qualitative approaches used for preclinical animal models. For example, unbiased methods to assess the value of quantitative models have been centered on calibration (model training) and (external) validation (ADA Consensus Panel, 2004). In this framework, calibration of quantitative models involves the construction and tuning of the model to meet certain defined constraints, while validation involves assessing the model's ability to predict novel behaviors. It has been suggested that a model, whether *in silico* or otherwise, should embody the key organizing and operating principles of the biological system in question while linking system-level behaviors with underlying biological mechanisms based on a comprehensive set of data across both time and physical scales (Young and Poon, 2001).

An example of a validated large-scale model of complex human physiology is the Archimedes model of diabetes (Eddy and Schlessinger, 2003a,b). At the cellular level, Christopher et al. (2004) developed and validated a model of the major intracellular pathways governing the cell fate of human cancer cells. Numerous other examples can be found in the literature, including PK–PD models that characterize human disease progression and response to drugs (Rajman, 2008). Such PK–PD quantitative models have been widely accepted by U.S. and European regulatory bodies as being valuable tools to aid pharmaceutical research and are considered central components of modern drug development and clinical trial design. Moreover, computational modeling has recently been considered as part of the FDA's Critical Path Initiative in an effort to streamline pharmaceutical drug discovery and development (FDA, 2004). However, the acceptance of such quantitative methodologies requires continued learnings (success and failure) from both pharmaceutical companies and regulatory bodies across multiple disease conditions and contexts. Moving forward, collaboration between academic, industrial, and regulatory bodies will be central for establishing best practices for *in silico* model validation approaches that appropriately weigh the benefits of new therapeutics for patients against the risks as well as the potential cost benefits for research organizations.

14.6. ADVANCING PERSONALIZED MEDICINE

The characteristics and behaviors of human physiology, known as *phenotypes*, are typically assessed by one or more measures recorded at a given moment or over time, perhaps in response to an environmental stimulus such as a drug or physical challenge. Comparison of phenotypes across the human population can give rise to various classifications or diagnoses, such as a normal healthy range, or a responder versus a nonresponder patient to a particular drug. However, most of these guidelines consider only one (univariate) or a few measures (multivariate) and often do not consider changes or fluctuations over time (i.e., static rather than dynamic). Such simplifications belie the complex nature of physiological systems. Moreover, as discussed earlier in the chapter, data integration at the systems level requires the explicit accounting of multiple factors over time to characterize a patient's health more completely.

One approach for improving care is via more complete and predictive assessment of health through the discovery and utilization of validated biomarkers. Biomarkers are physiological measures indicative of current and/or future medical conditions and/or responses, whether normal or aberrant. The use of biomarkers to aid in diagnosis and treatment is well established. Classic examples include the use of low-density lipoprotein cholesterol to assess cardiovascular health and risk, or the concentration of glucose for a diagnosis of diabetes.

Significant advances in medical knowledge and technologies have created new biomarker opportunities that have the potential for enhancing drug discovery and development in parallel with improving health care fundamentals. Recent biomarker efforts have focused on a wide range of physiological readouts widely characterized as "omics," including proteomics, metabolomics, genomics, transcriptomics, and epigenomics. Besides being used for diagnostic and prognostic purposes, such biomarkers (typically referred to as a *type 1 biomarker*) can be used to determine to which drug a patient is most likely to respond. More broadly, the utilization of diagnostic tools to enhance the administration of therapeutics has been coined *theranostics* (Picard and Bergeron, 2002). The use of biomarkers to enhance drug selection and dosing regimens for an individual patient promises to enable a new era of personalized medicine, improving efficacy and limiting toxicities and adverse events. However, to achieve these goals, there remain significant challenges, some of which can be met by systems biology.

Normal healthy behaviors as well as disease conditions are highly variable, in part due to genetic variation. Of course, it is now recognized that the genetic diversity of the human population enhances survival of the species in the face of environmental challenges. Such diversity also significantly complicates the study of human physiology and pathophysiology and their relationship to inherited genetic variants. The mapping of the human genome and the study of human genotypic diversity, or the variation of DNA sequences across the species, is a rapidly advancing field with profound implications for medical knowledge and drug discovery and development (a field known as *pharmacogenomics*). For example, the identification of single-nucleotide polymorphisms (SNPs), or single-nucleotide DNA sequence variations that occur in at least 1% of the population, has the potential to greatly affect our understanding of human physiology and disease.

Some SNPs have been shown to be highly predictive of certain human diseases and response to treatments; their discovery may lead to greater understanding of the molecular causes of disease. For example, the risk for developing age-related macular degeneration (AMD) was found to be approximately two- to seven-fold higher in those with a common variant in the complement factor H (CFH) gene, depending on whether a person is homozygous or heterozygous for the variant (Edwards et al., 2005; Haines et al., 2005; Klein et al., 2005). This risk allele was estimated to account for 20 to 50% of the overall risk of developing AMD. Based on these and other insights, recent studies have explored AMD disease mechanisms and shown systemic complement activation in the circulation of AMD patients, suggesting that systemic activation is manifested in the aging macula (Scholl et al., 2008). These insights could lead to novel personalized therapies that target specific aspects of the alternative pathway of complement (Rohrer et al., 2009; Tortajada et al., 2009).

Other genetic polymorphisms have also been utilized to personalize treatments. For example, the appropriate dose of anticoagulants, such as warfarin, can be guided by a person's *CYP2C9* and *VKORC1* genes (Daly, 2009). However, although extremely powerful for some medical conditions, most human diseases are polygenic, making their prediction and understanding via genetic testing alone more challenging (Kraft and Hunter, 2009). Moreover, the predictive nature of individual genotypes will probably vary, depending on the disease condition and outcomes of interest.

Although clearly a powerful prognosticator for certain diseases, a person's genotype is not always as predictive as perhaps widely believed. For example, genetically identical monozygotic twins showed only 15% concordance for development of rheumatoid arthritis (RA) (Silman et al., 1993). This concordance rate reflects the maximal direct genetic contribution to RA development, given that both genotype and similar environmental factors experienced by most identical twins probably contribute to disease development. Hence, it is likely that genetic testing alone may not suffice to meet the far-reaching goals of personalized medicine.

Given these limitations, personalized medicine cannot rely on genotypic information alone. Clearly, environmental factors are important contributors to the development of many diseases by, among other effects, stably altering DNA expression patterns. The emerging field of *epigenetics* is focused on understanding stable alterations of DNA expression patterns, not the genome itself, that occur due to environmental influences during development as well as in fully mature individuals (Jaenisch and Bird, 2003). A growing number of molecular mechanisms have recently been discovered that can alter gene expression patterns, DNA methylation and histone modification being perhaps the most extensively studied to date (Feinberg, 2008). The complexity of such molecular adaptations to environmental stimuli is of fundamental interest to the understanding of both health and disease, and represents an opportunity for significant scientific advancement. The National Institutes of Health (NIH) recently made a significant commitment to fund and prioritize research in this field by including *epigenomics* research as an NIH Roadmap initiative (http://www.nih.gov/news/health/jan2008/od-22.htm). Moreover, the NIH's Genes, Environment and Health Initiative (GEI) is focused on understanding the development of diseases such as diabetes, childhood asthma, obesity, and autism, as the result of interactions between environmental exposures and genes (http://www.nih.gov/news/pr/sep2007/nhgri-04.htm).

Given these complex properties of physiological systems, it is clear that traditional reductionist approaches alone will not suffice to advance medical knowledge and treatment approaches, slowing the identification and validation of novel biomarkers. That is, the dynamic interplay between genotype, the environment, and time-varying gene expression patterns gives rise to complex physiological behaviors for which narrowly focused experimental observations are grossly inadequate, especially when the aim is to understand system-level physiologies. A major challenge to the use of biomarkers is therefore to accurately characterize dynamic physiological behaviors and, simultaneously, to gain insights into the cause-and-effect relationships in physiological networks. According to the FDA guidance, biomarker validation requires "an established scientific framework or body of evidence that elucidates the physiologic, toxicologic, pharmacologic, or clinical significance of the test results" (http://www.fda.gov/cder/guidance/6400fnl.pdf). Systems biology is suited to deciphering these system-level properties by integrating molecular, cellular, and organ-level functions into a unified framework. To this end, mathematical analyses and modeling can help address both short- and long-term cellular behaviors in concert with molecular experimentation (Polyak et al., 2009). Such quantitative analyses can discern the manners in which dynamic, adaptive behaviors give rise to robust healthy behaviors in addition to robust disease patterns. Moreover, these insights will help identify the best approaches for distinguishing clinical phenotypes via multifactorial, dynamic biomarkers.

14.7. IMPROVING CLINICAL TRIALS AND ENABLING MORE COMPLEX TREATMENT APPROACHES

As discussed in earlier chapters, systems biology approaches can be applied to improve the success rate of drugs entering clinical studies by enhancing trial design, execution, and analysis. Despite significant increases in scientific knowledge, current success rates in clinical studies are at historic lows. For example, recent estimates suggest that on average only 8 to 11% of new molecular entities entering clinical studies will be approved by regulatory agencies and enter the marketplace despite increased spending (Gilbert et al., 2003; Kola, 2008). During the 1980s, the success rate for new molecular entities was 15%, a rate higher than current success rates (Gilbert et al., 2003; Kola, 2008). The success rate of novel compounds has been shown to depend on the targeted disease, with higher success rates (20%) in infectious and cardiovascular diseases and lower rates (5 to 8%) in diseases of the central nervous system and oncology (Kola, 2008).

A compound can fail, for a variety of reasons, at any of the clinical stages during the critical path to approval. Several recent studies (Elias et al., 2006; Kola and Landis, 2004) have shown that the attrition rate in phase III trials is 42 to 43%, while the most frequent cause of failure is a lack of efficacy or differentiation from existing treatments. These high failure rates, particularly in late-stage, large-scale pivotal studies, significantly increase costs for pharmaceutical companies, necessitating new approaches to reduce attrition and increase the number of new safe and effective compounds that reach the marketplace.

To address the declining productivity in the pharmaceutical industry, the FDA's Critical Path Initiative calls for new approaches to streamline the pathway to drug approval (U.S. Department of Health and Human Services, 2004). Among several opportunities to enhance the efficacy and safety of drugs entering clinical studies, the FDA highlighted model-based drug development (MBDD) with quantitative modeling as an emerging approach for improving decision making and the acquisition of knowledge from clinical studies. Over the last two decades, novel clinical trial modeling and simulation approaches have been utilized by pharmaceutical companies and have been credited with significant cost and time savings as well as improved decision making (Lalonde et al., 2007). Not only do these modeling and simulation approaches enhance clinical designs, they also enable earlier unbiased, rigorous assessment of drug candidates and intervention strategies, allowing some compounds to be prioritized while others may be abandoned (Pallay and Berry, 1999).

The complexity of clinical studies requires significant domain knowledge in their design, implementation, analysis, and reporting to reduce risk of failure. Sheiner (1997) elegantly presented the "learn" and "confirm" notions for clinical studies, where the aims of human trials generally cycle between phases of (1) discovering a drug's dose–response relationship, including efficacy and toxicity, in subgroups of patients, to (2) validating these hypotheses in subsequent trials. It has been shown in numerous studies that model-based data integration and analysis improve this learn-and-confirm process. As has been shown in several studies (Rajman, 2008), the systems approach of data integration and quantitative modeling can facilitate the more rapid acquisition of knowledge and improve decision making when faced with data of complex time-varying disease processes, multiple time scales and clinical endpoints, prior knowledge from other studies, and heterogeneous clinical subjects. A major challenge for the pharmaceutical industry is therefore to advance clinical trial modeling and simulation approaches across various disease areas spanning early preclinical and phase I to IV studies. To be fully embraced, these analytic approaches must be well validated and comprehensible to decision makers and researchers of diverse backgrounds at both pharmaceutical companies and regulatory agencies.

Traditional PK–PD modeling studies have relied on empirical approaches, where the underlying mechanisms are either not well understood or not incorporated into the model. In an effort to enhance the predictability and utility of models, recent MBDD efforts aim to integrate mechanistic biological and pharmacologic knowledge from prior preclinical and clinical studies. More broadly, to enhance the efficiency of drug development, MBDD can integrate and model data spanning multiple domains, including trial performance metrics, PK–PD disease models, commercial factors and the competitive landscape, clinical trial design and execution parameters, analytic models for data analysis, and quantitative decision criteria (Lalonde et al., 2007). Development, analysis, and simulation of these sophisticated models benefit from systems-level approaches that are focused on understanding emergent complex behaviors across multiple dimensions and scales. Analysis and simulation of such models can help test key hypotheses regarding the compound, its effect on the disease, and the likelihood for success of candidate clinical trial designs.

Although typically more challenging to develop, the use of mechanistic-based models have shown significant value to pharmaceutical companies by helping to reduce costs and improve the efficiency of clinical development. For example, a recent study employing a systems modeling approach reported the development and application of a mechanistic disease model in combination with drug pharmacokinetics (Marathe et al., 2008). In particular, this model represented key cellular processes describing bone metabolism, drug (denosumab) pharmacokinetics, and the drug's effects on the RANK–RANKL–OPG pathway. In contrast to an indirect, empirical PD model also developed, the authors showed that the mechanistic PD model had the advantage of being able to investigate the impact of changes in cellular physiologies on drug responses. This capability allowed the investigators to simulate changes in disease physiology associated with multiple myeloma and to assess the potential impact on both short- and long-term drug responses. Moreover, such a mechanistic model can be used to understand how patient variability and heterogeneity could affect drug responses, leading potentially to novel biomarkers to identify patient responders and the development of enhanced treatment regimens.

Recently, a modeling and simulation study served as key confirmatory evidence to support regulatory approval of a new compound, gabapentin, for the treatment of postherpetic neuralagia (Miller et al., 2005). The dilemma in this case was that there were no replicate clinical data to support efficacy at the sought-after drug doses. To support approval, the application sponsors used modeling and simulation to demonstrate the exposure–response relationship across all doses. In this way, the sponsor won regulatory approval and avoided a second well-controlled clinical investigation as initially suggested by regulators, saving the sponsor significant time and resources.

In addition to supporting multiple aspects of traditional clinical design and analysis, there are also opportunities for systems biology to transform clinical investigation into a more efficient process by enabling more sophisticated, streamlined studies, such as adaptive trials. Adaptive trials generally seek to use accumulated data to make specific modifications and/or decisions for an ongoing clinical trial without undermining the trial validity or integrity (Chow et al., 2005). In essence, adaptive trials aim to utilize knowledge gained as soon as possible in a rational, preplanned manner. To improve patient care during trials, reduce development times, and cut costs, Gallo et al. (2006) recommend three adaptive approaches: phase I dose-finding studies, seamless phase II/III designs, and sample size reestimation.

Adaptive trial design requires careful planning and regulatory review, including trial logistics and statistical approaches. Integral to these adaptive approaches are quantitative modeling. For example, the continual reassessment method used for dose-finding studies (O'Quigley et al., 1990) uses quantitative models to represent the dose–toxicity and/or dose–efficacy relationships. Using the current state of knowledge, Bayesian models are typically used to quantify these relationships: namely, at the start of the trial the historical information regarding the drug effects informs the prior, or initial, model. During the trial, data collected determine the likelihood function, and together these data determine the updated real-time model called the *posterior*. Such statistical techniques are generally applied to models with few parameters to ensure identifiability.

Extension of such inferential modeling approaches to larger mechanistically focused models faces several challenges associated with parameter estimation, parsimony analysis, and model selection (Baker et al., 2005; Balsa-Canto et al., 2008). Parameter sensitivity analyses can provide insights into parameter uncertainty and the impact of model uncertainties on model predictions (Gutenkunst et al., 2007). Emerging approaches, such as model-based experiment design, can be used to design the next optimal experimental procedure to generate the most informative data for parameter estimation and model refinement (Balsa-Canto et al., 2008; Gadkar et al., 2005a,b). For example, these approaches can help identify when to collect certain measurements in order to best refine the model and associated predictions. The prudent and measured application of such systems biological modeling and analysis approaches to the clinical setting could further increase the productivity of clinical drug development.

14.8. COLLABORATION AND TRAINING FOR SYSTEMS BIOLOGISTS

Significant advancements in systems biology and its application to drug discovery and development are under way in industrial, academic, and governmental centers around the world. Further advancement in the field will be achieved through concerted coordination and cooperation across these sectors and geographic boundaries. In this section we focus on several challenges associated specifically with educational and technological developments in the field.

Educating future systems biologists represents a significant ongoing challenge. The successful application of systems biology to drug discovery and development requires knowledge spanning multiple disciplines. For example, interdisciplinary training in biology, genetics, chemistry, pharmacology, computer science, physics, engineering, and mathematics are central for the application and thorough understanding of systems biology. Currently, graduates from each of these disciplines share little common ground, impeding scientific collaboration and cross-fertilization. Interdisciplinary education appears, however, to be at odds with recent educational and research trends, which tend toward extreme and narrow specialization. The requirement in systems biology for broad knowledge clearly represents a challenge, as it requires novel educational programs that effectively combine teaching and research opportunities involving multiple disciplines. Such extensive training may not be fully attained in undergraduate programs alone, requiring advanced graduate programs and continuing education opportunities for professionals.

New programs have been initiated in several institutions to address the unique requirement for systems biologists. For example, a novel integrated educational approach has been initiated at Princeton to educate system-level biologists (Wingreen and Botstein, 2006). Namely, coursework begins in the first year of college by integrating multiple disciplines, such as mathematics, physics, chemistry, and biology—subjects traditional taught in separate courses—into a standard training program. However, cross-disciplinary education does present some risks. For example, will broad-based programs provide enough in-depth education in core subdisciplines? Will graduates effectively compete with other students who have completed traditional, single-discipline programs? Do broadly focused undergraduate programs necessitate ongoing graduate studies, and may this requirement be an impediment to attracting young students into this emerging field? Will broadly educated researchers be able to secure competitive research funding that traditionally favors more narrowly focused research? Answers to these questions will emerge over time, and new educational approaches will no doubt be devised to meet these challenges.

Enhanced cooperation among government, academia, and industry is needed to help meet many of the educational needs for systems biologists. The design of, and commitment to, novel academic programs by educational institutions should be further encouraged and funded by governmental agencies and supported by industrial entities. Besides initiating new departments, academic researchers can further encourage cross-department research and educational programs. Valuable training can also occur through industrial internship programs for both undergraduate and graduate students. In a similar vein, research collaboration between industry and academic groups can help align academic training and research with essential problems facing industry, further shaping educational programs to meet future industry needs.

Integral to training initiatives, students, as well as professionals, require tools for enhanced productivity and collaboration. Over the last decade, there has been a rapid proliferation of modeling and simulation software tools aimed specifically at systems biology research. Many of these tools have been developed by academic centers with government support and are widely available to the research community. Most of these software tools are highly specialized, focused on specific systems biology applications. For example, over 70 software systems address modeling and simulation of dynamic intracellular pathways [e.g., Virtual Cell (http://www.vcell.org), E-cell (http://www.e-cell.org), and Silicon Cell (http://www.siliconcell.net)]. Selecting the appropriate software tool is therefore not a simple endeavor. The available simulation tools can be differentiated by their ability to simulate discrete stochastic, spatial, and/or continuous deterministic processes. In addition to simulation, many tools include a variety of analytic capabilities, such as model sensitivity and stability analyses. Other software packages focus on clinical trial design and pharmacokinetics–pharmacodynamics. It is also important to consider the quality of the software documentation, user support, and ongoing development status of the application.

While these software tools address very well a host of research problems, the vast array of software tools available is not necessarily a sign of success for the field. Indeed, there have been many duplicate efforts, making inefficient use of talented researchers and financial resources, perhaps reflective of a lack of broader coordination. Numerous tools may require substantially more training than fewer, more comprehensive software packages. Moreover, the sharing of systems biology research and models becomes more difficult if each research group employs its own customized software tool. Efforts to standardize research methods and tools are therefore of paramount importance for the efficient exchange of knowledge in systems biology. Some progress has been made in this area, as reflected in the wide adoption of Systems Biology Markup Language (SBML) (http://www.sbml.org) (Hucka et al., 2003) and Cell Markup Language (CellML) (http://www.cellml.org). These software coding languages enable efficient exchange of quantitative models across software packages by creating standard machine-readable formats for representing models. Standard scripting languages allow the description of systems of biochemical reactions typical of cell signaling pathways, metabolic pathways, biochemical reactions, and gene regulation.

Standardized languages for encoding models have enhanced model sharing and publication. In fact, a number of consortiums have begun collating diverse biological models. These shared models can be more easily interrogated by other researchers, allowing more efficient extension of prior work. One example is JWS Online (http://jjj.biochem.sun.ac.za/), which allows access to a database of curated biological system models, enables Web-based simulations, and facilitates reviews of manuscripts containing mathematical biological models. Similarly, the BioModel Database (http://www.ebi.ac.uk/biomodels-main/) is a free centralized database of curated published models of biochemical and cellular systems.

Given the diverse background of researchers in the field of systems biology, there is a fundamental need for forums that enable effective communication of research progress recognizing the diversity of the participants' areas of expertise. In this respect, the sustained growth of systems biology is fed by the growing number of international journals related to the field, including *PLoS Computational Biology*, *IEEE Proceedings: Systems Biology*, *In Silico Biology*, *Molecular Systems Biology*, *BMC Systems Biology*, and *IET Systems Biology*. The advancing opportunities for publication of systems biology research in high-impact journals is bound to enhance research efforts and hasten achievements in this rapidly developing field. Moreover, international meetings enable efficient exchange of ideas. For example, the International Conference on Systems Biology, an annual meeting begun in 2000 by Hiroaki Kitano (Sony Computer Science Laboratories, Inc.), is rapidly becoming the premiere conference in this field, with a steadily growing number of attendees every year. Other related meetings focus more specifically on industrial applications, including modeling and simulation of clinical trials.

14.9. CONCLUSIONS

In this chapter we reviewed current and future opportunities and challenges for systems biology. Based on a strong foundation of successes in both basic biologic research and clinical applications, new and exciting applications for systems biology are emerging as researchers aim to more fully understand biological phenomena simultaneously at both the mechanistic and the patient levels. The further adoption of such new modeling and analytic approaches requires careful validation as well as clear communications with decision makers and researchers of diverse backgrounds at both pharmaceutical companies and regulatory agencies. The application of systems biological modeling and analysis in both the laboratory and clinical settings will further increase the productivity of drug discovery and development promising to increase drug efficacy, reduce toxicities, and enable more personalized patient care.

REFERENCES

Ahn, A.C., Tewari, M., Poon, C.S., and Phillips, R.S. (2006a). The clinical applications of a systems approach. *PLoS Med 3*, e209.

Ahn, A.C., Tewari, M., Poon, C.S., and Phillips, R.S. (2006b). The limits of reductionism in medicine: Could systems biology offer an alternative? *PLoS Med 3*, e208.

American Diabetes Association (ADA) Consensus Panel. (2004). Guidelines for computer modeling of diabetes and its complications (Consensus Statement). *Diabetes Care 27*, 2262–2265.

Araujo, R.P., Liotta, L.A., and Petricoin, E.F. (2007). Proteins, drug targets and the mechanisms they control: the simple truth about complex networks. *Nat Rev Drug Discov 6*, 871–880.

Atkinson, M.A., and Leiter, E.H. (1999). The NOD mouse model of type 1 diabetes: as good as it gets? *Nat Med 5*, 601–604.

Baker, C.T.H., Bocharov, G.A., Ford, J.M., Lumb, P.M., Norton, S.J., Paul, C.A.H., Junt, T., Krebs, P., and Ludewig, B. (2005). Computational approaches to parameter estimation and model selection in immunology. *J Comput Appl Math 184*, 50–76.

Balsa-Canto, E., Alonso, A.A., and Banga, J.R. (2008). Computational procedures for optimal experimental design in biological systems. *IET Syst Biol 2*, 163–172.

Beckers, J., Wurst, W., and de Angelis, M.H. (2009). Towards better mouse models: enhanced genotypes, systemic phenotyping and envirotype modelling. *Nat Rev Genet 10*, 371–380.

Carlson, J.M., and Doyle, J. (2002). Complexity and robustness. *Proc Natl Acad Sci USA 99*(Suppl. 1), 2538–2545.

Chassagnole, C., Jackson, R.C., Hussain, N., Bashir, L., Derow, C., Savin, J., and Fell, D.A. (2006). Using a mammalian cell cycle simulation to interpret differential kinase inhibition in anti-tumour pharmaceutical development. *Biosystems 83*, 91–97.

Chopra, P., and Kamma, A. (2006). Engineering life through synthetic biology. *In Silico Biol 6*, 401–410.

Chow, S.C., Chang, M., and Pong, A. (2005). Statistical consideration of adaptive methods in clinical development. *J Biopharm Statist 15*, 575–591.

Christopher, R., Dhiman, A., Fox, J., Gendelman, R., Haberitcher, T., Kagle, D., Spizz, G., Khalil, I.G., and Hill, C. (2004). Data-driven computer simulation of human cancer cell. *Ann NY Acad Sci 1020*, 132–153.

Csete, M.E., and Doyle, J.C. (2002). Reverse engineering of biological complexity. *Science 295*, 1664–1669.

Csete, M., and Doyle, J. (2004). Bow ties, metabolism and disease. *Trends Biotechnol 22*, 446–450.

Daly, A.K. (2009). Pharmacogenomics of anticoagulants: steps toward personal dosage. *Genome Med 1*, 10.

Eddy, D.M., and Schlessinger, L. (2003a). Archimedes: a trial-validated model of diabetes. *Diabetes Care 26*, 3093–3101.

Eddy, D.M., and Schlessinger, L. (2003b). Validation of the Archimedes diabetes model. *Diabetes Care 26*, 3102–3110.

Edwards, A.O., Ritter, R., 3rd, Abel, K.J., Manning, A., Panhuysen, C., and Farrer, L.A. (2005). Complement factor H polymorphism and age-related macular degeneration. *Science 308*, 421–424.

Elias, T., Gordian, M., Singh, N., and Zemmel, R. (2006). Why products fail in phase III. *In Vivo 24*, 49–54.

Endy, D. (2005). Foundations for engineering biology. *Nature 438*, 449–453.

Feinberg, A.P. (2008). Epigenetics at the epicenter of modern medicine. *J Am Med Assoc 299*, 1345–1350.

FDA (2004). *Challenge and Opportunity on the Critical Path to New Medical Products*. U.S. Department of Health and Human Services, Food and Drug Administration, Washington, DC.

Fitzgerald, J.B., Schoeberl, B., Nielsen, U.B., and Sorger, P.K. (2006). Systems biology and combination therapy in the quest for clinical efficacy. *Nat Chem Biol 2*, 458–466.

Gadkar, K.G., Gunawan, R., and Doyle, F.J., 3rd (2005a). Iterative approach to model identification of biological networks. *BMC Bioinf 6*, 155.

Gadkar, K.G., Varner, J., and Doyle, F.J., 3rd (2005b). Model identification of signal transduction networks from data using a state regulator problem. *Syst Biol (Stevenage) 2*, 17–30.

Gallo, P., Chuang-Stein, C., Dragalin, V., Gaydos, B., Krams, M., and Pinheiro, J. (2006). Adaptive designs in clinical drug development: an executive summary of the PhRMA Working Group. *J Biopharm Statist 16*, 275–283; discussion, 285–291, 293–278, 311–272.

Gilbert, J., Henske, P., and Singh, A. (2003). Rebuilding big pharma's business model. *In Vivo 21*(10), 1–10.

Gutenkunst, R.N., Waterfall, J.J., Casey, F.P., Brown, K.S., Myers, C.R., and Sethna, J.P. (2007). Universally sloppy parameter sensitivities in systems biology models. *PLoS Comput Biol 3*, 1871–1878.

Haines, J.L., Hauser, M.A., Schmidt, S., Scott, W.K., Olson, L.M., Gallins, P., Spencer, K.L., Kwan, S.Y., Noureddine, M., Gilbert, J.R., et al. (2005). Complement factor H variant increases the risk of age-related macular degeneration. *Science 308*, 419–421.

Horrobin, D.F. (2003). Modern biomedical research: an internally self-consistent universe with little contact with medical reality? *Nat Rev Drug Discov 2*, 151–154.

Hucka, M., Finney, A., Sauro, H.M., Bolouri, H., Doyle, J.C., Kitano, H., Arkin, A.P., Bornstein, B.J., Bray, D., Cornish-Bowden, A., et al. (2003). The systems biology markup language (SBML): a medium for representation and exchange of biochemical network models. *Bioinformatics 19*, 524–531.

Jaenisch, R., and Bird, A. (2003). Epigenetic regulation of gene expression: how the genome integrates intrinsic and environmental signals. *Nat Genet 33*(Suppl.), 245–254.

Johnson, J.I., Decker, S., Zaharevitz, D., Rubinstein, L.V., Venditti, J.M., Schepartz, S., Kalyandrug, S., Christian, M., Arbuck, S., Hollingshead, M., et al. (2001). Relationships between drug activity in NCI preclinical *in vitro* and *in vivo* models and early clinical trials. *Br J Cancer 84*, 1424–1431.

Kaznessis, Y.N. (2007). Models for synthetic biology. *BMC Syst Biol 1*, 47.

Kitano, H. (2004). Biological robustness. *Nat Rev Genet 5*, 826–837.

Kitano, H. (2007). A robustness-based approach to systems-oriented drug design. *Nat Rev Drug Discov 6*, 202–210.

Klein, R.J., Zeiss, C., Chew, E.Y., Tsai, J.Y., Sackler, R.S., Haynes, C., Henning, A.K., SanGiovanni, J.P., Mane, S.M., Mayne, S.T., et al. (2005). Complement factor H polymorphism in age-related macular degeneration. *Science 308*, 385–389.

Kohn, K.W. (1999). Molecular interaction map of the mammalian cell cycle control and DNA repair systems. *Mol Biol Cell 10*, 2703–2734.

Kola, I. (2008). The state of innovation in drug development. *Clin Pharmacol Ther 83*, 227–230.

Kola, I., and Landis, J. (2004). Can the pharmaceutical industry reduce attrition rates? *Nat Rev Drug Discov 3*, 711–715.

Kraft, P., and Hunter, D.J. (2009). Genetic risk prediction: Are we there yet? *N Engl J Med 360*, 1701–1703.

Kunkel, E.J., Dea, M., Ebens, A., Hytopoulos, E., Melrose, J., Nguyen, D., Ota, K.S., Plavec, I., Wang, Y., Watson, S.R., et al. (2004). An integrative biology approach for analysis of drug action in models of human vascular inflammation. *FASEB J 18*, 1279–1281.

Lalonde, R.L., Kowalski, K.G., Hutmacher, M.M., Ewy, W., Nichols, D.J., Milligan, P.A., Corrigan, B.W., Lockwood, P.A., Marshall, S.A., Benincosa, L.J., et al. (2007). Model-based drug development. *Clin Pharmacol Ther 82*, 21–32.

Lauffenburger, D.A. (2000). Cell signaling pathways as control modules: complexity for simplicity? *Proc Natl Acad Sci USA 97*, 5031–5033.

Laurent, L.C., Nievergelt, C.M., Lynch, C., Fakunle, E., Harness, J.V., Schmidt, U., Galat, V., Laslett, A.L., Otonkoski, T., Keirstead, H.S., et al. (2010). Restricted ethnic diversity in human embryonic stem cell lines. *Nat Methods 7*, 6–7.

Leiter, E.H., and von Herrath, M. (2004). Animal models have little to teach us about type 1 diabetes: 2. In opposition to this proposal. *Diabetologia 47*, 1657–1660.

Mahmood, I. (1999). Allometric issues in drug development. *J Pharm Sci 88*, 1101–1106.

Marathe, A., Peterson, M.C., and Mager, D.E. (2008). Integrated cellular bone homeostasis model for denosumab pharmacodynamics in multiple myeloma patients. *J Pharmacol Exp Ther 326*, 555–562.

Michelson, S., and Cole, M. (2007). The future of predictive biosimulation in drug discovery. *Expert Opin Drug Discov 2*, 515–523.

Miller, R., Ewy, W., Corrigan, B.W., Ouellet, D., Hermann, D., Kowalski, K.G., Lockwood, P., Koup, J.R., Donevan, S., El-Kattan, A., et al. (2005). How modeling and simulation have enhanced decision making in new drug development. *J Pharmacokinet Pharmacodyn 32*, 185–197.

Novak, B., and Tyson, J.J. (2004). A model for restriction point control of the mammalian cell cycle. *J Theor Biol 230*, 563–579.

O'Quigley, J., Pepe, M., and Fisher, L. (1990). Continual reassessment method: a practical design for phase 1 clinical trials in cancer. *Biometrics 46*, 33–48.

Pallay, A., and Berry, S.M. (1999). A decision analysis for an end of phase II go/stop decision. *Drug Inf J 33*, 821–833.

Picard, F.J., and Bergeron, M.G. (2002). Rapid molecular theranostics in infectious diseases. *Drug Discov Today 7*, 1092–1101.

Polyak, K., Haviv, I., and Campbell, I.G. (2009). Co-evolution of tumor cells and their microenvironment. *Trends Genet 25*, 30–38.

Rajman, I. (2008). PK/PD modelling and simulations: utility in drug development. *Drug Discov Today 13*, 341–346.

Roep, B.O. (2007). Are insights gained from NOD mice sufficient to guide clinical translation? Another inconvenient truth. *Ann NY Acad Sci 1103*, 1–10.

Roep, B.O., and Atkinson, M. (2004). Animal models have little to teach us about type 1 diabetes: 1. In support of this proposal. *Diabetologia 47*, 1650–1656.

Roep, B.O., Atkinson, M., and von Herrath, M. (2004). Satisfaction (not) guaranteed: reevaluating the use of animal models of type 1 diabetes. *Nat Rev Immunol 4*, 989–997.

Rohrer, B., Long, Q., Coughlin, B., Wilson, R.B., Huang, Y., Qiao, F., Tang, P.H., Kunchithapautham, K., Gilkeson, G.S., and Tomlinson, S. (2009). A targeted inhibitor of the alternative complement pathway reduces angiogenesis in a mouse model of age-related macular degeneration. *Invest Ophthalmol Vis Sci 50*, 3056–3064.

Scholl, H.P., Charbel Issa, P., Walier, M., Janzer, S., Pollok-Kopp, B., Borncke, F., Fritsche, L.G., Chong, N.V., Fimmers, R., Wienker, T., et al. (2008). Systemic complement activation in age-related macular degeneration. *PLoS One 3*, e2593.

Sheiner, L.B. (1997). Learning versus confirming in clinical drug development. *Clin Pharmacol Ther 61*, 275–291.

Shoda, L.K., Young, D.L., Ramanujan, S., Whiting, C.C., Atkinson, M.A., Bluestone, J.A., Eisenbarth, G.S., Mathis, D., Rossini, A.A., Campbell, S.E., et al. (2005). A comprehensive review of interventions in the NOD mouse and implications for translation. *Immunity 23*, 115–126.

Silman, A.J., MacGregor, A.J., Thomson, W., Holligan, S., Carthy, D., Farhan, A., and Ollier, W.E. (1993). Twin concordance rates for rheumatoid arthritis: results from a nationwide study. *Br J Rheumatol 32*, 903–907.

Singh, S.S. (2006). Preclinical pharmacokinetics: an approach towards safer and efficacious drugs. *Curr Drug Metab 7*, 165–182.

Stelling, J., Sauer, U., Szallasi, Z., Doyle, F.J., 3rd, and Doyle, J. (2004). Robustness of cellular functions. *Cell 118*, 675–685.

Tortajada, A., Montes, T., Martinez-Barricarte, R., Morgan, B.P., Harris, C.L., and de Cordoba, S.R. (2009). The disease-protective complement factor H allotypic variant

Ile62 shows increased binding affinity for C3b and enhanced cofactor activity. *Hum Mol Genet 18*, 3452–3461.

von Bertalanffy, L.V. (1968). *General System Theory: Foundations, Development, Applications*. George Braziller, New York.

Wiener, N. (1965). *Cybernetics: or, Control and Communication in the Animal and the Machine*. MIT Press, Cambridge, MA.

Wingreen, N., and Botstein, D. (2006). Back to the future: education for systems-level biologists. *Nat Rev Mol Cell Biol 7*, 829–832.

Yang, K., Hitomi, M., and Stacey, D.W. (2006). Variations in cyclin D1 levels through the cell cycle determine the proliferative fate of a cell. *Cell Div 1*, 32.

Young, D.L., and Poon, C.-S. (2001). Soul searching and heart throbbing for biological modeling. *Behav Brain Sci 24*, 1080–1081.

Systems Biology in Drug Discovery and Development, First Edition.
Edited by Daniel L. Young, Seth Michelson.
© 2012 John Wiley & Sons, Inc. Published 2012 by John Wiley & Sons, Inc.